AF214315

Our American Red Cross

Stories from those who served

presented by

Association of Retirees from the American Red Cross

ASSOCIATION OF RETIREES FROM THE American Red Cross

TURNER PUBLISHING COMPANY
Paducah, Kentucky

TURNER PUBLISHING COMPANY
Publishers of America's History
412 Broadway•P.O. Box 3101
Paducah, Kentucky 42002-3101
(270) 443-0121

Publisher's Editor: Dayna Spear Williams
Designer: David Hurst

Copyright © 2000 Turner Publishing Company
All rights reserved
Publishing Rights: Turner Publishing Company

This book or any part thereof may not be reproduced without the express written consent of the publisher.

This publication was produced using available and submitted materials. The author and publisher regret they cannot assume liability for errors or omissions.

Photos on pages 96-100, 102 are used with permission of The American National Red Cross. Other photos and clippings were submitted by American Red Cross retirees.

Library of Congress Catalog Control No. 00135752
ISBN: 1-56311-488-7
LIMITED EDITION

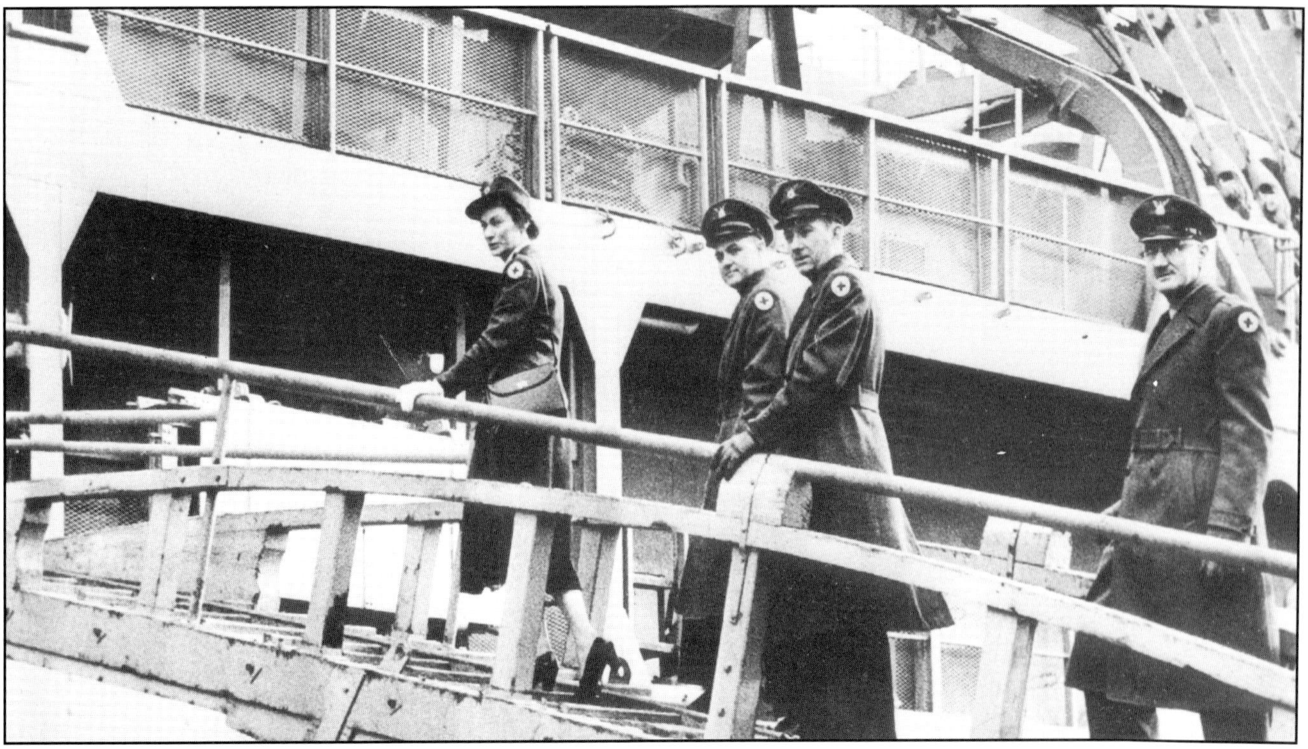

Red Cross team boards the USNS General W.C. Haan, December 12, 1956.

Our American Red Cross

Table of Contents

Introduction ... 10

Publisher's Message ... 11

Membership and Benefits of the ARARC ... 12

An Overview of the American Red Cross ... 15

Red Cross Memories ... 25

Katie's Story ... K.H. Van Hogendorp ... 26
Hollywood Celebrities and the Cherry Blossom Dance... M.T. Joyal ... 52
Hospital Ship ... P. Steffey ... 53
Recreation ... E.H. Smith ... 54
Midway Kansas Chapter ...G.A. Savage ... 54
Can't You Tell Time? ... M. Robinson ... 55
A Memorable Red Cross Experience ... J.R. Russell ... 55
World War II in India and Germany ... C. Ross ... 56
Field Director in Phu Bai, Vietnam ... M. Fredericksen ... 57
Nearly Trapped by Big German Push ... J. Willicombe, Jr. ... 58
Custody Assistance ... D. Fannin ... 59
Serving Troops in Greece and Turkey ... B.W. Evans ... 60
How I Lent President Kennedy My Hands ... N.T. English ... 61
VJ Night in Manila, PI ... E.R. Denman ... 62
Clubmobile Days at 1st Cavalry, Korea ... L. Davidson ... 62
The Commodore ... G.W. Colle ... 64
Mabel Boardman ... G.W. Colle ... 65
Leper Colony ... L. Allen ... 66
The Mission Service Center ... 66
American Red Cross Community Support ... E.B. Waite ... 66
I Remember ... E. M. Sweet ... 67
Working with Military Families ... G. Longoria ... 67
From Disaster Exercise into Genuine Disaster ... H.L. Ettlin ... 68
A Red Cross Career ... J.R. Russell ... 68
Pianist in Vietnam ... M.V. Bain ... 70
Emergency Loans and Alleged Emergencies at Home ... W.D. Conn ... 70
Blood Bank ... R. Furse ... 71
Japanese Brides ... M. Minamoto ... 71
Flower Children ... M. Klass/M. Grandcolas ... 72
The Bradshaws' Release... L. Allen ... 72

American Red Cross Presidents ... 95

American Red Cross Retirees ... 103

Red Cross Profiles ... 117

Index ... 144

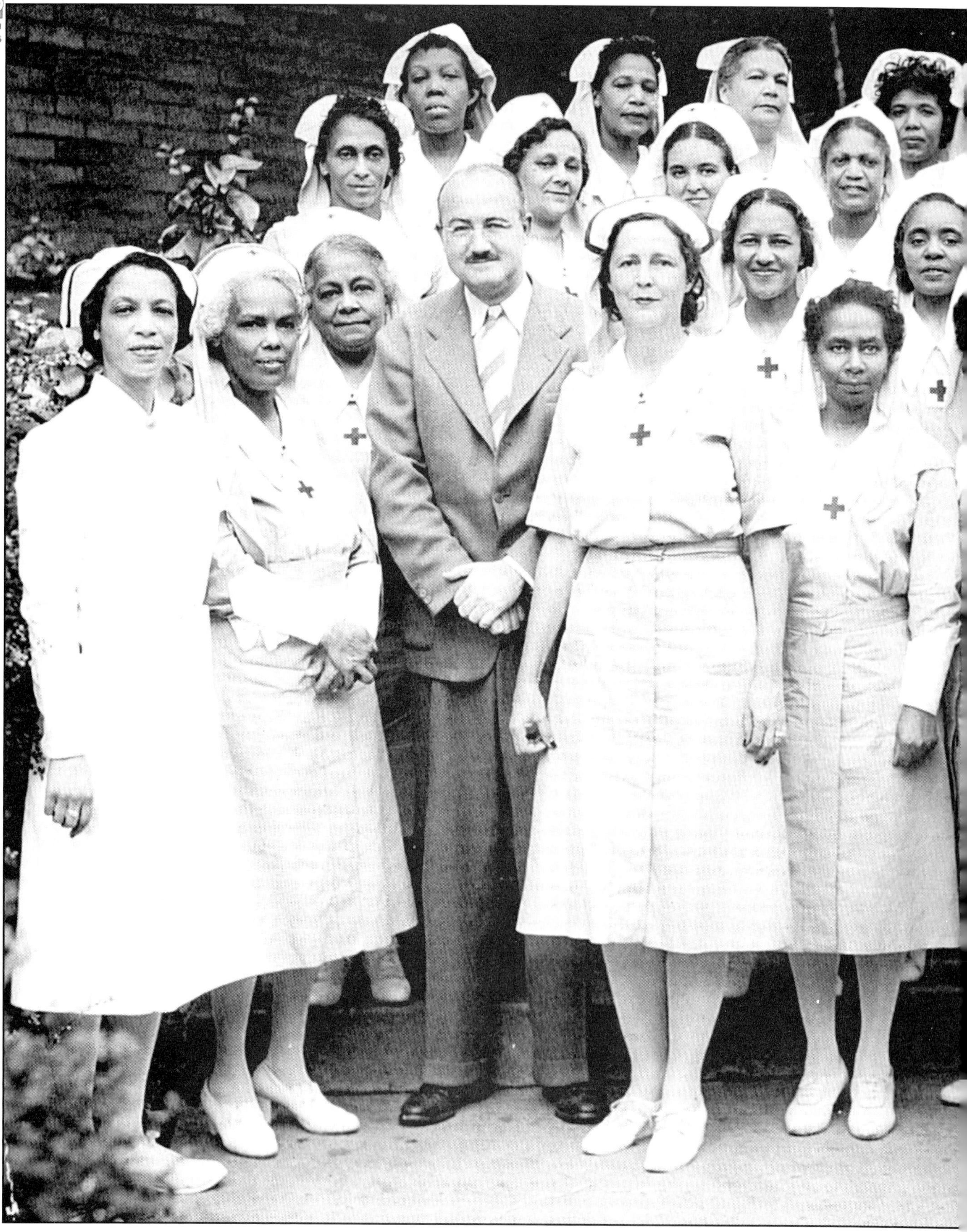

Gray Ladies trained by Thelma Radden

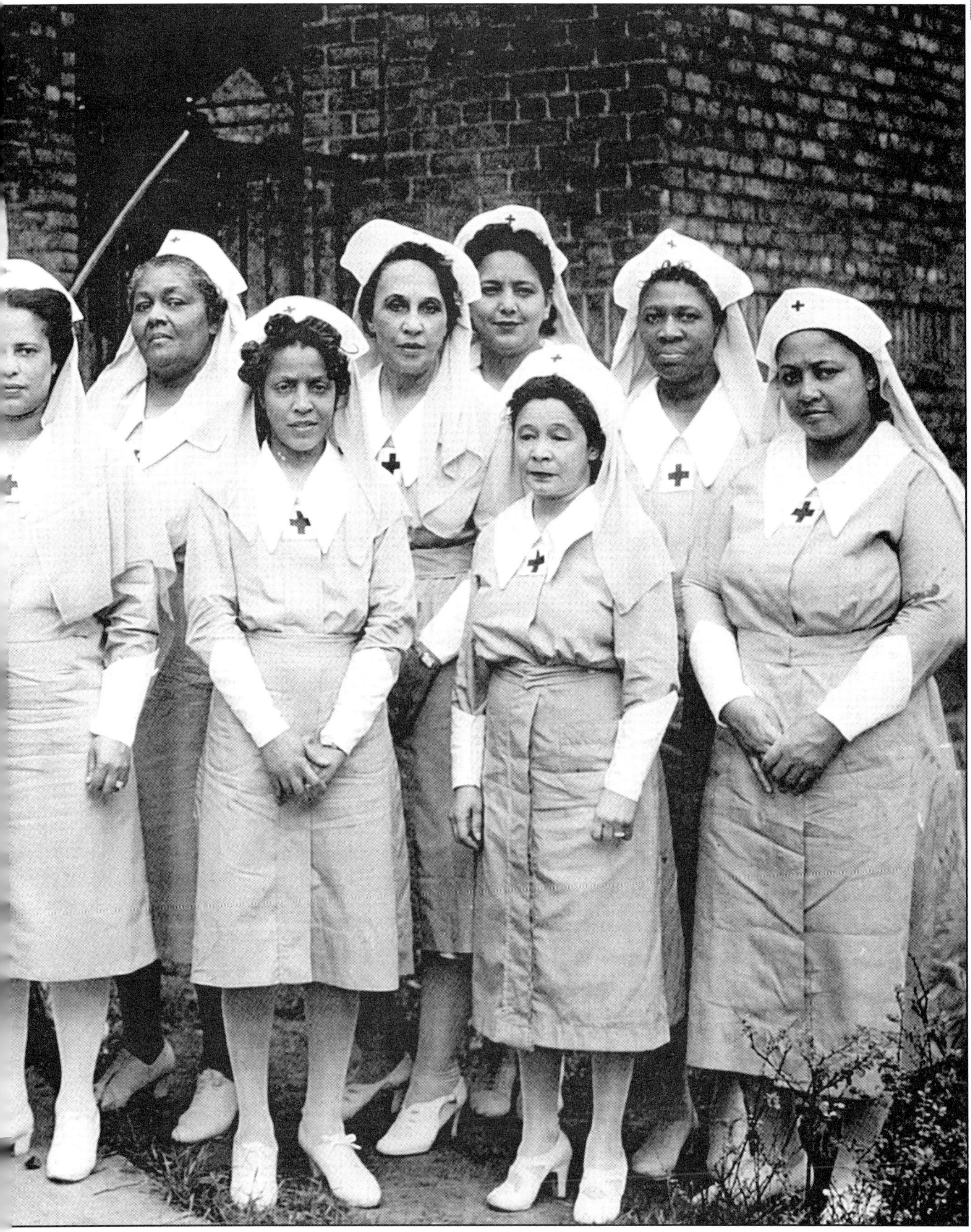

Vietnam

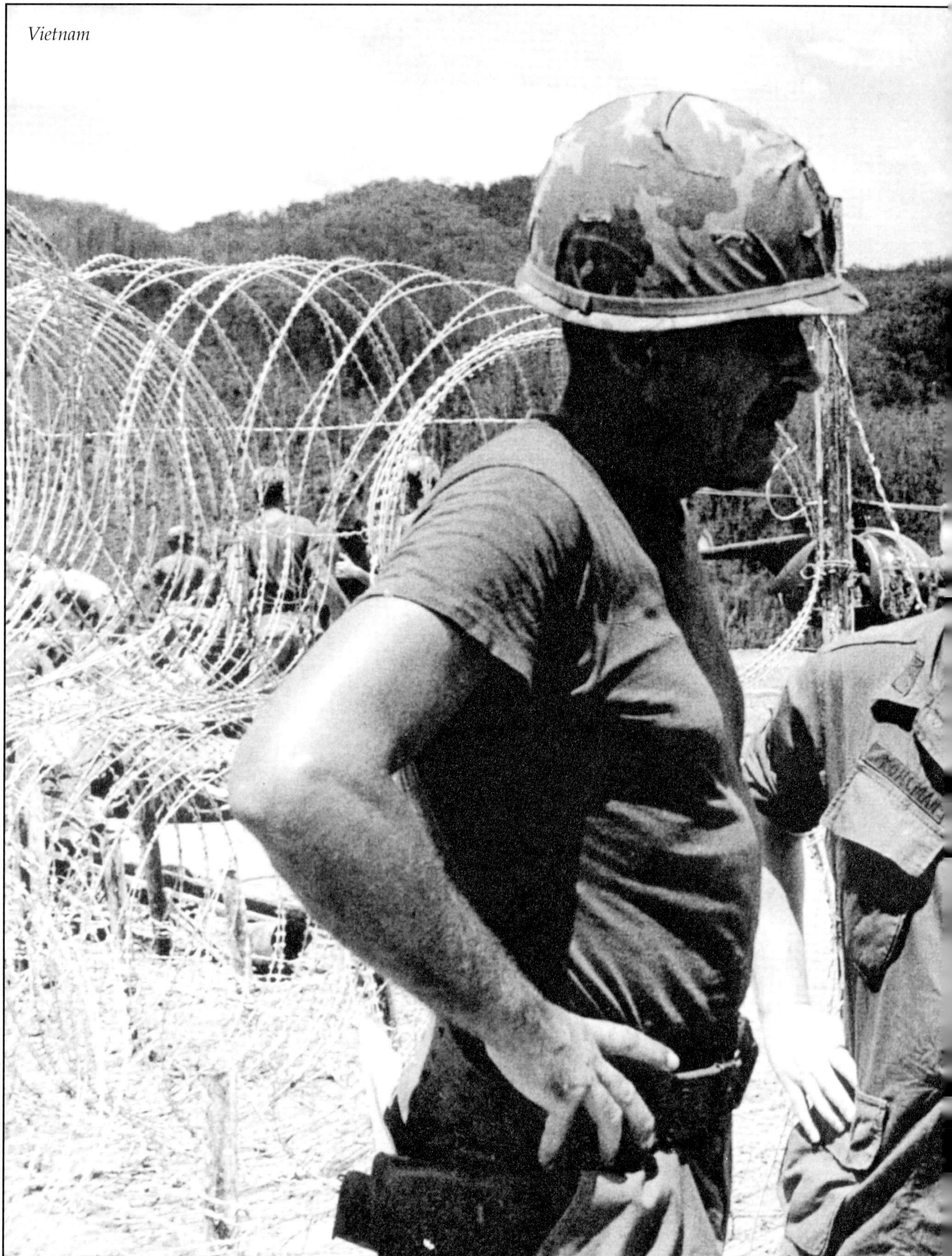

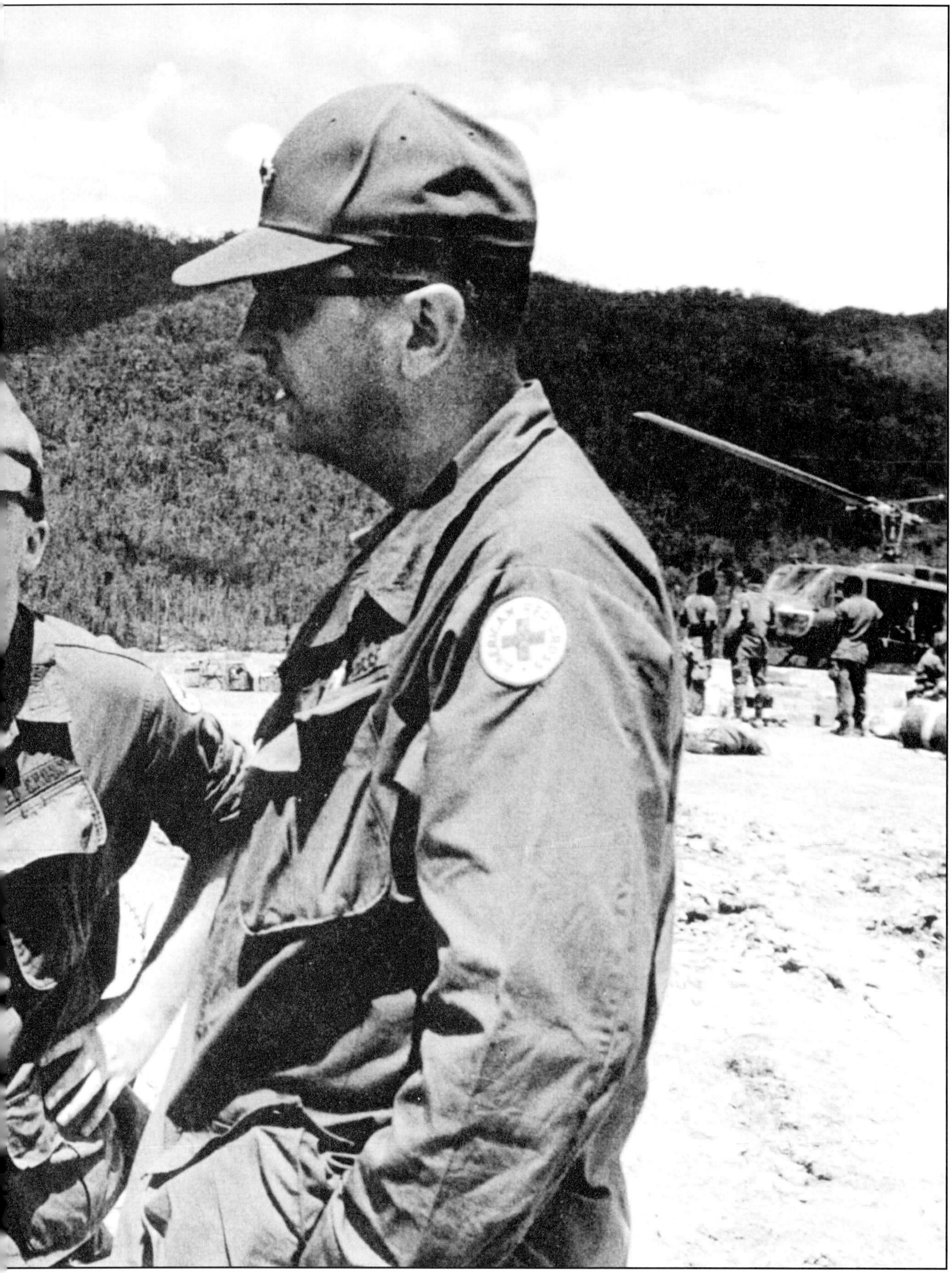

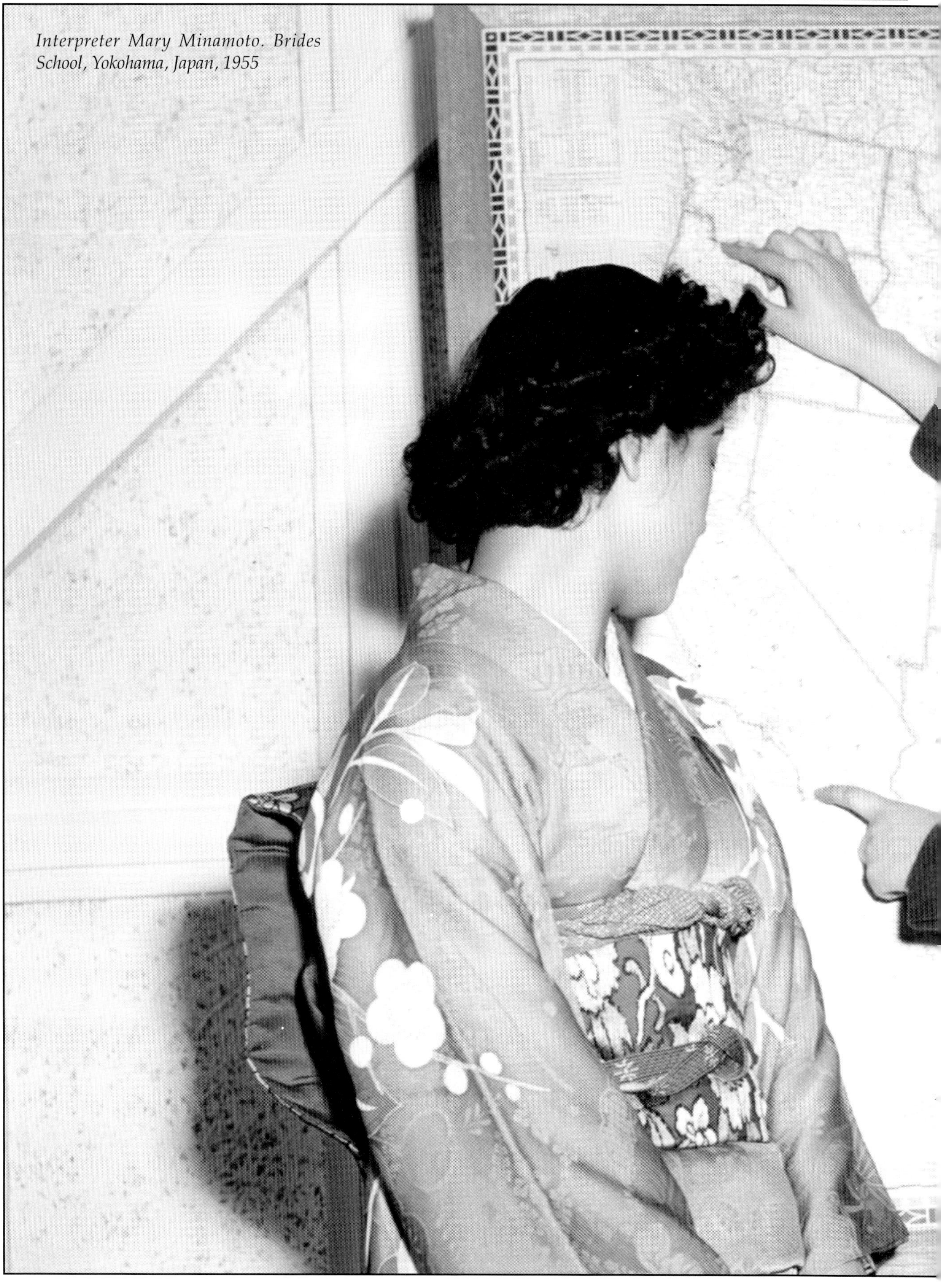

Interpreter Mary Minamoto. Brides School, Yokohama, Japan, 1955

ASSOCIATION OF RETIREES FROM THE
American Red Cross

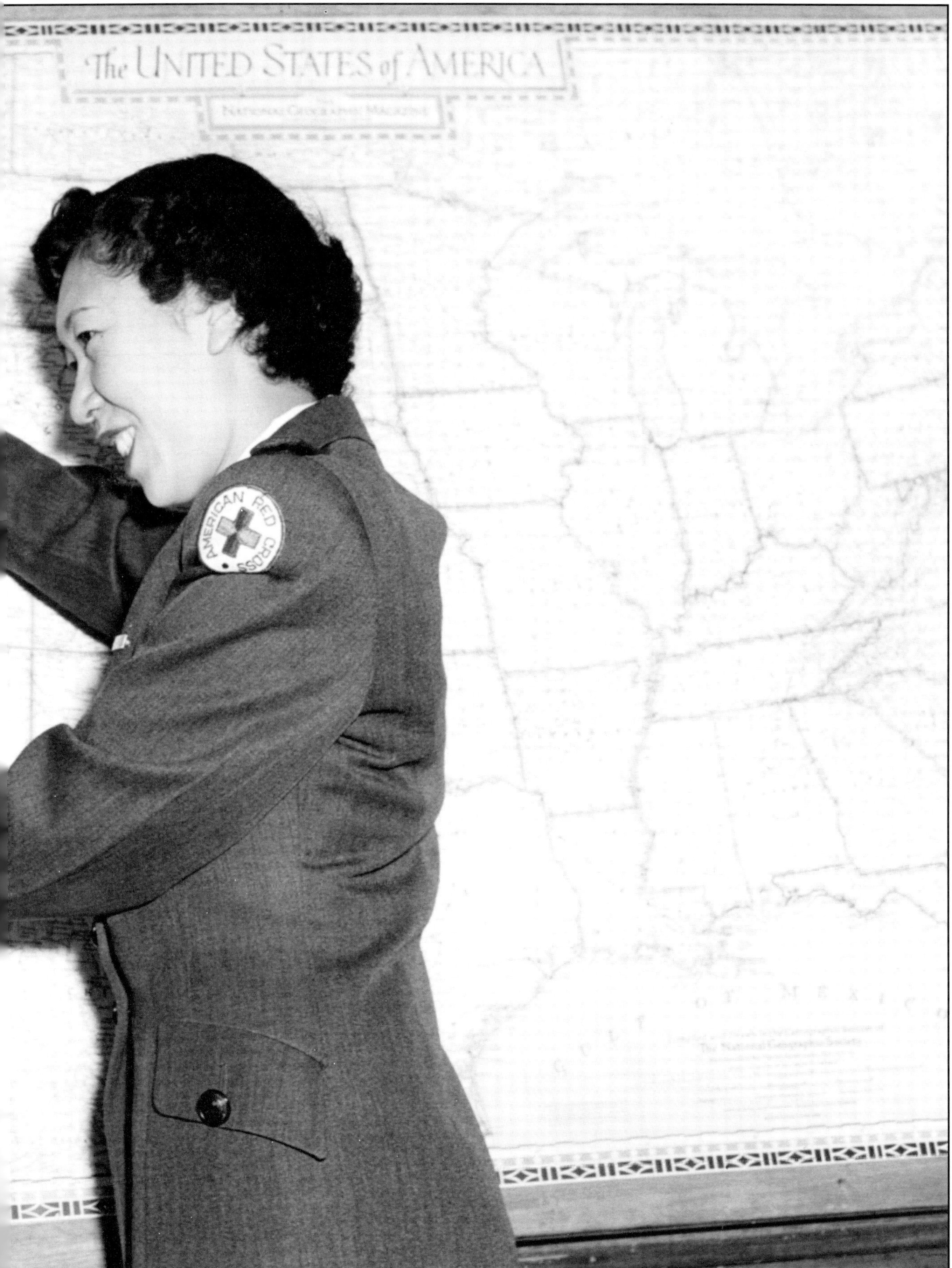

ASSOCIATION OF RETIREES FROM THE

American Red Cross

Retirees from the American Red Cross have a unique opportunity in this book to share with you some of their adventures gathered during the years they wore their Red Cross uniforms or Red Cross insignia, fulfilling their duties both at home and overseas.

Some served as caseworkers or field staff with the Armed Forces within the United States or at overseas military bases. Some worked to provide on-the-scene disaster relief to those afflicted by fire, flood, and earthquake. Some taught health and safety courses in first aid, CPR, and water safety. Some staffed hundreds of bloodmobiles and donor centers that provided a safe and adequate supply of blood and blood products. All were Red Cross staff, and all were guided by the principles of the American Red Cross.

As you turn these pages and read of experiences of these members of the Red Cross family, you may be reminded of interesting, challenging, and sometimes harrowing experiences in your own career. The personal profiles, photographs, and memories of these Red Cross retirees should enlighten and inspire you. No one who reads this book will come away unmoved by the selfless dedication and hard work of those who have carried the Red Cross banner over the years.

Share these stories with your friends – they are the stories of your American Red Cross in action as seen through the eyes of dedicated Red Cross retirees.

Marjorie L. Miller

Marjorie L. Miller
President
Association of Retirees from the American Red Cross

8111 Gatehouse Road, 2nd Floor Falls Church, VA 22042 Phone: 703-206-7184

PUBLISHER'S MESSAGE

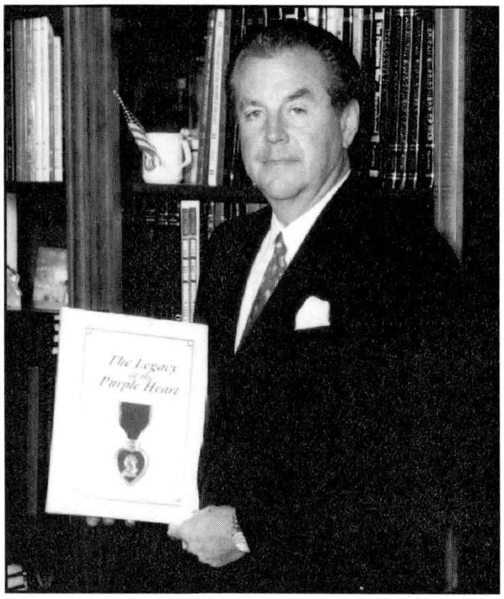

The American Red Cross. The name itself invokes images of brave men and women who risked their lives to serve in war zones, disaster areas, hospitals, offices and training centers, in the name of impartial, humanitarian benevolence, both nationally and internationally.

Special thanks belongs to Betty Wagner of the Association of Retirees from the American Red Cross. Without her assistance and continued support, this project would not have become a reality. Appreciation also goes to each member of the Association of Retirees, who, with forethought and a desire to remember the past, painstakingly prepared their profiles, photos and personal experience stories for publication.

Turner Publishing Company has published over 800 military, law enforcement, fire department and specialty titles, including such titles as *American Ex Prisoners of War, Battle of the Bulge, American Defenders of the Bataan and Corregidor, Gold Star Wives of America, Pearl Harbor Survivors, The Purple Heart Legacy* and many more. In the spirit of true patriotism, Turner now proudly presents to you *Our American Red Cross: Stories From Those Who Served.*

Sincerely,

Dave Turner, President
Turner Publishing Company

MEMBERSHIP AND BENEFITS OF ARARC AND UNIT MEMBERSHIP

Who Can Join...

Anyone who is - or will become - a retiree of the American Red Cross should be a member of ARARC and one if its local units.

Voting Membership is open to all retired and vested members of the Red Cross Retirement System. This includes the beneficiaries of deceased retirees who were members of the system.

Non-Voting, Associate Membership is open to other current Red Cross staff (including Reserves) and volunteers, and current contributors.

Unit Membership is open to Red Cross chapters, biomedical regions and field stations that participate in the American Red Cross retirement system.

What Are the Benefits of Joining a Unit...

Local membership helps retirees and current staff and volunteers to stay in contact with their fellow retirees in the nearby areas. Local membership provides opportunities to socialize as well as to work together on service projects. Many units operate personally supportive programs that assist Red Cross retirees who live alone or require special care from members of our unique family. These programs often also focus on assisting spouses of deceased Red Cross retirees.

Why It Is Important to also Join ARARC...

When the local units are joined together in the national organization, this enables the local unit members to be part of a concerted and effective voice with the Red Cross Management, our Retirement System, the Benefits Office, and others in matters important to retirees. Building a strong national organization and presence requires local members to also be members of the national ARARC on an annual basis.

The ARARC is working on a stronger relationship with the Retirement System and Benefits Office to assist in more effectively communicating its advantages as well as responding to the collective and individual needs and concerns of the retirees. The more our ARARC numbers increase the more likely we will be recognized as credible and worth listening to.

We must be more than a collection of individual units and its local members to be heard. It is a known fact that power is in numbers, which in this case represents the number of ARARC members and will be the strength of our national retirees organization.

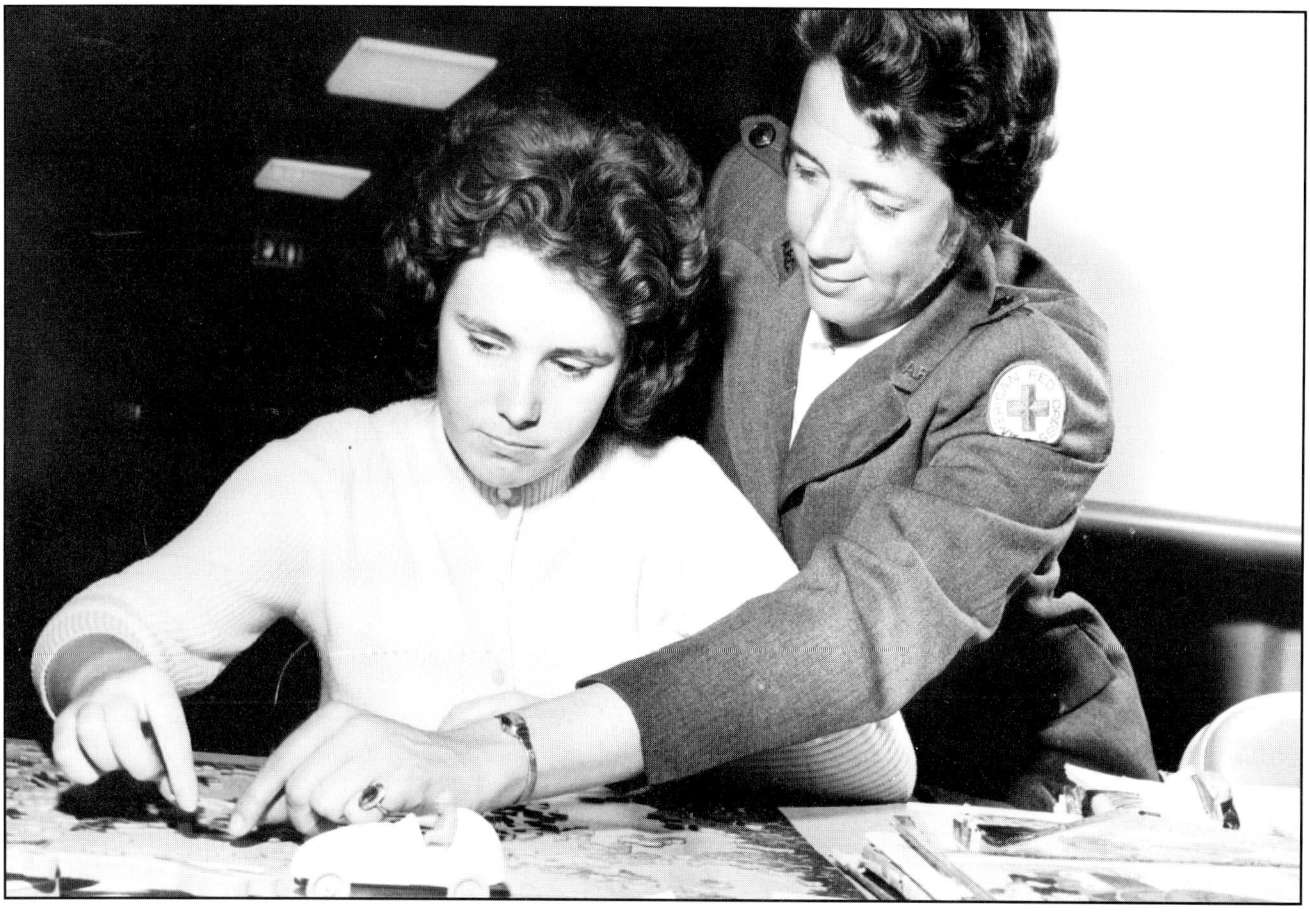

Red Cross Worker, Ann Woessner Priem

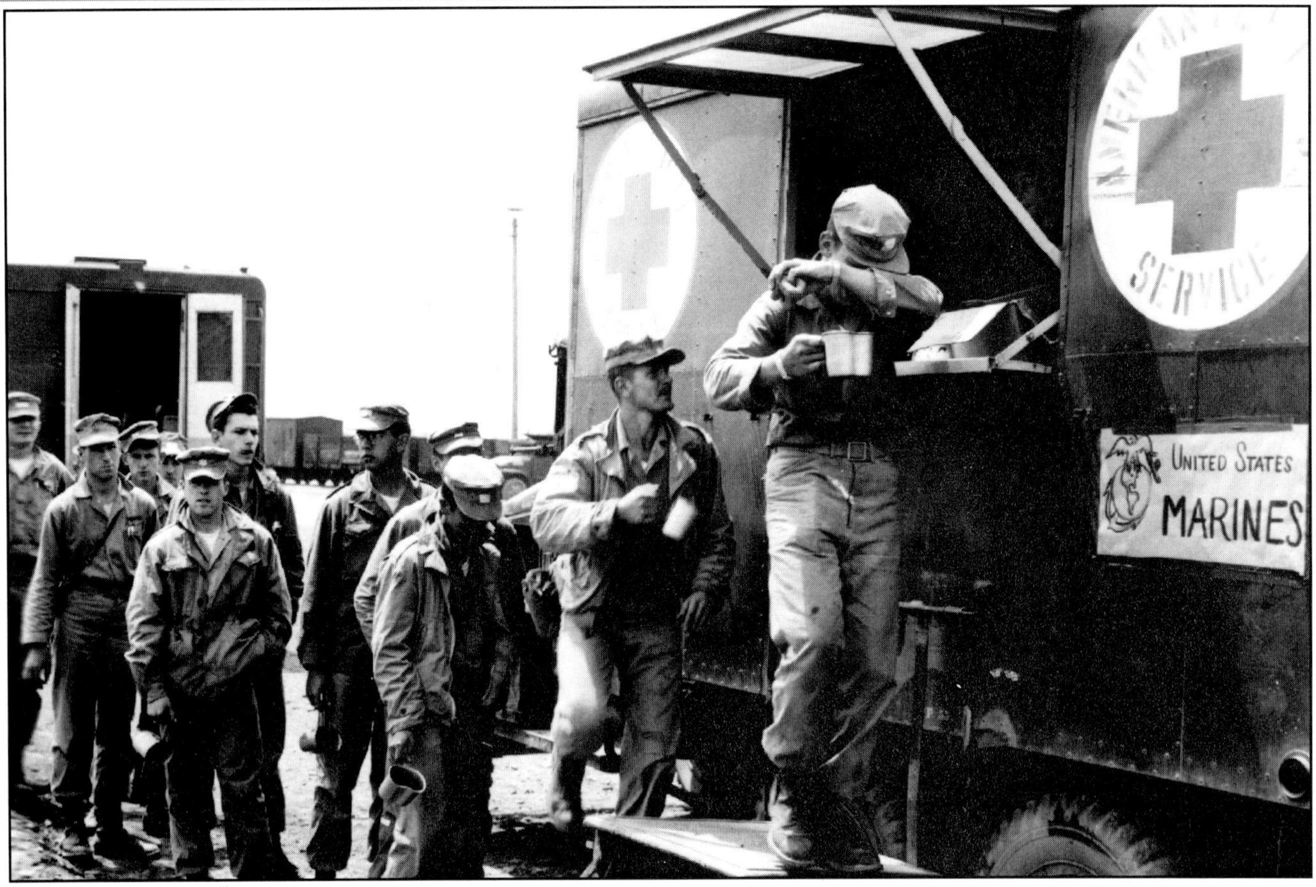

Members of the Marine Regimental Landing Team-5 being served hot coffee and doughnuts from a Red Cross Clubmobile at Inchon Harbor, prior to departure.

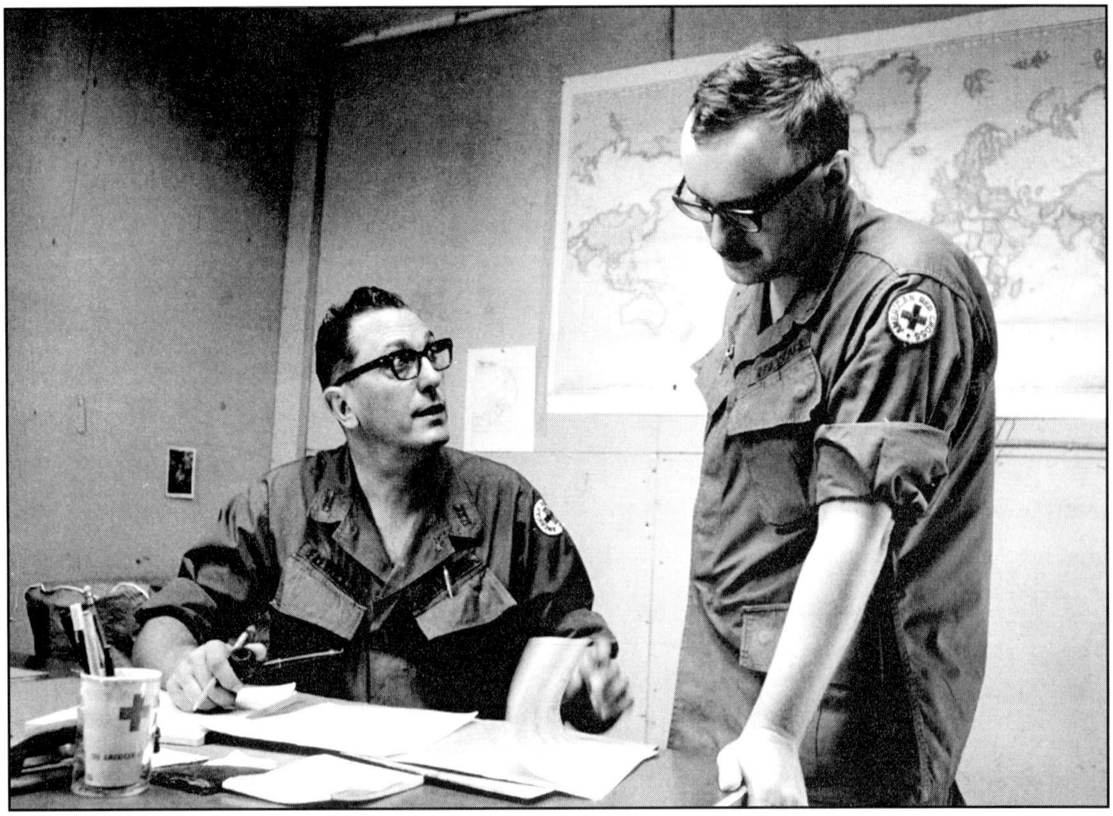

Mel Fredricksen, left, in Vietnam

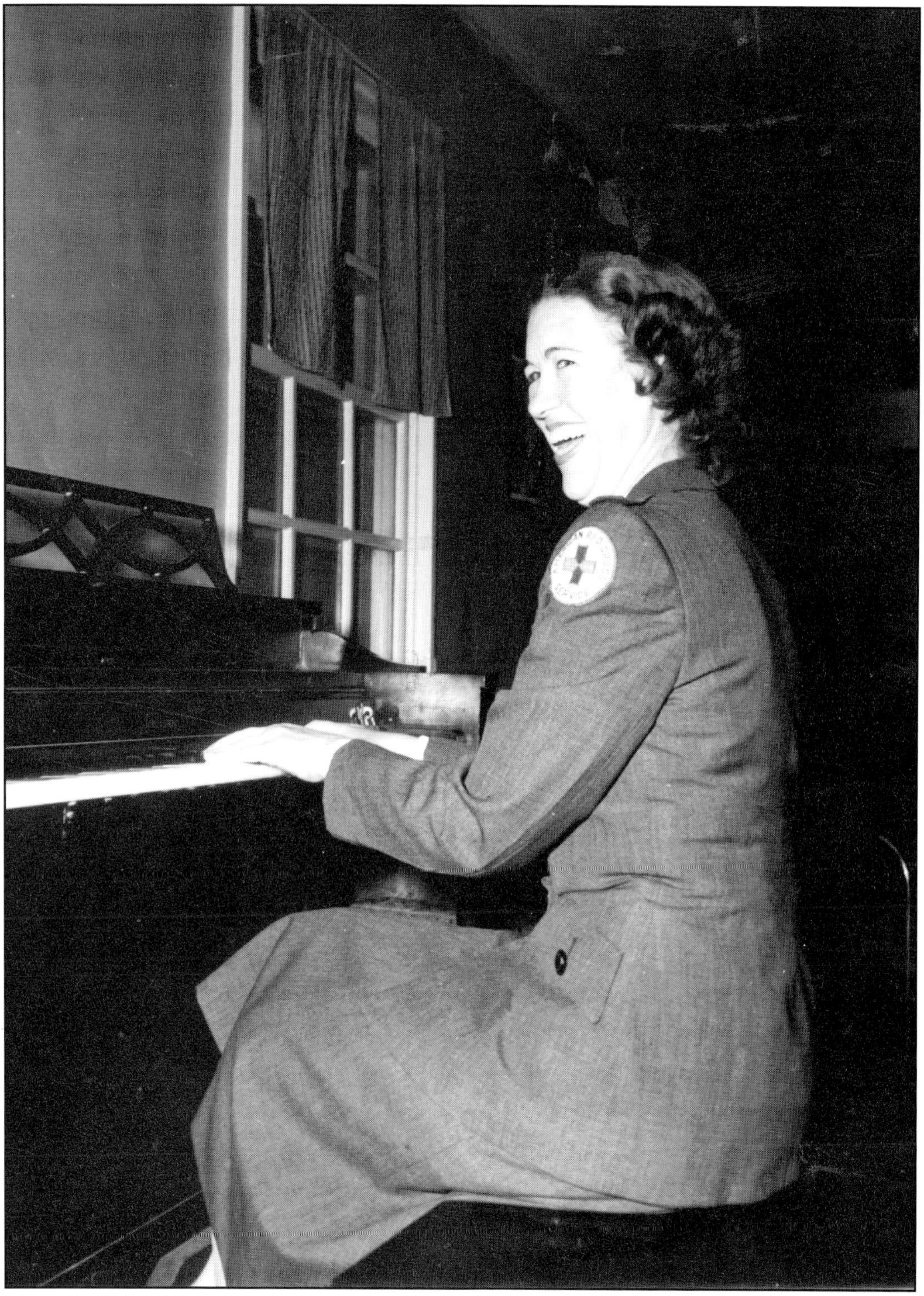

Mildred B. Powell, SRAO Center, Chateauroux, France

A History of the American Red Cross

The emblem of the Red Cross internationally symbolizes a dedication to humanity, unity and neutrality. By its very appearance, it encourages peace and universality. A wonderful example of unified voluntary service, the International Red Cross was established through the efforts of Henry Dunant to provide impartial care to the wounded in war. In August 1864, twelve governments signed the First Geneva Convention Treaty, in Geneva Switzerland. Great Britain, Saxony, Sweden and the United States were not included.

Dunant's observation of and compassion toward 40,000 wounded soldiers who suffered in the Battle of Solferino in northern Italy, moved this Swiss businessman to write a pamphlet entitled, *A Memory of Solferino*. In this influential piece, he asked:

> Would it not be possible to found and organize in all civilized countries permanent societies of volunteers which in time of war would render succor to the wounded without distinction of nationality?

Thereafter, the "Committee of Five" was formed (now known as the International Committee of the Red Cross). These compassionate humanitarians played the biggest part in getting the International Red Cross established.

In 1901, one of the first (of two) Nobel Peace Prizes was awarded to Henry Dunant for his humanitarian efforts. Although he died poor in 1910, his birthday, May 8, is still celebrated as World Red Cross Day.

Less than 20 years following the establishment of the International Red Cross, Clara Barton's vision helped shape the American Red Cross. She is an important figure in the early history of the American Red Cross, which was modeled after the International Red Cross. Although she did not originate the Red Cross idea, she was the first person to establish a lasting Red Cross Society in America. Barton became president at its formation with eleven members serving on the executive board.

Clarissa Harlowe Barton was born December 25, 1821 in Oxford, Massachusetts. She became a teacher at age 17 and later a copier in the U.S. Patent Office, before she permanently entered volunteer service at age 40. Her benevolence became legendary in the Civil War when she assisted by nursing and feeding as an independent volunteer. She could not work with the

International Red Cross because she was a woman, so she again volunteered independently in the Franco-Prussian War (1870-1871). Margo (Kitty) Antoinette, her first volunteer, traveled with Clara to the German border to aid civilians who had suffered from the bombings and other war-related traumas.

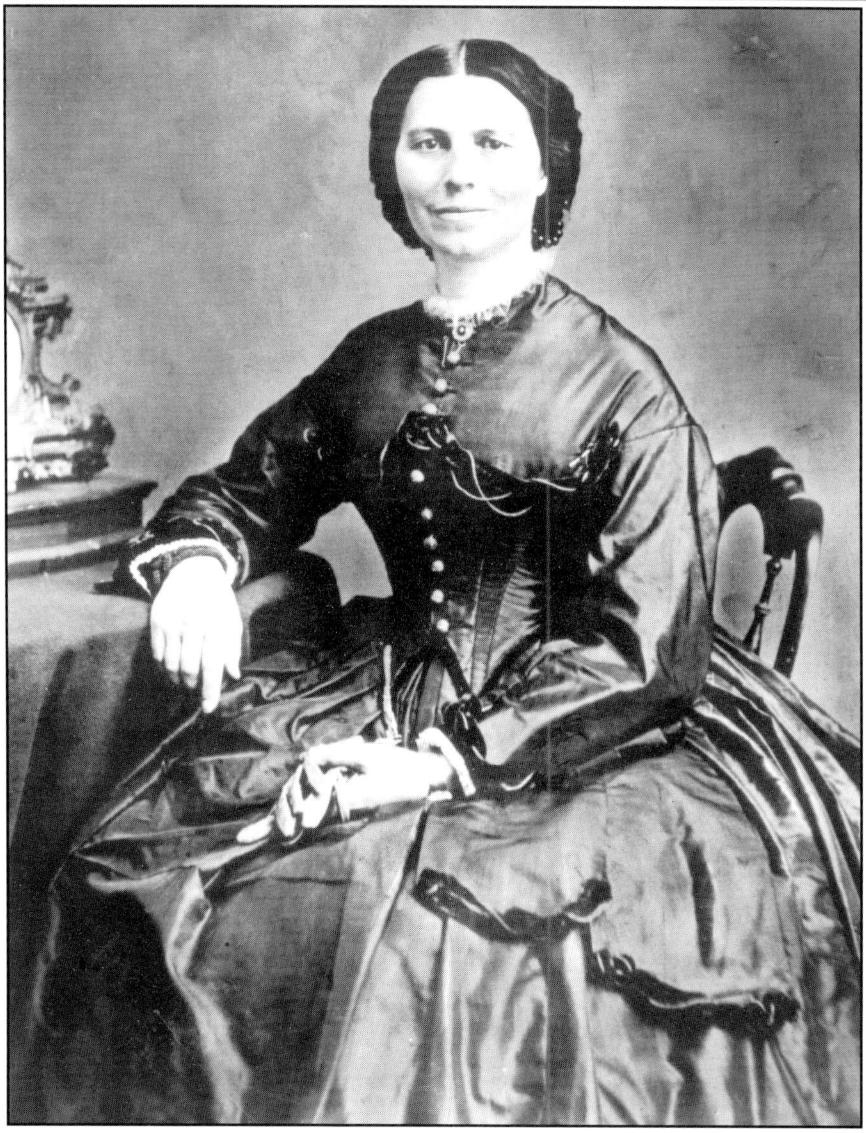

Clara Barton, president of the American Red Cross, June 9, 1881 - June 16, 1904

Relentlessly, Clara lobbied for the U.S. ratification of the Geneva Convention (First Treaty of Geneva). At last her efforts were rewarded when it was signed in March 1882. She said that serving in time of disaster, calamity as well as in war was the foundation of all American work for the Red Cross.

The United States the thirty-second nation to sign the First Treaty of Geneva. This meant that the United States would agree to protect and aid the wounded in wartime without respect to nationality.

During the Michigan Forest Fires of 1881, Dr. Julian B. Hubbell was sent by Clara Barton as the first American Red Cross field representative. While still a young man, he had asked her how he could help her in her humanitarian efforts, and she advised him to become a doctor.

The steamboat, *Josh V. Throop*, was another "first" in Red Cross history. It was the first inland vessel to fly the Red Cross flag and carry emergency supplies to victims of the Ohio and Mississippi River floods.

This led to the first known Red Cross youth activity. A group of six children put on a play in Waterford, Pennsylvania, and raised $50 for the Red Cross. When the children mailed their contribution they wrote, "Sometime again when you want money to help you in your good work, call on the Little Six."

After the reincorporating in 1900, the Red Cross began in 1904 to experience growing pains stemming from loose financial management. An investigation was launched and President Theodore Roosevelt withdrew his official support. Through all of this, Barton resigned and handed the baton to Mabel Thorp Boardman. This was a major turning point for the expansion to disaster relief, a commitment to humanity in war and peace. The Red Cross

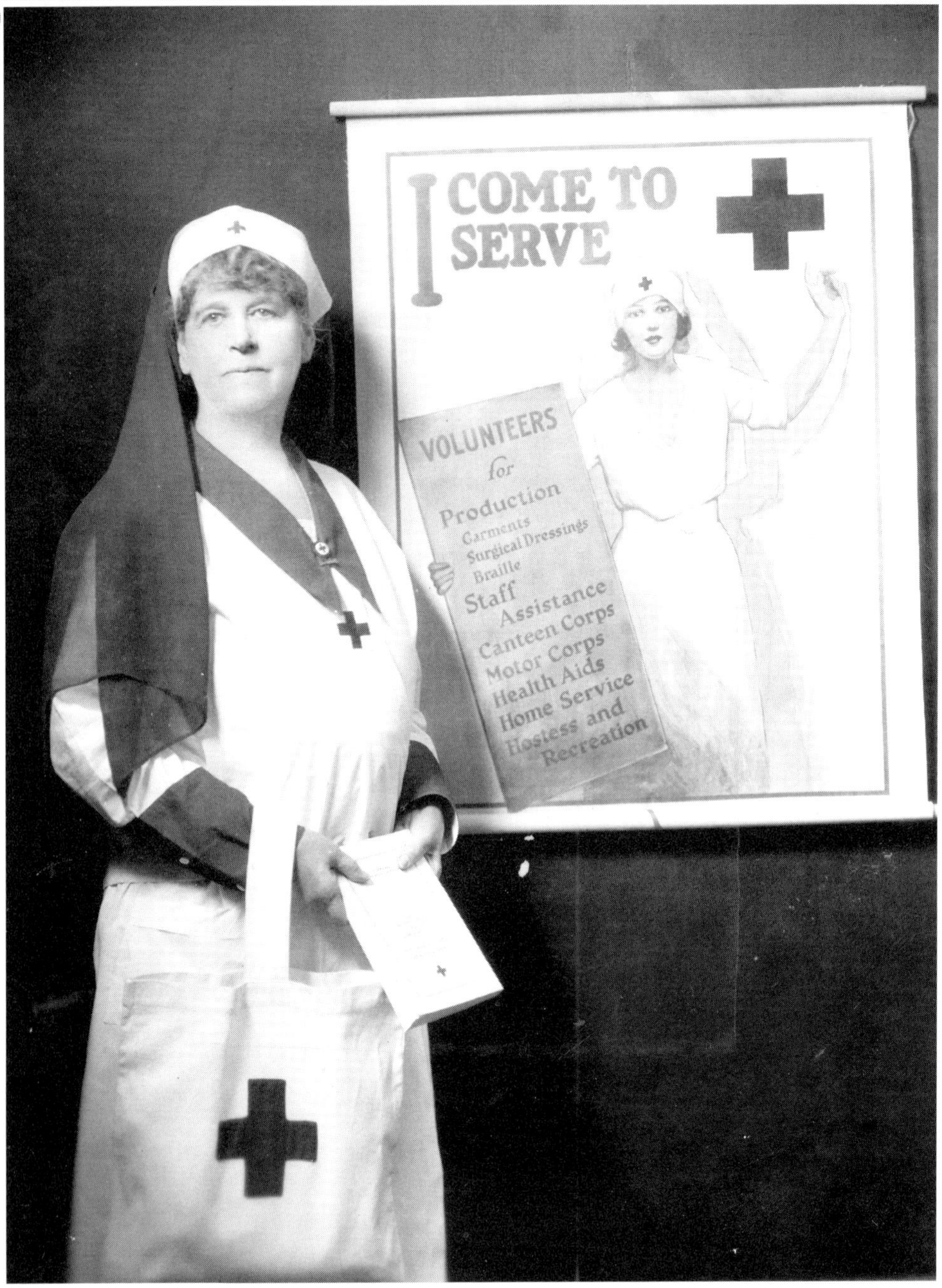
I COME TO SERVE
VOLUNTEERS
for
Production
Garments
Surgical Dressings
Braille
Staff
Assistance
Canteen Corps
Motor Corps
Health Aids
Home Service
Hostess and
Recreation

Mabel T. Boardman, wearing volunteer uniform

expanded much in disaster relief thereafter: Michigan fires; Ohio and Mississippi River floods; Johnstown flood; Russian famine; Georgia Sea Islands; Armenian massacres; San Francisco earthquake; Galveston, Texas hurricanes; Cherry, Illinois mine disaster; and many others.

Mabel Boardman brought about a revised charter in 1905. During World War I, the War Council was presidentially appointed to "run" the organization, and Mabel Boardman became second in command. She became secretary in 1919 and continued until 1944. She was honored by President Franklin D. Roosevelt for her services.

The American Red Cross had experienced a complete turnaround from the days of their financial crisis when President Taft passed a law that the only agency authorized by the U.S. government to offer services to wounded military personnel was the American Red Cross.

Expansion was also part of the growing process. In 1881, the first Red Cross chapters had been organized for local involvement. After 1905, state and territorial branches were organized to keep the disruptive local autonomy from threatening the internal unity of the organization. In 1909, chapters began to report directly to Red Cross National Headquarters to confirm that their activities were coordinated with those of the national organization.

The World War I era focused on fundraising in a few distinct manners. Posters by famous artists such as Alonzo Earl Foringer were part of the patriotic war drives. His oil painting, *The Greatest Mother on Earth*, was the most famous. His model was sculptress Agnes Tait, who was painted to be a "modern madonna" stretching her hands to everyone in need, "knowing no favorite, yet favoring all..."

During the war the Red Cross coffers shot up from $200,000 to $400 million. And another fund-raiser that perpetuated this effort was the Red Cross Annual Roll Call membership drives. One-year memberships were just $1, while a lifetime membership went for $25.

In 1915, groundbreaking for the permanent national headquarters, designed by Trowbridge and Livingston, took place at Seventeenth and "D" Streets in Washington, D.C. Half of the $800,000 cost was taken care of by congressional appropriation and the other half by private sponsors such as James A. Scrymser, Mrs. Russell Sage, Mrs. E.H. Harriman, and the Rockefeller Foundation.

It was President Woodrow Wilson who visualized the American Junior Red Cross and within 18 months of its announcement, 11 million volunteers offered services. These services produced 10% of the 371 million relief articles between 1918 and 1919.

First Aid's introduction in 1908 as well as the Rural Nursing Service in 1912, paved the way for the millions of volunteers who joined the Red Cross

Mrs. Harry Wiese, Red Cross Gray Lady, helps PFC Orville Janowski of Muskegon, MI, make a recording to send home.

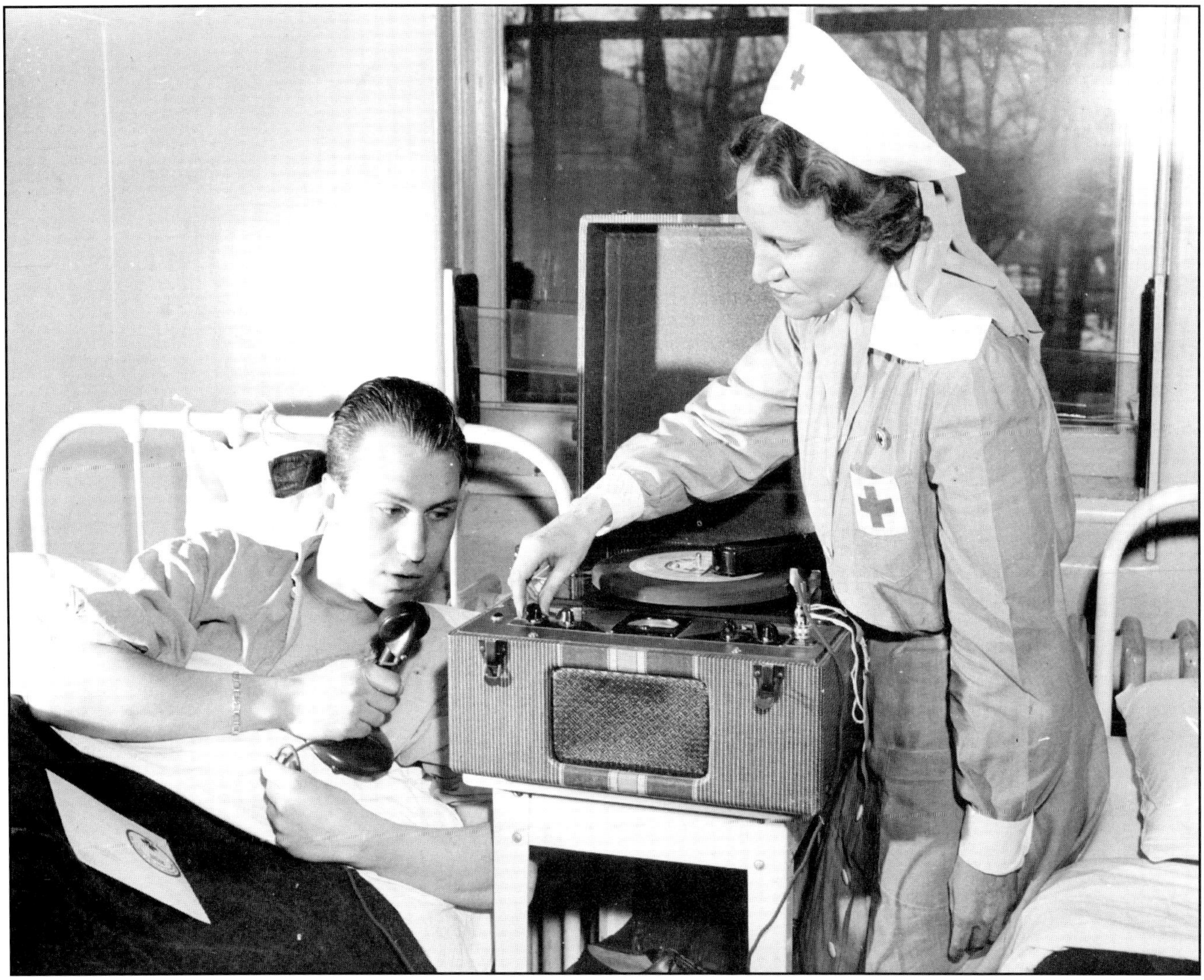

during the war. The number of chapters grew from 562 to 3,724 chapters and 17,000 branches, and it grew from 500,000 members to 31 million.

Judge John Barton Payne, appointed chairman of the Red Cross in 1921, is remembered for his efforts to bring volunteers and paid staff to work together more harmoniously. He died following an appendectomy complicated by pneumonia in 1935.

About the time Judge Payne was serving as chairman, the Gray Lady Service was founded in 1918 at Walter Reed Hospital in Washington, D.C. and by 1938, uniforms were worn nationwide. The Gray Ladies provided non-medical assistance, such as occupational therapy in Army and Navy hospitals and veterans' hospitals.

In 1912, Jane Delano left her position as superintendent of the Army Nurse Corps to become a fulltime Red Cross volunteer. She organized and directed the Red Cross Nursing Service, saying, "I would rather live on a crust and serve the Red Cross than do anything else in the world."

Following the First World War, the Red Cross began to assist with veterans' readjustment to civilian life. The Russian Civil War saw Red Cross volunteers rushing to the Trans-Siberian Railway to provide assistance to the sick and wounded. Disasters such as highway fatalities; the Chinese famine;

June 1934. The Red Cross Public Health Nurse is recognized by her uniform and Red Cross symbol as a firm friend in time of injury or illness.

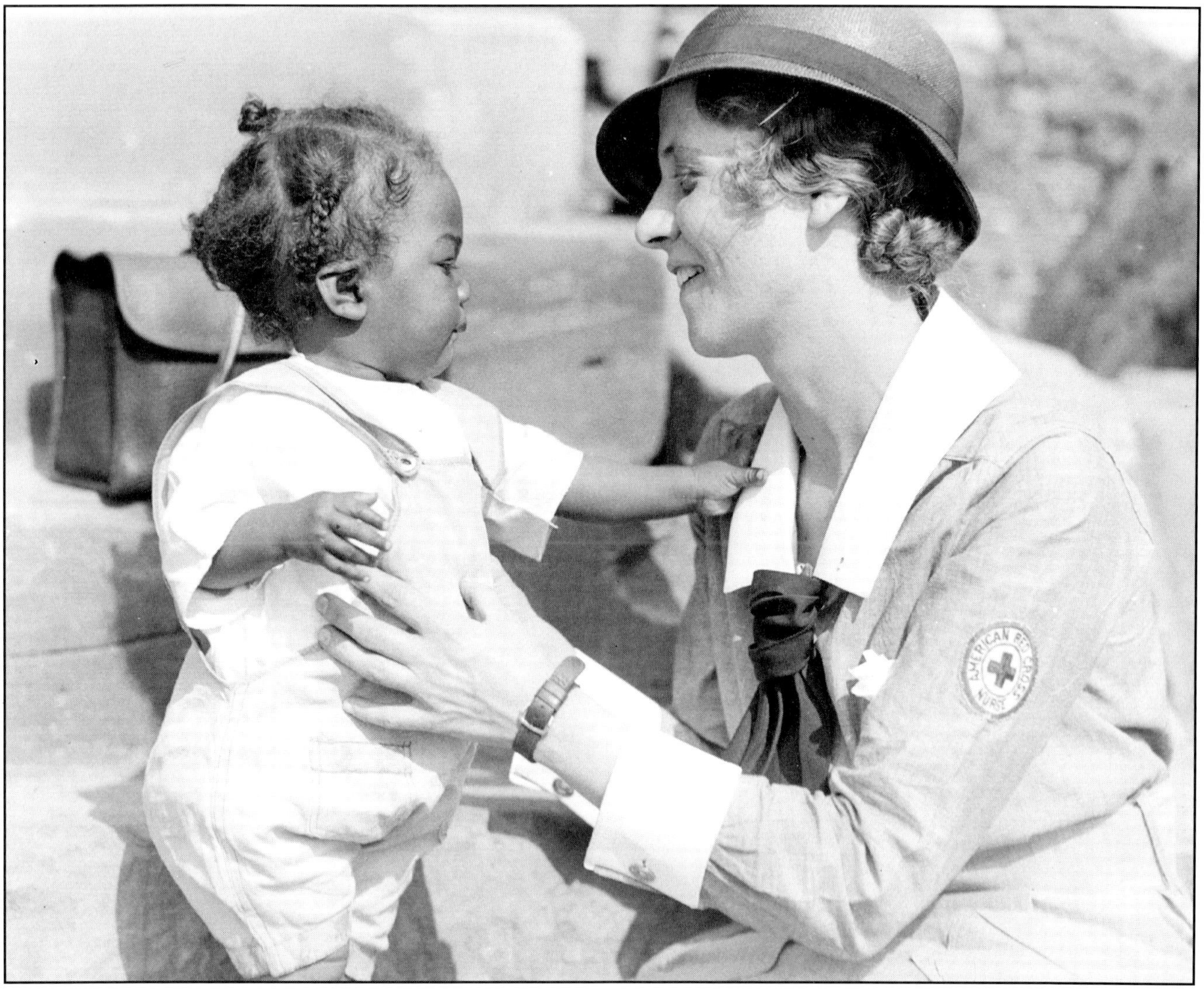

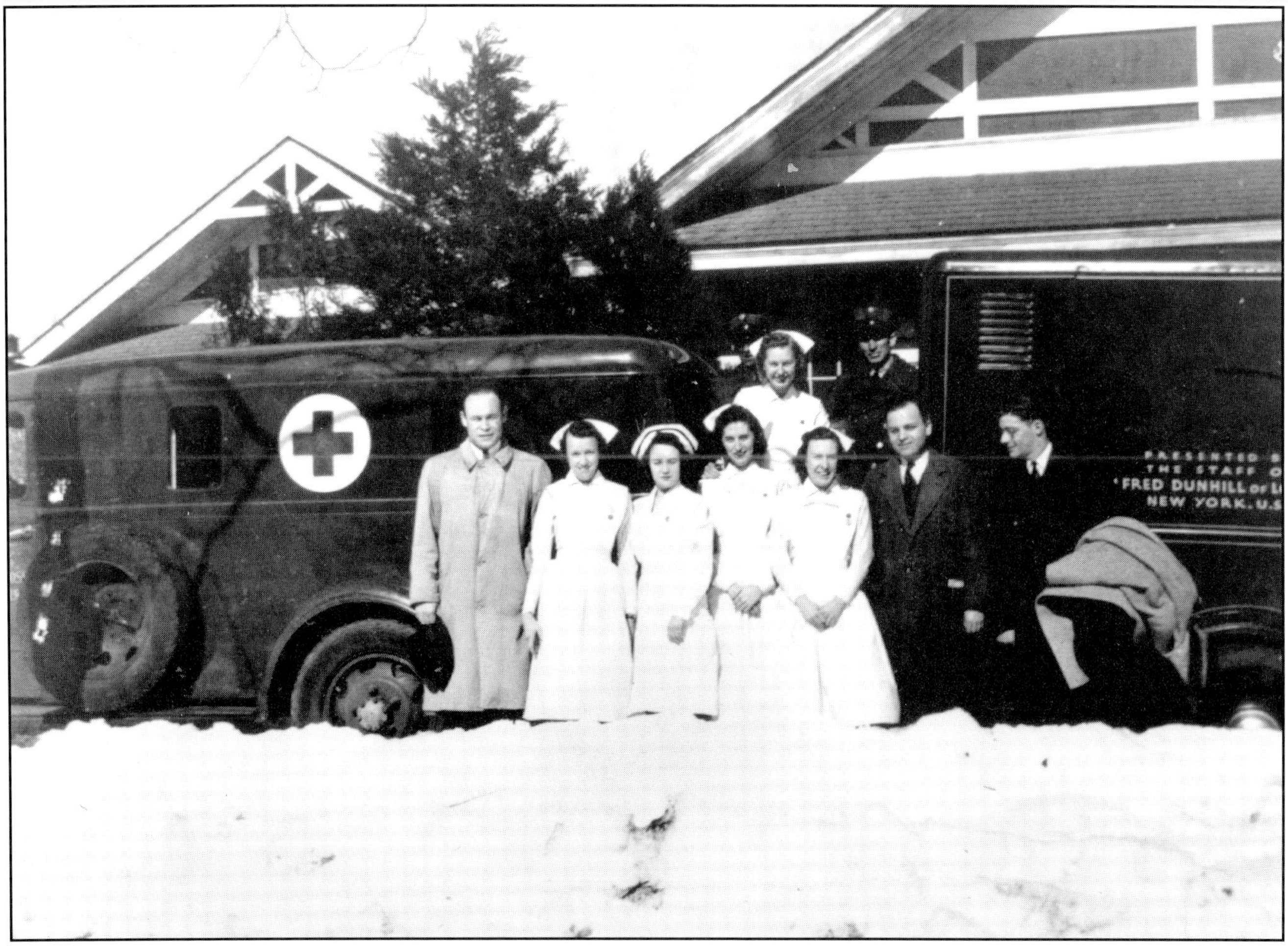
PRESENTED B
THE STAFF O
FRED DUNHILL of L
NEW YORK, U.S

September 1940. Dr. Charles R. Drew (left) is shown with doctors, nurses, and drivers from a mobile unit of the New York Presbyterian Hospital. The first of its kind, the unit was to collect blood plasma for Britain. Dr. Darrell Shaw, second from right, is the only other identified.

the Tokyo and Yokohama earthquake, fire and typhoon; the flood in Mississippi; and the 23-state drought gave the Red Cross plenty to do until the 1940s. A new memorial building was erected in 1930 on "E" Street NW, Washington, DC, to honor the heroic women of World War I.

World War II and the 1940s and 50s provided opportunities for the Nurse's Aide Corps, the Gray Lady Service, the Junior Red Cross, the Hospital and Recreation Corps and others. Blood drives sent blood donations up from 2,735 monthly pints to 53,770 pints. This blood was given to soldiers at the front and also civilians in need. The dried plasma became especially necessary at Pearl Harbor. The Red Cross also assembled food packages (also known as POW packages) for 1.3 million Allied and 115,000 American prisoners; 26 million by 1944. "Blood means life" was the slogan for the National Blood Program in which the American Red Cross collected nearly five million pints of blood for the armed forces.

During the Korean War at General MacArthur's request, the Red Cross began to provide recreation club services for all United Nations troops.

Jesse O. Thomas helped open professional ranks to African Americans when, on May 1, 1943, he was named special assistant to the director of domestic operations of the American Red Cross. He was able to be a liaison for blacks to the Red Cross, starting more effective integration of African Americans into Red Cross volunteer work.

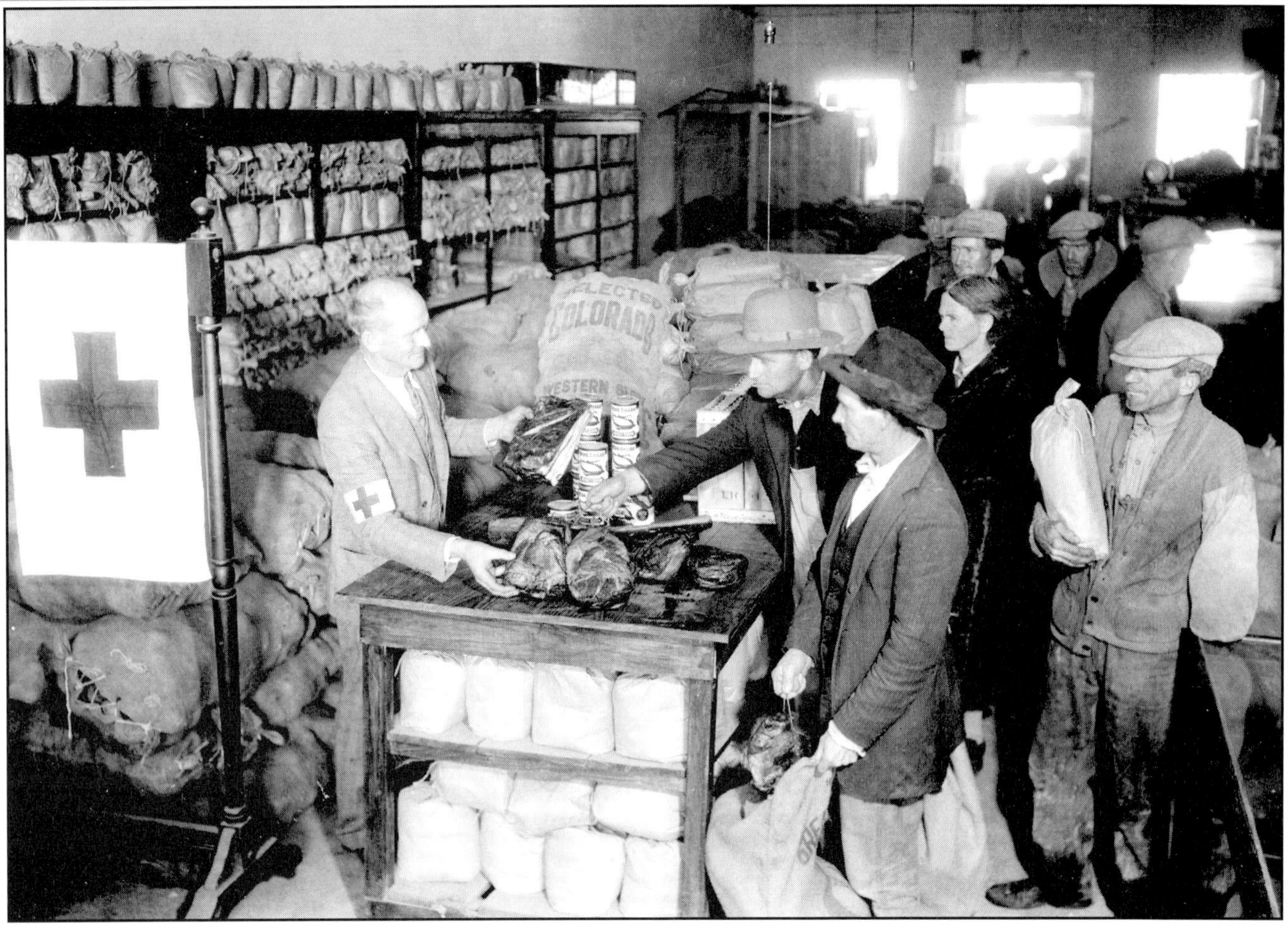

Lonoke Arkansas, 1930, drought. Relief to hundreds of thousands of victims of the great drought was provided by the Red Cross in terms of food, clothing, and seeds. This operation cost more than $11,000,000.

A study performed in 1956 revealed that many young people looked on the Junior Red Cross as "a sissy organization" and "mostly for girls." So in 1964, Red Cross Youth replaced the Junior Red Cross, moving toward the principle of "one Red Cross" and encouraging more participation from youth, boy and girl alike.

Dr. Jerome Holland was the first African American to be appointed chairman of the American Red Cross by President Carter in 1979. He was elected to the American Red Cross Board of Governors in 1973, and re-elected in 1974 and 1979.

New technologies enabled the American Red Cross to be more effective in the 70s. CPR (cardio-pulmonary resuscitation) was introduced by the American Red Cross in 1974. They worked closely with the American Heart Association to teach CPR. Also, improved medical technologies helped the American Red Cross donate blood more efficiently with computerized blood inventory and rare donor registry.

During the Vietnam War the American Red Cross sent paid staff to assist servicemen. The 1980s brought the 100th Anniversary of the American Red Cross (May 1981), increased health services to minorities, a tissue program, AIDS/HIV testing and aquatics programs. The Charles Drew Biomedical Institute was founded in 1994 to help ensure the quality of blood, tissue and plasma supplies through courses in management development, quality, biomedical technology, education and training.

The American Red Cross has a lasting legacy of humanitarian service, unity, universality, independence and neutrality world-wide. Not only has its participants nobly served the wounded on battlefields internationally, but they have also gone the second mile in providing relief to many areas ravaged by natural disasters. Following are some disasters in which the American Red Cross has served in the last century: Hurricane Hugo; Hurricane Andrew; the Midwest flood; various tropical storms and hurricanes; the Oakland Hills, CA fire; the Oklahoma City bombing; African Relief Campaign, the Armenian earthquake; and the massacre of Tutsis.

The Armenian earthquake in 1988 necessitated the largest disaster relief operation to date. This earthquake measured 6.9 on the Richter scale and shook for 40 seconds. It left over 25,000 people dead, thousands more injured and some 500,000 homeless.

The American Red Cross volunteers' efforts sometimes have gone unnoticed and without thanks. Yet their legacy lives on, especially in the hearts of those whose loved ones have been assisted and whose lives have been saved through Red Cross efforts, many times rendering their services in the face of danger. The American Red Cross personnel should be commended and honored for more than a century of outstanding humanitarian service.

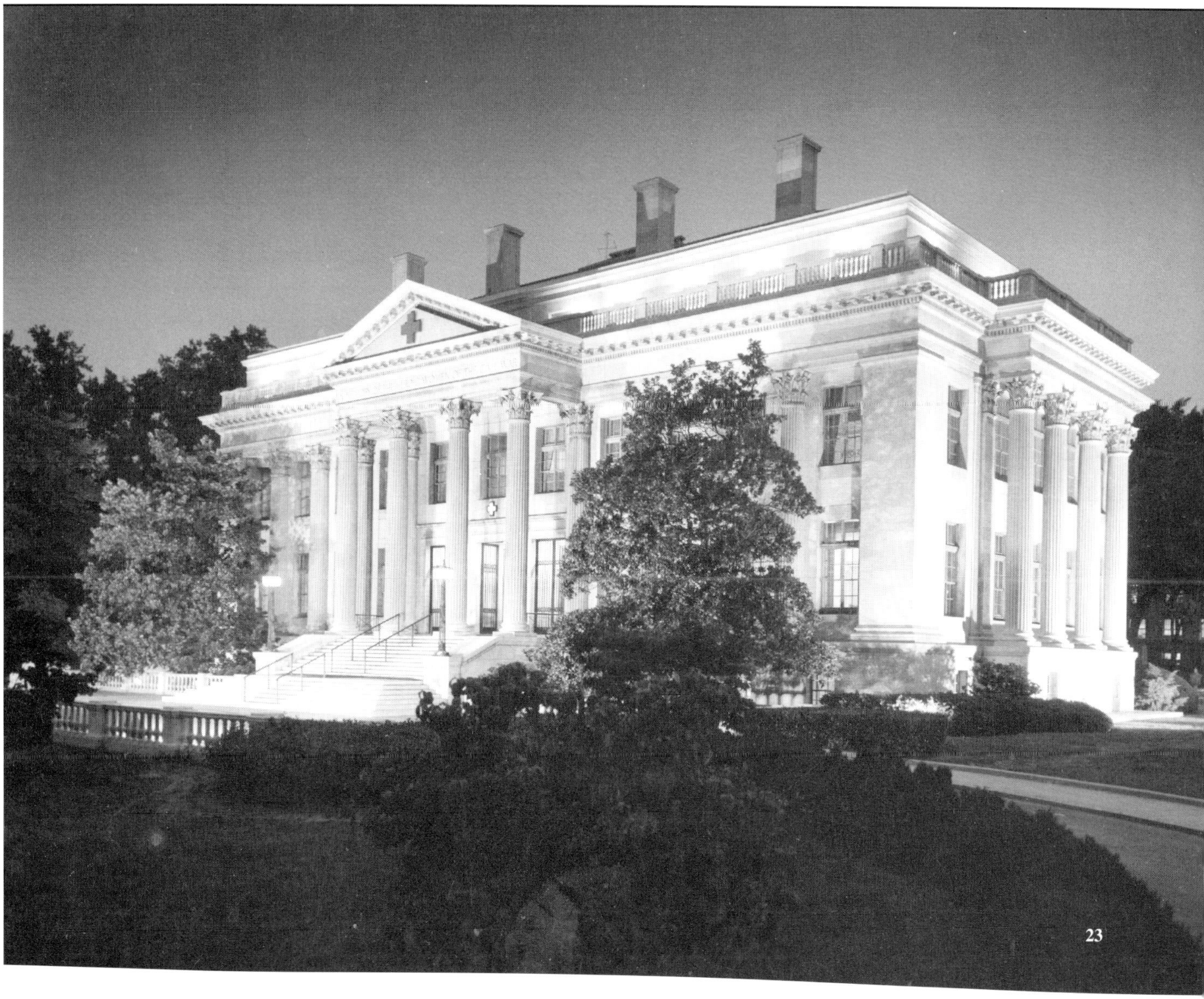

American National Red Cross Main Building at night, 1971

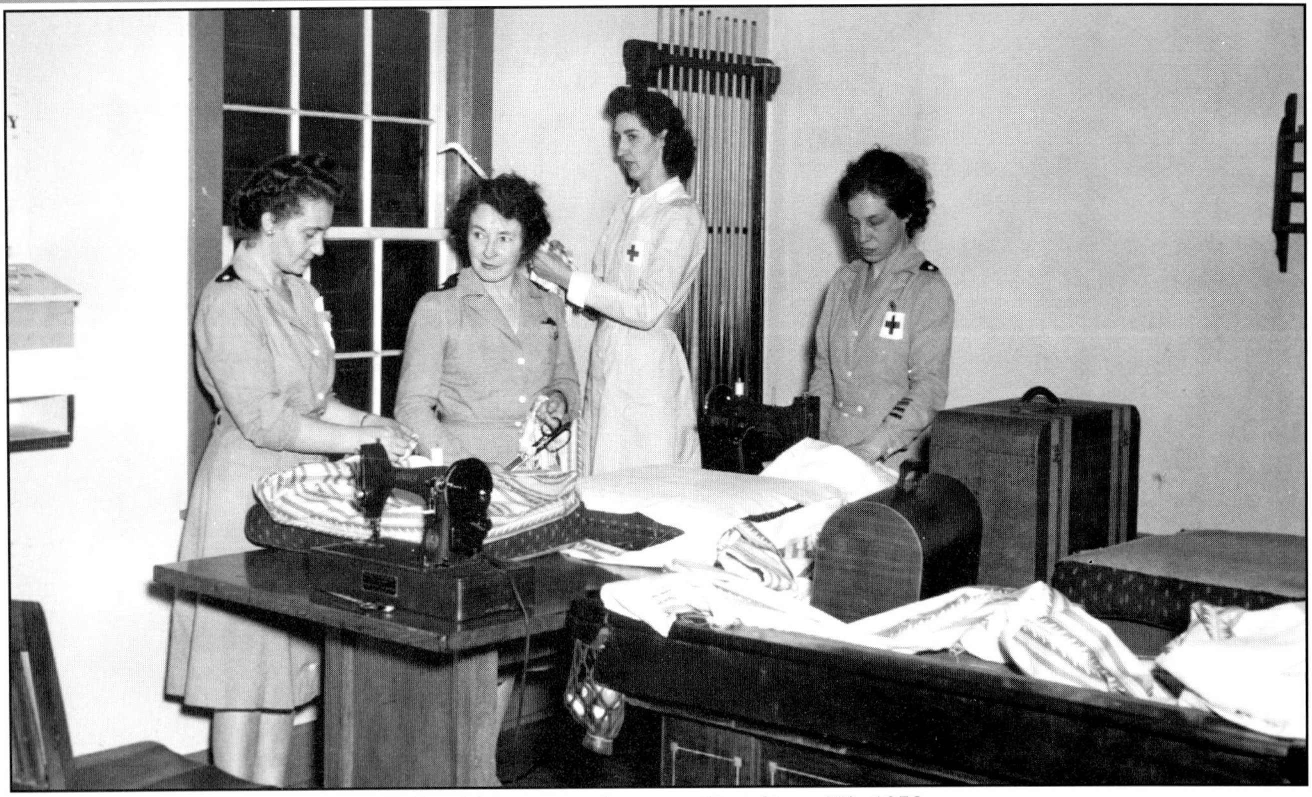

Refurnishing recreation room, Fort Story, VA, 1950

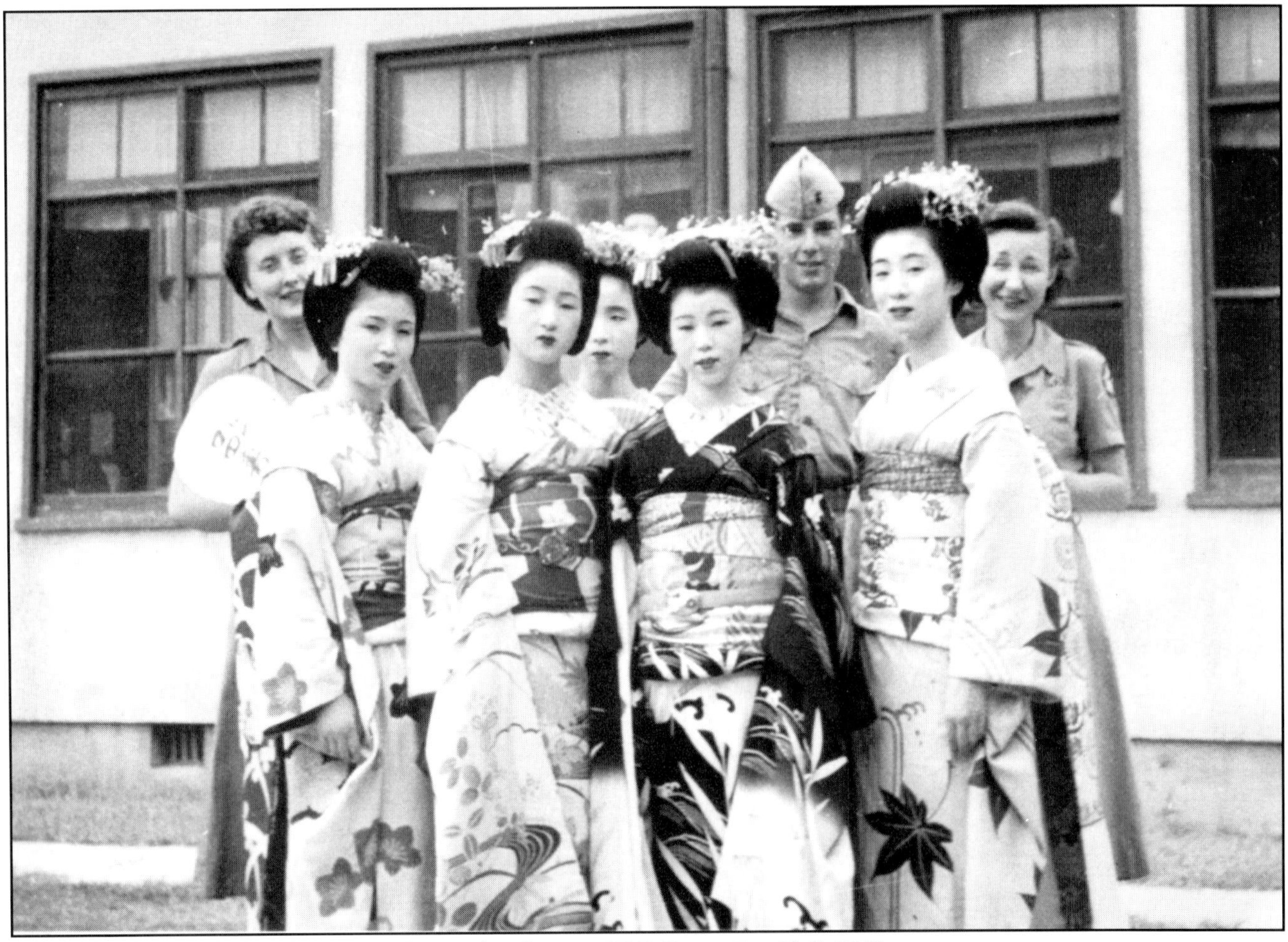

Recreation dances, ARC, Recreation Hall, 1951

American Red Cross Memories

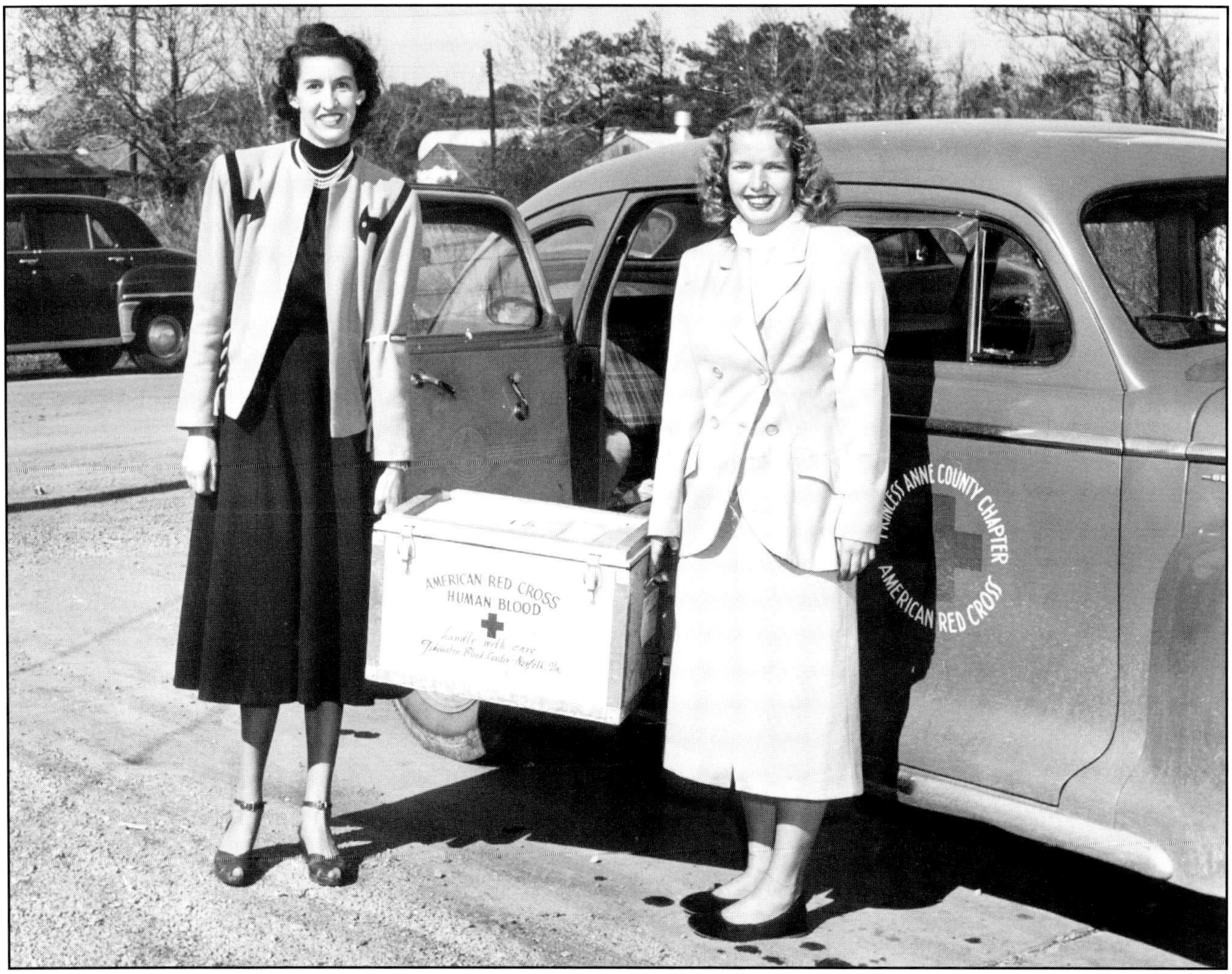

Pearl Duty Mallory and Marjorie Ferrar, Motor Corps, delivering blood to Virginia Beach Hospital, 1951.

KATIE'S STORY

by Katherine van Hogendorp

LEAVE TAKING

Was I being followed? Frantically I walked as fast as I could for several blocks. I saw a bus and quickly got on. I wanted to be as far away as possible from American University. After about an hour, I spotted an empty-looking tavern. I got off the bus and hurried inside.

"May I use your phone?" I asked a sleepy-looking attendant. He nodded his head. Hastily I dialed the number of my sister with whom I lived in Baltimore, praying that she not only would be home, but also would not question my call and simply reply, "Yes."

She answered, and in as calm a voice as I could muster, I said slowly, "Just wanted to verify my date with you and Harry (her husband). Isn't it dinner at seven tonight at the Mayflower?" It was obvious she was puzzled by my question. I held my breath while waiting for an answer. It finally came! "Yes, of course." Thank God she sensed the urgency of the call.

It was December of 1943, the period when Hitler was pushing back our forces in Europe, and the Japanese, at an alarming rate, were advancing and capturing our bases in China. Troopships, traveling through the Mediterranean on their way to the European Theater, were constantly torpedoed. Our losses were mounting.

I had volunteered and signed an agreement with National Red Cross to go overseas anywhere American troops were stationed and to remain for the duration of the war. Two weeks of orientation at the American University were to be followed by six weeks of training at a U.S. military base.

Once Red Cross volunteers arrived in Washington, we were warned that at any time we could be called for overseas duty. The signal would be simply a particular kind of tap on the shoulder. Further instructions would be found in one's footlocker which was placed under the bed in the dormitory. Extreme precautionary measures were in order. We were to trust no one, not even our fellow volunteers. Above all we were to disassociate ourselves as much as possible from our families, our friends and the general public. We were constantly reminded, "Loose lips sink ships."

When the inevitable shoulder tap occurred, one would leave Washington within 24 hours for an undisclosed destination. If this person had made a previous engagement on that particular day, it should be kept, and conversation was to be as normal as possible. No phone calls were allowed. Furthermore, the selected individuals would be closely observed until time of departure. Debarkation, obviously, was highly secret.

The batch of volunteers, of which I was a part, slept in one large room, with cots close to each other. A lone ceiling lamp was our only light. Having been spoiled at home by having my own bedroom, I found it an unpleasant adjustment to be in such crowded quarters. That dreary light was often turned on during the night, and frequently there was loud conversation.

Most of the day was taken up with briefing on war activities, lectures on survival under adverse conditions, and practice in packing a footlocker, musette bag and a small suitcase - our only possessions for the duration of the war. Everything had to go in them - mostly clothes for hot and cold climates - and was inspected and approved or eliminated.

One day at an opening lecture, I was seated next to an unusually attractive young woman. She looked like a movie actress. She was a delightful companion, and while waiting for the lecture to begin, we talked about the adjustments we had to make since arriving in Washington. Her pet peeve was having to stand in a long line to use the bathroom. Little did we know this would be daily routine for an indefinite length of time.

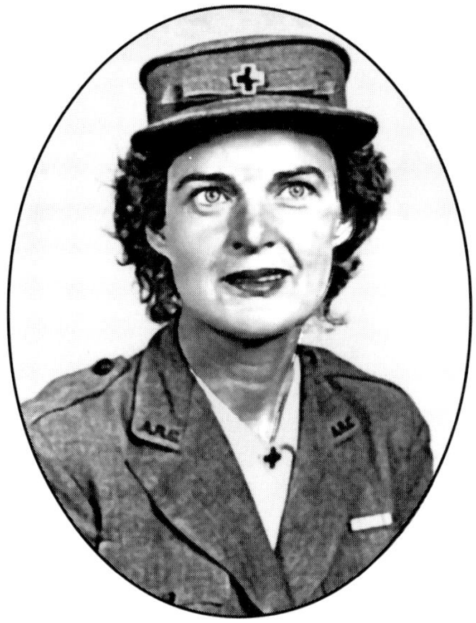

Katie in uniform

We planned to have dinner together that night. One hour into the lecture, our director made an announcement. "We have been hounded by the press ever since this group started. I have decided to grant fifteen minutes to the photographers for picture-taking. Miss Madelaine Carroll has agreed." Sitting next to her, I heard her say, "No closer than five feet, and only from the right side." A real professional!

On the eighth day after my arrival in Washington, I was tapped! I could not believe it. There must be a mistake. I hadn't even had a First Aid course! What would be my responsibilities? How would I know what to do? Would there be somebody to guide me? Was I supposed to do what I thought was necessary? The shoulder tap happened during a lecture. My throat became dry. My heart pounded. My family - I might never see them again. How did I ever get into this mess? Maybe I can just back out of the whole thing. I had volunteered for service because my two brothers were drafted and I wanted to go to war with them. Now they were 4-F and I was going off all alone.

Following the phone call to my sister, I returned quickly to the dormitory. There in my footlocker were the instructions. I was to be as casual as possible with my roommates. There were to be no farewells. I was to be packed and dressed in my newly issued winter uniform - the heavy overcoat would never have fitted in the footlocker - and to wait at a side entrance of the university at exactly midnight.

Feverishly I began to pack the footlocker with summer and winter uniforms and the required items from home, always aware of the training we had been given. "Tightly roll everything so that not even a pencil can be pushed between articles." Then I tackled the musette bag - the survival kit to be carried on one's back at all times. In it were medications and other items necessary to keep one alive for a period of time if circumstances resulted in an air crash or shipwreck. In this bag I included a good-luck charm - a little bottle of perfume called, "Je reviens" - I will come back.

A light snow fell as I made my way to the Mayflower Hotel. I had the feeling again that I was being followed. Somehow I didn't care. I was soon going to be reunited with my loved ones. My sister Annie and my brother-in-law Harry were there already. We embraced in silence, except for the pounding of our hearts. They had sensed the impending journey and the need for secrecy. We tried to make light conversation at dinner, and the drinks Harry ordered to lesson the tension only served to heighten it.

I waved good-bye to them as they walked slowly to the train at Union Station. They turned around, and my sister and I ran to each other and embraced once again. Then they turned and disappeared from my sight. My tears blurred my vision.

At the same station several hours later, I boarded a completely darkened train, arriving somewhere hours later. We were transferred to unlighted trucks which finally reached the gates of an embarkation camp. A soldier sitting next to me said, "Once we enter these gates, the only way to get back home is to cross the ocean and return." It was too late now to change my mind. Having said farewell to what I knew and loved, I was prepared to go.

The only sound was the crunching of our boots in the heavy snow. It was bitterly cold. We walked to barracks carrying our heavy musette bags and suitcases. An easterly wind blew in my face, causing warm tears to roll down my cheeks. It was New Years Eve, 1943.

This was the embarkation camp where, in a short time, we would learn some of the rigors of war and lose any sense of individuality or privacy we ever had before. It was a rugged experience, and if I had doubts before about my decision to go overseas, they were minuscule in comparison to my thoughts at this base of operations. Fortunately, we were there for only a week.

For some reason or other it was necessary for this contingent to march every day in heavy winter gear, carrying the musette bag strapped on the back, a newly-issued metal helmet and a small suitcase. The snow fell relentlessly. One particularly cold, windy day when we marched, GIs stationed on this base came out of their barracks and handed us chocolate bars to give us energy. It was one of the few humane gestures that occurred.

The sleeping quarters at the American University were luxurious compared with the over-crowded barracks here. I was assigned an area six by four feet. All possessions were stored under one's bunk. The back of an aluminum pan served as a mirror. Lights stayed on 24 hours a day. The latrines were in a separate building, and they had NO DOORS on them. Showers, minus curtains, were in one large room. The walk there and back at 6:30 in the morning was a guarantee you were fully awake. It wasn't unusual to stand in line for a half-hour with your canteen at chow time.

Shots for typhoid, hepatitis, yellow fever, etc. were given every day of that last week. On the last day, whatever was still needed as booster shots, was administered. I had nine, given in both arms. The following day I was unable to raise either of my arms.

It's amazing how the body, or the spirit, or both finally adjust - or maybe just give in. I think the Armed Forces accomplished probably what they had set out to do. Leave-taking from that camp into the unknown wasn't as hard as I expected.

CROSSING

The night was moonless. It seemed darker than usual—scary. There were no visible lights. Water lapped lazily against a pier. Suddenly, there was the sound of soldiers' heavy footsteps climbing a gangplank! We must be boarding a ship. The hours before had been spent on blacked-out trains and windowless vehicles. Secrecy was paramount. We had no idea where we were or where we were going - just sheep following the leader.

This converted troopship, I found out later, was the former Empress of Japan, one of the fastest vessels afloat. Because of her speed, it had been decided she would travel without convoy, taking the southern route around Africa.

Once aboard ship, we found the accommodations were miserable. Sixteen of us - nurses and Red Cross volunteers - were crowded into a cabin designed for four! Time schedules had to be arranged for getting up in the morning and for bunking in at night so we wouldn't bump into each other. In order to feed everyone, chow lines started at daybreak and continued until midnight.

Fortunately, there was some outstanding talent among the draftees on board, and before long a topnotch show was put together. I was a singer and was included in the program - a godsend for me. It not only relieved the tension, which seemed to build up relentlessly, but it also was relief from sitting on a hard deck all day. And that depended on whether you were lucky enough to find a space. The show was given twice daily, and always to a different group of GIs. The response was overwhelming. It was, after all, the only means of diversion. A week or so before landing, it became necessary to put on our show six times a day in order to accommodate the large numbers of troops aboard. For me it never became a burden, because of the GIs' overwhelming response. They whistled; they cheered; they applauded even before you started to perform. Civilian audiences back home were never like this.

The captain spoke to us daily over loudspeakers, warning us of impending danger. "It is highly suspected that enemy submarines are on our tail," he said. "Even a cigarette butt thrown overboard could be enough to give the enemy a clue to our location. You will be allowed on deck from sunrise to sunset. During the evening hours the outside of the ship will be completely darkened." He warned us to stay fully clothed, to wear our Mae West life jackets, and to carry musette bags 24 hours a day.

Almost 20 days had passed since that lonely night when we boarded this blacked-out ship. It was some time around then when Bob Clark made his proposition. "Have you ever seen the breathtaking constellation, The Southern Cross?" he asked in a half whisper. He looked at each of us, his three new buddies, huddled together as we had been almost every day on the over-crowded deck.

Bob had been a graduate student in astronomy before he was drafted. He continued, "You can see this beautiful Southern Cross in the sky only in the region of the equator. Heaven knows where we are headed, but by the temperature and direction the ship follows, I figure we are south of there now. I have a plan - we may never have another chance. Tonight, let's sneak out on deck, take a quick glance, and then find our way back inside."

Terry interrupted, "You're crazy. You know what will happen if we're caught? We'll be demoted, and they'll put us down in the brig."

Sandy followed, "Katie and I volunteered. How will it look if we're caught? They might think we are spies!"

Bob said, "Look, how do we know how long this war will last, or whether we'll live through it?"

Finally, he convinced us. We all decided to take the chance. Bob showed us the exit we would use, and we rehearsed in whispers his detailed plan. It sounded so simple, yet so frightening.

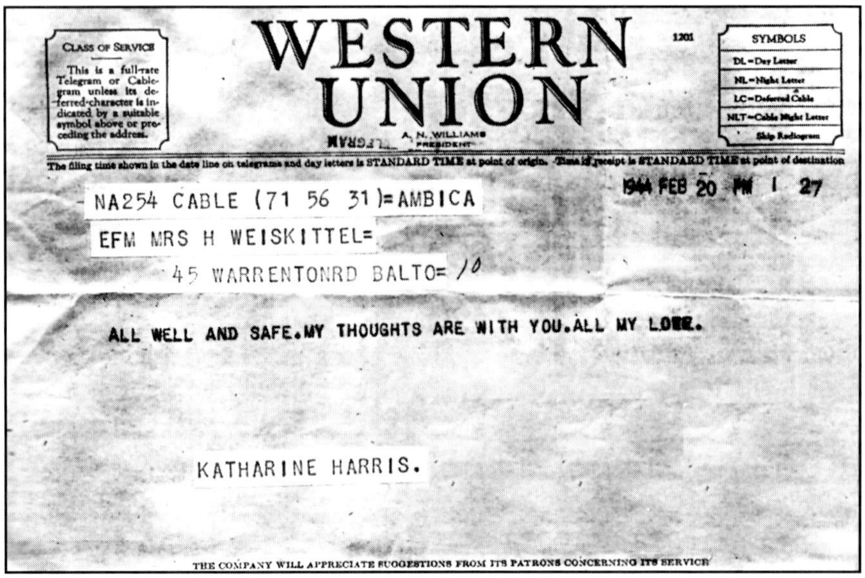
CLASS OF SERVICE
This is a full-rate Telegram or Cablegram unless its deferred character is indicated by a suitable symbol above or preceding the address.

WESTERN UNION

A. N. WILLIAMS PRESIDENT

SYMBOLS
DL=Day Letter
NL=Night Letter
LC=Deferred Cable
NLT=Cable Night Letter
Ship Radiogram

NA254 CABLE (71 56 31)=AMBICA 1944 FEB 20 PM 1 27

EFM MRS H WEISKITTEL=
45 WARRENTONRD BALTO= 10

ALL WELL AND SAFE.MY THOUGHTS ARE WITH YOU.ALL MY LOVE.

KATHARINE HARRIS.

THE COMPANY WILL APPRECIATE SUGGESTIONS FROM ITS PATRONS CONCERNING ITS SERVICE

Telegram home

At the appointed hour, one minute between each of our exits, I stealthily slid beyond the first maze of curtains, then the second then the third and finally the fourth. I was outside! The complete darkness of night startled me. We had been in the light for so long, even in our cabins, which were lit 24 hours a day. The air was fresh and warm. What a joy to feel a gentle breeze brush against my cheek!

I edged myself against the wall about three feet until I felt the welcome hand of one of my new-found buddies. My heart pounded as I lifted my eyes to behold this beauty of beauties stretched along the sky - The Southern Cross. The four stars that framed it were unusually large and bright. They seemed to float directly above me. I smiled in the darkness. What a good omen this must have been for sailors lost at sea! Suddenly, the voice of a guard sounded, "Who are you? Don't move or I will shoot!"

Immediately Bob answered. "There are four of us - we're GIs and Red Cross." He gave our names, our ranks, and then pled with the guard. "Please let them go. It is all my fault. It was my idea." He explained the reason for his curiosity, mentioning his studies in astronomy at the university.

The guard questioned him in more detail, and finally said, "I was a graduate student too, when I was drafted. You took a helluva chance, but I'm going to let you go and hope you won't get caught. But one of you better cover your florescent wristwatch."

ARRIVAL

On the 28th day, we landed in Bombay, India. We were shown three differently worded telegrams, from which we were allowed to select one to send home. My choice was "ALL WELL AND SAFE. MY THOUGHTS

ARE WITH YOU. ALL MY LOVE, SIGNED KATHARINE HARRIS"

It didn't sound like me, and surely wasn't what I would have chosen to say. However, I thought it was the best of the three.

After the war ended and I returned home, I learned about my family's reaction to this news. They felt certain this message was some sort of code - that I was trying to tell them something. Discussions were had with friends, and one of them even contacted a "code-breaker" in Washington.

After several days we embarked on a "troop train" for our week-long journey to Calcutta. This was our introduction to the great land of "Mystery and Romance," which the GIs before long changed to "Dysentery and No Chance."

Three times a day the train came to a halt, and the guys on kitchen duty prepared meals beside the tracks. The smell of food traveled fast, like all smells in India. As we formed our habitual chow line, we were approached by the local village inhabitants, the inquisitive and the hungry. Emaciated women in ragged saris carried hollow-eyed babies and cried, "Bakshish, bakshish!" (money), the word that would follow Americans wherever they went in India. Sometimes a group of monkeys or the ubiquitous sacred cows appeared. As we pulled away, we watched in horror the natives fighting over our garbage. I quit complaining after that.

Several weeks of orientation in Calcutta increased our awareness of some of the physical hazards involved in living in India. Survival in this over-populated, poverty-stricken country seemed formidable. Sacred cows roamed the streets. Children, and sometimes adults, relieved themselves whenever and wherever the urge prompted them. It was not uncommon to see natives who had died, lying in the streets or on the sidewalks, their bodies waiting to be picked up at the end of the day. Indians cooked over open burning fires, using dung for fuel. Once you've inhaled that odor, you never quite forget the sickening sensation it leaves.

CHAKULIA

My new assignment was handed to me. I took off in a C45, the only passenger aboard. There were no seats, but the heavy parachute I was wearing and a strap to hold on to kept me inI had experienced so many doubt's these last seven weeks, I felt reluctant to leave the plane. It seemed to be my last escape. I had finally reached my destination. Now there really was no turning back!

A cheery voice greeted me. "I'm Pat McDonald from Greeneburg, PA. I have the room next to you." Pat continued, "You know we're in a jungle. You've got to wear slacks and boots after sunset, and always carry a flashlight. The base is darkened at night. You never know what's around. An elephant wandered in the other night. Come on, I'll show you around the base."

She showed me a number of runways in the process of being built. The army engineers were feverishly working to complete them . There were endless barracks, mess halls, a hospital, officer's club, and a large Red Cross Club, recently completed for enlisted men.

Having been told of the secrecy on this base, I was surprised to hear some native villagers had been hired. They had been born into the caste system, which must have been a forerunner of our unions. Each employee, according to his caste, had been taught to perform only one function. He dared not intrude on the responsibility of another employee. He may have been trained to dust a room, but it was another person's duty to sweep the floor.

A young officer, named Charlie, drove me to my quarters in a jeep, which had painted on its bumper, "Miss Carriage." I later learned every moving vehicle on that base carried a name. Charlie left me, saying, "Enjoy your stay! If you're not happy with your quarters, maybe I can get you a room at our guest house, 'The Waldorf Hysteria.'" I stood and stared at the low building in front of me. It was called a "basha hut," and this was to be my home for an indefinite period -for as long as the war lasted, or as long as I lasted.

My room was one of four to be shared with three other Red Cross workers. The hut was made of concrete, obviously slapped together in a hurry, over which hung a shabby looking thatched roof. Surrounding the building was a four foot path made of small stones, which, later I was told, discourages snakes from crossing. Timidly, I entered a doorway measuring about three by four feet - one of two entrances. The

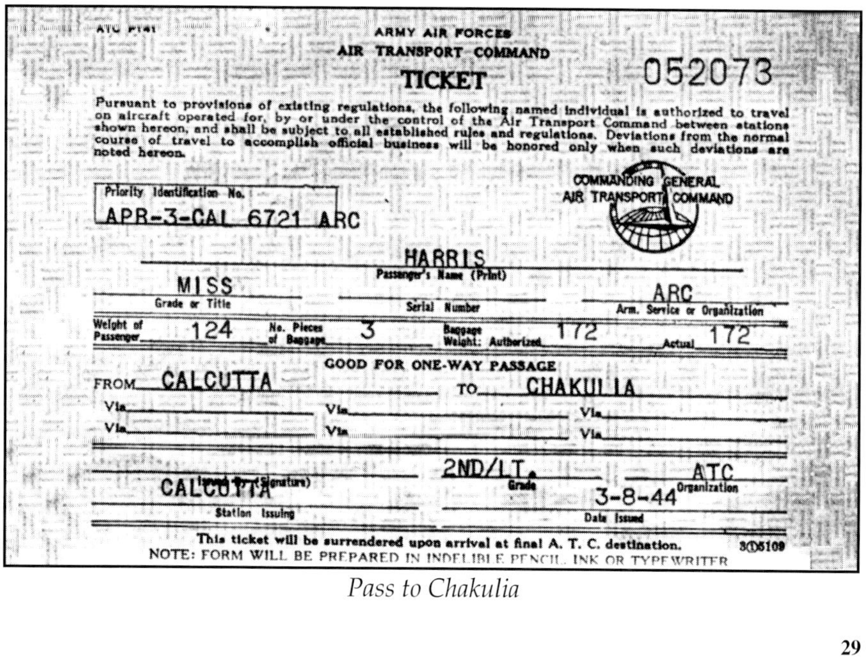
ATC F141
ARMY AIR FORCES
AIR TRANSPORT COMMAND
TICKET 052073

Pursuant to provisions of existing regulations, the following named individual is authorized to travel on aircraft operated for, by or under the control of the Air Transport Command between stations shown hereon, and shall be subject to all established rules and regulations. Deviations from the normal course of travel to accomplish official business will be honored only when such deviations are noted hereon.

COMMANDING GENERAL AIR TRANSPORT COMMAND

Priority Identification No. APR-3-CAL 6721 ARC

Passenger's Name (Print): HARRIS
Grade or Title: MISS
Serial Number:
Arm, Service or Organization: ARC
Weight of Passenger: 124 — No. Pieces of Baggage: 3 — Baggage Weight: Authorized 172 — Actual 172

GOOD FOR ONE-WAY PASSAGE

FROM CALCUTTA TO CHAKULIA
Via — Via — Via
Via — Via — Via

(Issued by) (Signature) — Grade: 2ND/LT. — Organization: ATC
Station Issuing: CALCUTTA — Date Issued: 3-8-44

This ticket will be surrendered upon arrival at final A. T. C. destination. 3(1)5109
NOTE: FORM WILL BE PREPARED IN INDELIBLE PENCIL, INK OR TYPEWRITER

Pass to Chakulia

other was even smaller and led to an outhouse affair. The air was stifling and steam was pouring off the walls.

Against one of the walls was a bed - four boards held together by heavy ropes over which was spread a muddy colored army-issue blanket to serve as a mattress. Why a blanket in temperatures ranging 100 degrees and up? Probably the idea of a behind-the-desk officer at the Pentagon in Washington. Four more vertical boards served as posters to hold up a limp mosquito net. A small mirror hung over a crudely made chest of drawers, and a simple wooden chair completed the arrangement.

Like everything else here, I soon found out the room was not mine alone. A hill of wet sand in the corner proved to be inhabited by a large family of giant termites, and in another corner a pair of busy tarantulas were staking out their claim.

That evening I had my first encounter with the little outhouse connected to the hut. Since there was no electricity I carried a flashlight, which I laid down beside me on the two-holer. In the shadow it cast, I noticed something in the corner that appeared to be one of a pair of galoshes. I shined the light on it and became rigid! It looked like a large, brown crab whose two claws slowly opened. Its long tail was arched over its head, pointed right at me. I was paralyzed with fright, but slowly rose. Still shining my light on it, I edged my way out, slamming the door behind me. An Indian guard told me it was a scorpion, whose bite one might not survive. He sounded an alert. Natives caught it and encircled its tail with a string. They hung it in a tree and walking around it, chanted mournful sounds. Everything in India is bigger except its people.

In bed that night I thought of the oft' spoken words, "It might not be much, but it's home." It was mine for almost two years, and I suppose after a period of adjustment I felt some small semblance of affection for it. However, when I finally left, I shed no tears. I didn't even look back.

RAISING MORALE

I found it hard to adjust to the unmerciful heat, especially at night. I would climb into my rope mattress bed, enveloped by thick mosquito netting. Once in, I turned and tossed until daybreak.

One night my new friend and coworker Pat and I decided to move our beds outside. "It can't be any worse than inside, Katie. Let's take a chance." She referred to the possibility of roaming wild animals. We still trembled when we thought of the wild elephant that caused such havoc on the base just the week before. It took three days before he was caught. Rifle shots just bounced off his hide.

"Good idea, Pat. Let's go to work!"

We had to dismantle the beds in order to get them through the small doorways. Amidst gales of laughter, we put them together again outside by the road. We decided to defy the bugs and snakes and try to get a good night's sleep. Psychologically we felt better, even though the temperature was about the same.

I heard Pat's voice, "Katie!"

"What Pat?"

"I was just thinking - you know, we volunteered for this."

"Shut up and go to sleep!"

We lay awake a long time outside. It was fun to go to bed under an Indian moon and sparkling stars and listen to the beat of the tom-toms in the far distance. I awoke quite early. The sky was blue and clear. I lay watching the birds, flying back and forth in all their freedom and abandon. The horror of war that surrounded us on earth seemed incongruous.

Suddenly we were aroused by the sound of marching boots. The GIs got quite a shock at the sight of the two little beds with sleeping beauties.

"Pull the sheet up, Katie! We're here to raise these guys' morale, but after all, there's a limit!"

There were wild cheers and laughter.

Most of the troops slept outside, and of course the natives did — very often without beds. We decided to stay out until the monsoons drove us inside.

These marching soldiers were part of the Corps of Army Engineers engaged in the construction of the base, and history-making long runways.

HARDSHIPS AT BASE

Those early days were rough before the 20th Bomb Command arrived with their B-29s. Rations were poor - Spam and K-rations. There was no refrigeration. Sometimes I'd take one look at the food and go back to my room and take a vitamin pill instead of eating. The heavily chlorinated water was warm and bitter. Water in outside tin tubs became too hot to bathe in. Connie Ascensio, our boss, hung a thermometer outside our club and it burst!

Among our early instructions, we were cautioned never to put on a shoe without turning it upside down and hitting it against the side of the bed or something hard. You never knew what could be hiding in there. In the early days I once forgot. I ended up in the hospital with a bite from the poisonous fangs of a six inch type of centipede. I never forgot after that. In fact, I continued the habit automatically for a period after the war.

Diarrhea and other tropical ailments were prevalent. There were frequent cholera epidemics. We were warned constantly to add special chlorinating pills to the water we drank and used for cleaning our teeth.

LETTERS FROM HOME

The close relationship with my family was sustaining, and it continued throughout my stay with letters. Letters arrived regularly expressing joy for my adventure and concern for my safety, my health, and even my love-life. News from home was so welcome.

My brother-in-law wrote to me after receiving my cable that I had arrived safely at my undisclosed destination.

March 14, 1944
Dearest Kakie,

Your cable and letters certainly brought good cheer to 45 Warrenton Road. Your Sis had been melancholy and depressed for sometime. That was hard on my whiskey stock. A.B.'s roaming around from room to room with a bottle in her hand was reminiscent of the old Peabody days and that famous degree.

The good news of your arrival was an occasion for a real celebration. Now we have settled to a more or less normal life, but always thinking of you.

Conditions at home have been unusually good. Lizzy, the cook, and Edith, the nurse, have worked out very well. Big Anne, temporarily has some free time on her hands. We are planning to go to New York on Thursday of this week for a few days.

Little Anne and Bebe are more wonderful and cuter than ever. Bebe has developed quite a personality. He seems to be everybody's pet, so I am forced to lavish most of my affection on my sweet little Annie.

Cod and Luce spent a couple of days with us. Annie was after Codie every minute. She certainly gave him a real workout and a few lessons in love making.

I wish, Honey, I had more interesting news to write about. Everything is about the same. No divorces or scandals to report.

We are always thinking about you and just waiting for the happy day when this whole terrible mess is over and our little Kakie will be with us again.

I will try to hide a few bottles from your sister so that we all can partake in an extra big celebration.

Much love,
Brother Harry

When I wrote to my sister that I was spending time with Joe Yagos, a tail-gunner whom I liked a lot, she panicked. And because she was unable to meet him, she worried and imagined nightmarish scenarios and lectured:

August 16, 1944

Dearest Kak,

Please don't think I'm crazy. I guess I'm still your old conservative sister, but although you are making a terrible sacrifice in uprooting yourself and giving your all to the war effort, don't let your standards of right and wrong be altered by the war. It's so easy in your circumstances to say - what the hell, everything's changed and the old standards by which I lived don't count. But you won't be living that life over there forever. And your own decency and self-respect are the greatest treasures you can have.

I hope Joe isn't married. If you don't know, you have a right to know. Another thing, if he is married, he went over there to fight for his country, his family and children. If he is unfaithful to them, he has already lost one thing he is fighting for. You have your whole life before you - don't let it be tainted forever, by what may prove to be a regrettable experience.

Well, now that that's over, I'll give you the local news. The weather has been most unpleasant for two weeks. Hot and humid, always soaring in the 90s and no rain. It is mean for us, but a temperate springtime for you, I guess.

There is a lot of Infantile around Baltimore, so I'm keeping the kids in the backyard.

Edith is acting queer; something ailing her all the time. I'm afraid she won't last much longer. H. thinks she is somewhat nuts.

Did you get Stell's perfume?

All our devoted love and a heartful of loving good wishes for the dearest Sis in the world.

Annya

When Joe's rotation took place a few months later he went to Baltimore to meet Harry and Annie. They really liked him. Joe told them about my bouts with illness and the deplorable conditions in India. He advised them to do everything they could to get me out of there. The alarm bells sounded, and my family sprang into action. My brother Charlie contacted Red Cross and pleaded for my transfer. I was furious with them all. Annie wrote me about my decision to stay put and included words of fondness for Joe.

January 19, 1945

Dearest Kakie,

I am thrilled with your decision to stay there at your post, although it will be a great personal happiness for me when

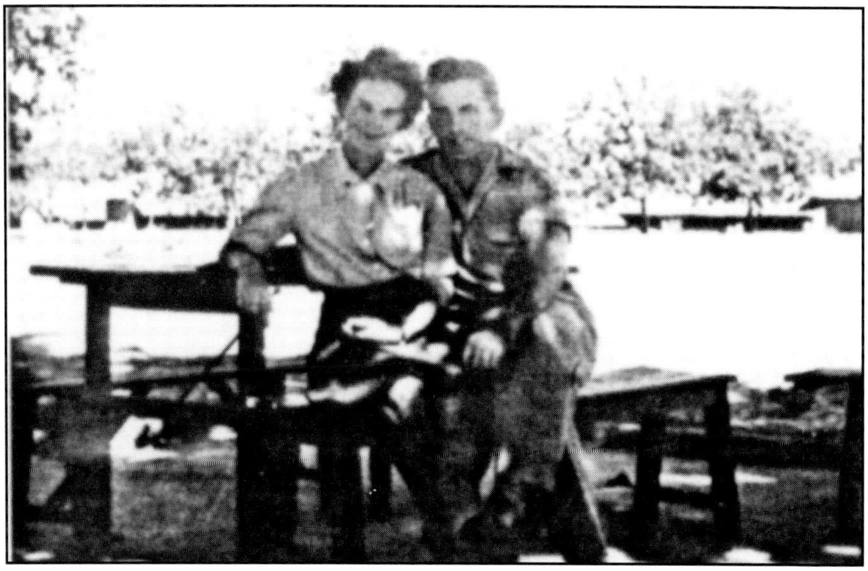

Katie and Joe Yagos

you return here, even though I know it will be a terrific adjustment for you to make after your life in the war. I am prepared to do all I can to help when that time comes. At the same time - I get much happiness in knowing you're happy where you are; that you "have found yourself" so wonderfully in your work - there is nothing so wonderful in life as in realizing you are achieving the maximum success with what talents God has given you. It is probably what everybody wants in this world, but not everybody, for lack of opportunity, and lack of ability and foresight, achieves. I knew in my heart the thing wouldn't defeat you. Our primary concern has been for your health; and what Joe said about the climate and its toll on you certainly can't be untrue. You mustn't blame Joe for our concern and our efforts through the Red Cross as to whether you should return to the States. Naturally living over here away from you, knowing you were in mental distress of the worst kind, and not being able to do anything about it, made Charlie and me anxious about you; but now we are happy - with you. However, don't you dare blame Joe for anything. Judging you from past experience, Kak, I know how easily some other dear guy - pilot or otherwise fox hole companion, can dim the pain of loneliness in your heart caused by parting with a former love. You must not be forgetful of Joe and what he meant to you in the early dark days over there. Much love, Darling, and fondest wishes for all your happiness and success - we eat up every word of your letters.

Your devoted

Annya

In November I received exciting news from my brother and his wife. They had become the proud parents of twin daughters, Janet and Judith. I wrote them immediately to tell them we were celebrating this birth on the other side of the world.

My Darlings!

Just received your letter. I'm spreading the good news over the base. Bought a box of cigars to hand out - had to get special permission. We are rationed to two a month. Also had message put on bulletin board with "Janet and Judith, Red Cross gals of War of 1944." There's a write-up about them in our base paper.

I'll be with you all in spirit on Christmas thinking of you all day.

Devotedly,

Kak

I never was far from my family in my thoughts, nor I in theirs. All joys and adventures and worries were shared.

THE B-29 SUPERFORTRESS

At first we were not quite sure what our duties involved. A sort of trial and error situation existed. We soon learned the needs changed as the war escalated.

One day some months after my arrival, rumors spread like wildfire. "It's coming today! The new plane will arrive at our base."

It started as a whisper in the distance. The sound of its four engines gradually increased to a roar. We looked upward and saw a magnificent aircraft circling to land. It was not only much larger and faster, but also capable of being airborne considerably longer than any existing plane. It carried a crew of thirteen.

This was the famous B-29 Superfortress, destined ultimately to drop the bomb that would bring the surrender of the Japanese Army and the end of World War II.

More planes arrived every day, and the long missions across the Himalaya Mountains into Burma, Indo-China and China became routine.

Up until this time our duties centered on activities in the large clubhouse for GIs, as well as daily visits to the sick in our hospital. As the war in this China-Burma-India theater escalated, so did the number of planes and missions.

HUMP-HAPPY BABY

I soon observed that the waiting period before an important event, especially if your life was at stake, can be a hectic and nerve-rattling experience. I refer to the crews of B-29s waiting on an airstrip for several hours before takeoff on a mission. This thought gave another Red Cross worker and me serious concern. We wanted desperately to be able to do something to relieve the tension of the long pre-mission wait. If only we could visit with the crews, exchange a few words of cheer with coffee and a snack! However, tight security surrounded the planes and the airstrips. Only flying crews, ground crews and official personnel were allowed anywhere near them.

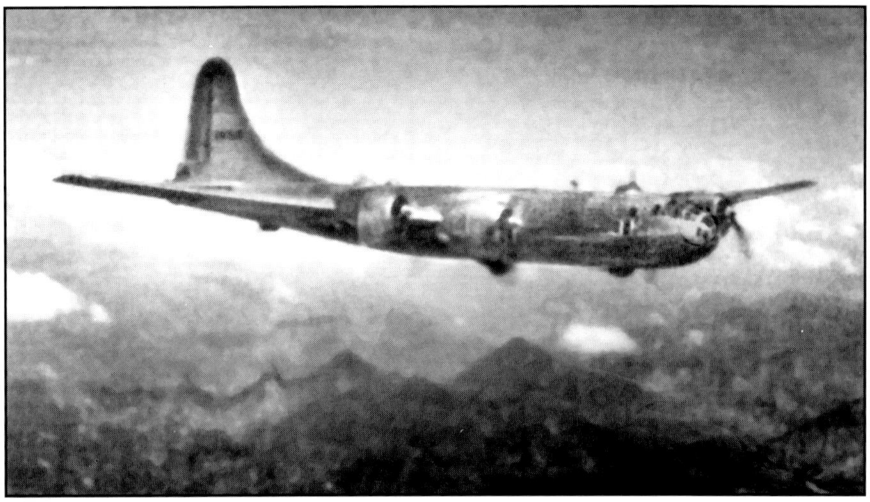

B-29, over the Hump

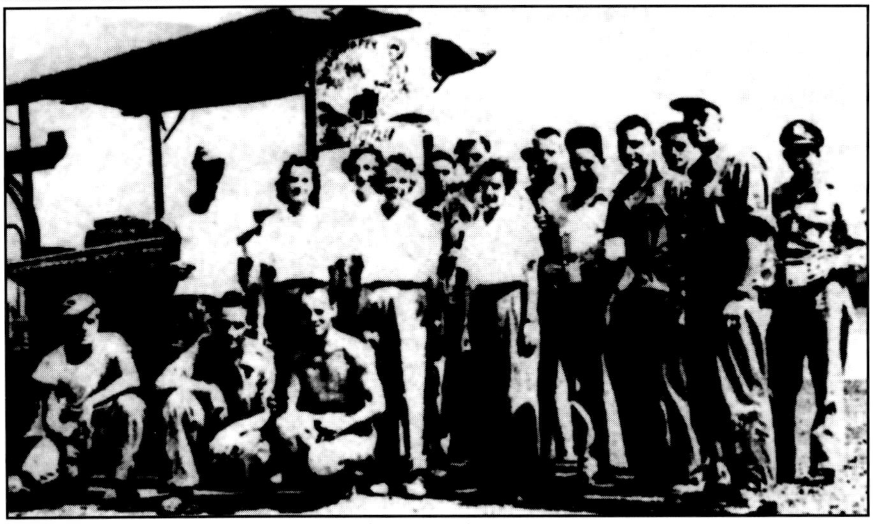

Hump-happy Baby in action

Finally, we were given permission to carry out our plan. We were warned, however, to be extremely cautious in conversations having anything to do with missions. "There's a spy out there somewhere, probably more than one. You can't be too careful," Lieutenant Brennan told us. There were no vehicles available for our new venture.

Several days later, however, after a long search, someone found the cab portion of a discarded British lorry, a kind of small truck, to which we attached an old dump cart. A heavy piece of canvas made a festive canopy from which we hung tinkling rickshaw bells. We covered a small inside table with a red-checkered tablecloth to create a homey atmosphere. All we needed was a name, and our cart full of doughnuts and coffee was ready for action.

Most of the B-29s on our base had a name and sometimes a picture painted on the side. Two of the more famous ones were "Hump-happy Pappy" and "Hump-happy Mammy." The "Hump" is a reference to the high Himalaya Mountains which had to be flown over on all the missions. "Pappy" and "Mammy" were popular funny paper characters from the cartoon known as Little Abner. Oh, what to name our little clubmobile? It didn't take long - "Hump-happy Baby"! Our gifted GI cartoonist from Hollywood painted an impish-looking baby with a small shock of hair, wearing a pair of diapers held together with a Red Cross pin. Our "Baby" pushed a baby carriage, piled high with donuts flying in all directions, up the sides of the high snow-capped Himalaya Mountains.

"Hump-happy Baby" had a distinguished career serving flight and ground crews through 12 - 24 hour days in temperatures ranging between 100 and 120 degrees. On one of those 120-degree days, a Coca-Cola bottle exploded in my hand when I took it out of a barrel of water and was about to hand it to a GI. I was given VIP attention at the hospital, Jim told me later the boys were going to recommend me for "The Purple Heart" - wounded in the line of duty. "Hump-happy Baby" served anti-aircraft forces stationed for miles around the base and visited most planes before take-off on a mission. It wasn't unusual to be awakened in the middle of the night to take "Baby" to the runway for last minute missions. The happy sound of her rickshaw bells, tinkling away in the darkness as she found her way down the runway prompted cheers from the crews, "Here comes 'Baby!'" She was on 24 hour call and became the symbolic friend of every GI.

Finally, she just fell apart, and at her dumping ceremony, she was cited by the Air Force for "service above and beyond the call of duty."

SONGS AT THE OUTPOST

One day a note was delivered to us at the club. It was from the office of our commanding officer, Colonel Blanchard. In it, permission was given for any of us to visit the outposts on the base. Somehow, it had never occurred to me that we had outposts, perhaps the most essential part of the base. I was very naive as far as military installations were concerned. The guys stationed out there were certainly among the unsung heros of the war.

The young GI, Hink, who delivered the note, said, "We'll pick you up any evening you can come. Just let us know."

"The club stays open often until nine in the evening. Will that be too late?"

"Oh, no. Can you come tonight?"

"Sure," Connie answered.

Hink picked up Connie, Pat and me and drove us for miles to an isolated spot. There was a group of small tents. We were ushered into one of them where a bunch of GIs were seated on the ground around a small fire.

"It gives light and keeps the bugs away," one of them said.

Hink introduced us and said, "That's Ken over there with the violin, and Joe with the guitar. They furnish the entertainment."

All sorts of goodies were spread out on a cloth. These specialties obviously had come from home. There was also XXX Rum, an alcoholic beverage, found in one of the villages. The bottle had a skull and crossbones on its label and had the kick of a mule. It wasn't long before this fireball found its way through the base.

One of the guys said, "Be careful, this Bamboo Juice really packs a whalop! The other night a new recruit tried some of that dynamite. He was the bashful type, but my, how he changed. He put on a great show - handsprings and that sort of thing. The next day he didn't remember a thing."

I sang several popular songs of

the early 40s, and we harmonized on some of the old favorites, "I've Been Workin' on the Railroad," "Dixie," and many others. Pat and I (after partaking of a little Bamboo Juice) sang a duet, probably the worst rendition of *The Indian Love Call* ever heard. They loved it because it made them laugh.

After that evening we joined them every few weeks. These boys seemed so grateful to have a few females around. They showered us with gifts. They always shared any special goodies sent from home. Having a violinist and guitarist was a great asset and kept us on key when we sang.

Often, on a Sunday, Father Adler would suggest we go to the Outpost to have a service. It, more or less, followed the same routine we used on the base. One time the little, old, unpredictable organ just decided to quit. We pumped and cursed (quietly) to no avail. I had planned to sing a solo. With no organ accompaniment, I decided I might just skip it. For some reason or other, I thought about home where I was a church soloist, and the renowned Virgil Fox was the organist. Always, he tried to drown me out. I chuckled at this thought, cleared my throat and happily sang away.

Each time we were invited to the Outpost, Hink would send us a gift and an invitation in rhyme.

At seven-thirty this Thursday night
We'd like to get together to enjoy a bite.
With good ole bamboo juice and a little swing
And maybe some doughnuts that you can bring.

We have a guitar player and a guitar
So if you can come, I'll get a car.
Music like ours is hard to beat And the jive we play is really a treat.

So, please do try to make this date.
We'll call for you, and won't be late.
Our morale will jump as high as the sky.
So again I say to you ... PLEASE TRY.

IMPROVISING EASTER

One night, Connie asked Pat and me to come to her room for a meeting after the club closed at nine. She did this frequently. We were able to have discussions there without interruptions. Also, we seemed better able to think seated on the floor, minus our stuffy boots worn since sunset.

"Easter is just about ten days off," said Connie. "What are we going to do to make it a happy day for these guys?" I spoke up. "Father Adler and the other two chaplains and I have already met. We're planning to have a short, outdoor sunrise service for everybody. Later on there will be Catholic, Protestant and Jewish services. Available choir members will sing something, and I'll do an Easter solo."

"Good, Katie. Now, how can we decorate the club? I wish we could have some Easter baskets or an egg hunt or something to make it fun."

"You know that Chinese restaurant in the village?" Pat asked. "I'll bet we can buy some duck eggs from them."

"But how would you color them?" Connie asked.

"Well, let me think about it a minute. I've got it. Remember those colored sheets of paper someone brought into the club? They were in a Christmas box sent to one of the boys. We could boil those sheets. That would color the water. Lower the eggs in the pan and - viola! - they're colored."

"Great idea, if they'll sell us the eggs," said Connie, "And what will we use for a basket and the nest?"

"Well, why not a helmet? We don't use them much for anything else, except sometimes in an air raid. Heaven knows there is plenty of dried grass around here. We can make a swell nest with it - hot and cozy."

Except for the 110 degree temperature, all went off well. We even had "Open House" at the club in the evening and served coffee and doughnuts. And we didn't forget to have "Hump-happy Baby" deliver some to the guys stationed at the outpost.

HOTHEAD IN A TRENCH

After settling into life at Chakulia, I thought sometimes about the luxuries at home, things I had taken for granted. My sister was great about mailing me things I wanted: my yellow sundress - the boys preferred dresses to uniforms; vitamins, and especially calcium; watchstraps, that consistently disintegrated; and "Venus" (kotex). I asked her to tell anyone who sent me a photograph to be sure to have it in a frame. Otherwise the picture would curl up in this heat and fall apart.

One time I received a package from my friend Martha. It contained a new product just developed in the States, a Toni Home-Permanent-Wave set. I contacted several GIs, former hairdressers, who were fascinated by this new "survival kit."

"Sure, Katie. We can follow these directions. It's easy. We'll put your hair up in these curlers and come back in an hour to take them down - simple!"

They finished and had just taken off when the alert rang out its ominous cry, starting at a low pitch and crescendoing to a shrill, deafening shriek. I made my way, as I had on numerous occasions during the past months, to the nearest slit-trench.

After about an hour, the increasing heat on my head prompted me to tell the boys about those "hot-rods" on my scarf enshrouded head. "Take a look under this scarf. My hair is all wrapped up, and when those guys take it down, I'll look like a Hollywood star - at least that's what the directions say. These perms are the newest thing back in the States. I'll be the only person on the base - probably in India - with a new perm! Can you imagine how glamorous I'll be? It's certain to raise the morale of the whole base. Maybe I won't have to work anymore. I'll just walk back and forth and listen to the whistles!"

The daytime alerts weren't as scary as the night ones, perhaps because you could see who your mates were. Sometimes, when I was the only female in the trench, I wondered who were more frightening - the Japs or the GIs. This was a large base with troops arriving every day, and only four Red Cross girls plus twenty or so nurses.

After some time in the trench I began to worry. "How many hours have we been here? I'm burning up! Those guys told me to go about my business and they would return at the right time to complete the job. I guess they are in another trench and have forgotten all about me."

The "All Clear" sirens began to ring - there was never a happier sound - and I was boosted to the surface ground. As I ran to my hut, I noticed that most of my trench mates were following me. "We want to have the first look at this new Hollywood star," they laughed.

Two excited hairdressers were waiting and shouted, "Hurry up, we're two hours overdue removing those damn curlers, and the special solution has to be applied."

Quickly I sat down on my rope bed, and my audience -increasing by the minute - gathered around on the floor, eager to witness this metamorphosis. With rapt attention their eyes focused on my head.

The hairdressers busied themselves mixing and applying the magic solution; then slowly they began to unroll the curlers. I was shocked by the expressions on the faces staring at me -surprise - disbelief - horror! The sudden silence brought chills to my spine.

"What is it?" I wailed.

It was then that I was handed a rod - complete with my hair!

Slowly I raised my hand to my scalp, and I felt only stubby little pieces of hair. Tears trickled down my cheeks. I thought to myself, "Good grief - I'm topless!"

I found out this wasn't such a bad thing after all. It turned out to be quite a morale booster. I was hounded by GIs who bribed me to take off the scarf I wore on my head. "I'll give you a pack of cigarettes!" This was quite a sacrifice, since the only ones available came from civilians who were rationed at home. "I'll chill your beer for you!" We had recently been issued a beer ration - three cans a month. Of course, there was no ice, but natives had taught us to wrap a can in wet straw and tie it on the limb of a tree. Condensation cooled it somewhat - a neat trick.

I finally gave up wearing the scarf. It just made life unbearable with soaring temperatures and the approaching, humid monsoon season.

One day, a couple of excited GIs came to the club and said, "Guess who's just arrived! Don Barkely - you know, he's the famous cartoonist from Hollywood! Come on, he wants to do a sketch of you."

"Oh, no! Not with my hair looking like this."

"Ah, come on, Katie, be a sport!"

I eventually gave in. We ran to the spot where he was sketching everyone. I dreaded this, but there was no way out.

Don made two unbelievably amusing cartoons of me. One of them made me look like a witch. I could have haunted a house. The boys asked me which broom I came over on, rather than which ship. Funny thing was, it looked a little like me. The boys carried them back to the club and hung them on the wall. The next day they told me all the rats had been frightened off.

AYAH

It all started one evening when we had had some problems with a couple of roughneck GIs at the club. Pat and I were both very uptight. We came back to our Basha to find our barefooted, ring-nosed ayah sashaying back and forth, and as usual, not doing anything.

Why was she there? I had told her so many times through our English speaking Gurkha guard never to come in the evenings. The room was too small for three persons. Besides, she didn't have any evening duties. During the day she did a little laundry and filled the outside tin tubs with water, in which we bathed. She oversaw a lower caste worker empty the latrine buckets and another one sweep the floor. That was all.

"*Salaam, Memsahib*," she said.

"*Salaam*. Oh, go to h—," I answered. "Don't worry, Pat. She can only say that *Salaam* stuff — doesn't understand word of English," I added.

Pat answered, "I don't trust this old bag. I think she's a *ghoul*."

"What's a *ghoul*, Pat?"

"A grave robber," she replied.

"I think she's a son of a b——."

One day several weeks later she didn't show up. We had been told to report immediately the absence of any native employee.

"Good morning. This is Katie." I told Lieutenant Brennan. "Our *ayah* didn't show up here today."

"We know all about her — trained by the Japs."

"But she doesn't speak English."

"Come on, Katie, don't be so naive. I just hope you were guarded in your conversation when she was around."

"Guarded? Well... yes, as far as missions were concerned," I said sheepishly.

FORBIDDEN MISSION

Living under wartime conditions, so far from home, sometimes drives people to do things they would not — should not — ordinarily do. I was no exception, and one morning I went for the ride of my life.

The sun had not yet risen, and in the predawn darkness I could barely make out the rows of airplanes silhouetted against the horizon. Even at dawn the air was hot and still; the tall, dry grasses around my hiding place were suffocating. The Air Force fatigues I was wearing clung to my body. My heart pounded. I glanced at my watch. Just five more minutes

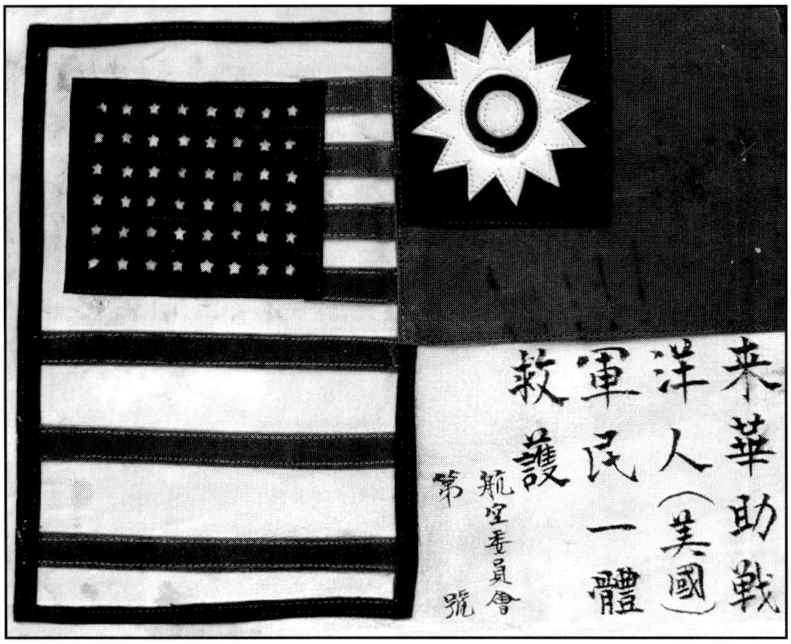

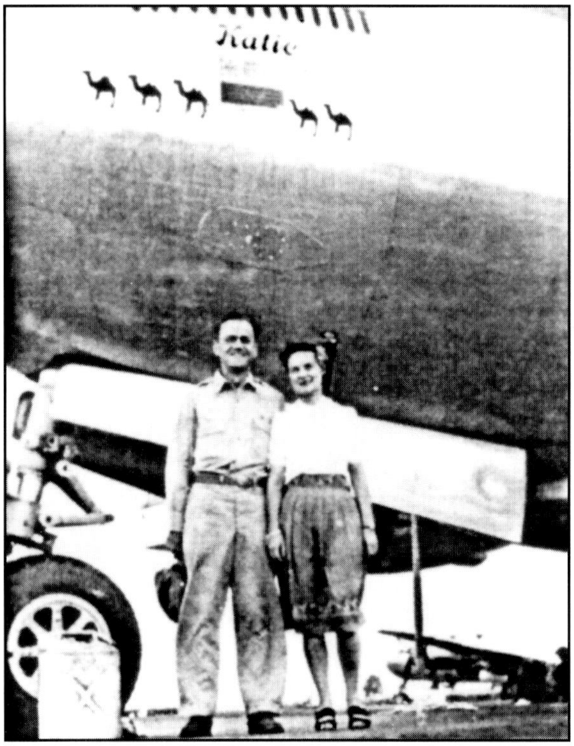

Above, Katie's ID patch Right, Ned Baugh and Katie by "The Katie," five missions

and the plane will start down the runway. It will slow down at this well-planned location and pick me up. I will be off to fly with my buddies over the mountains to Burma.

I had spent several sleepless nights worrying over this momentous decision to join the crew on a highly secret mission. There were severe consequences if I were caught. As a trusted American Red Cross volunteer stationed at this base I had gained the respect of my co-workers as well as the officers in command of the base. How would they react? If I were caught, I would surely be dismissed and sent home, welcome as that could be after a year and a half in this godforsaken country. With strict security measures in force at the base, the crew would be severely disciplined for taking me on a mission. These men were among my closest friends, and the pilot, Ned Baugh, and I had shared more than a casual relationship. I was honored when they decided to name their B-29, "Katie," after me. It took very little persuasion when they suggested that I join them on this special, reconnaissance mission. They gave me Air Force fatigues with leather American and Chinese flags attached to the back. Chinese characters below the flag spelled out, "I am a friend. Take care of me. America will pay you." I had confided only in my immediate superior, who , though skeptical, promised to keep my secret and even fill in with my duties for the day.

The bright lights of the plane beginning to taxi down the runway alerted me. I sneaked out of the tall grasses as the plane slowed down. A small, rope ladder was lowered; Joe, the tail gunner, appeared in a flash. He helped me with my footing as Bill, the navigator, grabbed me by my arms and hoisted me aboard. I joined the crew in a loud cheer as we rounded the runway for takeoff.

Our plane, a B-29 bomber, quickly soared into the sky. Only the pilot and copilot had seats. The rest of us, crew, photographers and I, knelt at the windows or sat on the floor.

We reached altitude as daylight broke. Far in the distance below I could see the rugged mountain range and snake-curling rivers of Burma. The purpose of the reconnaissance mission was to take pictures of Rangoon, the principle port of Burma, then occupied by the Japanese. Rangoon was to be the next target of a bombing mission.

We circled the port several times and the photo crew completed their shots. Then we banked and turned in the direction of our base.

After landing, Ned suggested that I debark at the end of the runway where the plane slowly turned to taxi back to headquarters. I hadn't thought much about this part of the scenario. This would be the most likely time I could be discovered. While the plane barely moved, I was lowered by two of the crew. As I ran toward the grasses my foot caught in a too-long trouser leg. I let out a gasp, and like a hunted animal, crawled to the safety of the high grasses.

I never got caught and promised not to reveal this memorable escapade for 25 years. I guess it's safe to tell it now. For a long time afterwards, I was haunted by the memory of knowing that this beautiful, tranquil countryside would be devastated the next day by hundreds of bombs, and that unknown numbers of innocent victims would die.

A CHRISTMAS TO REMEMBER

"Christmas is everywhere December 25, but it sure doesn't seem like it in this stifling jungle!" Joe Varney, a young sergeant complained. "Did you hear that Tom Snyder passed out in that hot Santa Claus suit? He was sitting on top of a jeep, bellowing 'Ho! Ho! Ho!' when he slid right down to the ground - passed out. But he wasn't hurt bad, just blood on his face and hands, poor guy, matched his suit."

The sagging branches of the Eucalyptus tree, trimmed with cans of C and K rations wrapped in red paper, just didn't look like or smell like an old-fashioned evergreen, Christmas tree.

My fellow Red Cross workers and I, along with entertainment personnel, hoped to save the day with an evening gala performance in our newly-constructed amphitheater. We had been fortunate to find some good instrumentalists among the troops on the base - former members of bands, orchestras and symphonies in the US. Ellen, Program Director for the Red Cross, and I planned to start things rolling by playing on two old upright pianos. Aware of some of the GIs' distaste for "high class" music, we decided to fool them. We started out with the first bars of a Grieg concerto, with the intention of suddenly switching to the heavy beat of Boogie!

We were minutes into the concerto, thrashing our arms in the air, when the all-familiar strains of loud sirens began to wail, and the whole base suddenly was in darkness.

"Katie! Katie! Put out your hand!" It was my good friend, Tommy.

"Is that you, Tom? Keep talking so I can find you." The night was pitch black. Naturally, that's the kind of night the Japs would hit.

"That's me all right. Hold on." I had touched his arm. We followed the voice of a lucky soldier who had located a trench near by. Quickly we slid down. Someone recognized my voice and said, "Gee, Katie, can't you play anything but that dumb classical stuff?"

Christmas was definitely on everyone's mind. Someone started, "I remember last Christmas .... " And so it went on with mostly happy memories. However, one guy began to cry and confessed to a crime that had never been revealed - and probably never would be.

There is something about the circumstances of being in a trench during an air raid that frees the mind of inhibitions. It's dark - no one can see you. You're scared - you may not come out alive, and someone has plenty of time to listen to you.

IN THE HOSPITAL

I found it increasingly difficult to combat the heat. Twice I passed out on the runway while dispensing coffee to the crews. The second time, after an examination at the hospital, I was admitted for Heat Prostration.

I was the only female patient, and because of that distinction, was given one of the few small cubbyholes, called "private rooms." The nurses' aids and orderlies were all GIs. I experienced no lack of visitors. Every GI who could walk came to see me. They said the sight of my silk nighties gave them a thrill. They spoiled me rotten bringing me gifts - candy, cigarettes, chewing gum and canned juices taken from their care packages from home.

One other occasion brought me back to the hospital. I was bitten by a mosquito which transmitted the dreaded disease, Dengue Fever. It was referred to as back-break fever, to which I had ample reason to agree. Convalescence was slow and agonizing. The GIs kept up my spirits with their visits and encouragement. At chow time, all plates were prepared alike - dehydrated eggs or spam, canned vegetables, canned gravy, and jello for dessert - all running together. I felt like throwing up every time I saw that plate. I lost a considerable amount of weight in the four weeks I was hospitalized. India - the land of romance and diarrhea. I've suffered from both, but right now, the latter took precedence.

SURE SHOT KATE

One day an emergency meeting was called for Red Cross personnel. Lieutenant Brennan's face was disturbed as he reported the physical condition of Mahatma Ghandi had taken a turn for the worse. The political and spiritual leader of India had been on a hunger strike for many weeks. This time his protest was not directed against the British, as it had been several times before, but rather to his own people. Despite his appeals for non-violence, the Hindus and the Muslims continued to fight each other.

There was a sense of urgency in Lieutenant Brennan's voice. "If Ghandi should die, the lives of Americans and British could be in grave danger. It has been decided that you must wear a holster carrying a .45-caliber revolver at all times until this emergency is over."

I thought of Abdul, our bodyguard who had been hired to protect the Red Cross hut during the night. He was a member of the tribe of fierce fighters, the Gurkha Guards of Nepal. His head was wrapped in a turban and around his waist hung the curved lethal Gurkha sword, which, when deftly swung, severs the head of the intended victim; Abdul's was marked by two nicks representing two beheadings. Would Abdul be a friend or foe?

The Lieutenant continued, "Report for target practice at once."

Three cans were placed on a mound some distance away. A tough sergeant addressed us, "You have five shells to hit three cans. This procedure will be repeated until you have succeeded. Now, Go for it!"

I had never held a pistol - not even a water one. It was mid-afternoon when the training started, and well after evening chow before I passed the test. In my weariness I decided to close my eyes and shoot at the target. I shot the first can, opened my eyes and missed the next two.

That night while we were at the Outpost the boys served us some of that powerful "bamboo juice" that really makes a man of you. The next morning at target practice with my .45 I nailed three cans. The boys gave me a "sharp shooter medal" and called me "Sure-shot-Kate."

Three days later, Gandhi was persuaded to end his fast. What a relief to hand over this heavy, awkward pistol! A .45 is a strange bedfellow. But I couldn't wait to write to my brother-in-law to tell him about my medal. I ended my letter with the words, "Now, I'm going duck shooting with you!"

FIREATER

He came to our base when we needed him most. We were desperate for relief from tension because of a devastating series of casualties. His name was Private Thomas Dever of Oregon. Featured "The Fireater," he was part of a show we put on to build morale.

Before an awe-struck audience, and with the relish of a good ole pie-a-la-mode, he swallowed tacks, annas (coins), and marbles. They were merely appetizers. For the main course he chose part of a victrola record, an electric light bulb, and double-edged razor blades. Private Dever topped off his meal by literally swallowing fire which blazed forth from his mouth. Several guys lit cigarettes from the flame. With the expression that follows a Thanksgiving dinner, he raised his shirt and patted his belly. It rattled!

We learned that doctors back home took X-Rays and saw all that stuff. I remember he ended his show by saying for $1,000 and a discharge from the army, he would uncover the mystery of his act and how he could "stomach it!"

I've seen fireaters since, but none as convincing as Private Dever. I wonder how his stomach is holding up.

CELEBRITY ROOMMATE

Gogo came to our base as a Red Cross replacement. She was the daughter of the famous designer, Madame Schapparelli. All she had to do was walk across the floor to raise the morale of the boys. She knew a lot of famous people. One day, the well-known author, Vincent Sheehan, came to see her. We entertained him in our Basha, for want of a better place.

Unfortunately it was the monsoon season. Our sad shack had many leaks in the ceiling. He had to wear his hat to keep from getting wet. The lights went out, and we brought out an old oil lamp which had a peculiar attraction for huge flying ants. They came in droves. He had to cover his glass of Bamboo Juice with his hand to keep from drinking them. He didn't stay long.

LILY PONS AND ANDRE KOSTALANETZ

Not many celebrities found their way to our isolated Air Force base. On one occasion, however, we had the good fortune to have famed orchestra leader Andre Kostalanetz, the first conductor to introduce classical music over the radio, and his wife at the time, Lily Pons, renowned coloratura of the Metropolitan Opera Company.

I was able to gather together a group of topnotch singers, selected from the ground and flying crews of the B-29s. Some were veterans of the concert stage and Broadway productions, while others were amateurs who enjoyed singing. We performed at regularly scheduled shows given in our outdoor amphitheater as well as at all religious ceremonies. Since there was little to do between the bombing missions, the members of this group found respite and relaxation in rehearsals. We worked up quite a repertoire, as well as a reputation on base.

Mr. Kostalanetz, accompanied by his wife and orchestra, was touring and entertaining American forces in the China-Burma-India theater. There was high anticipation on the day of their arrival, and even more excitement when the great conductor, hearing about our chorus of singers, asked permission for them to sing several numbers in his show, scheduled for that evening.

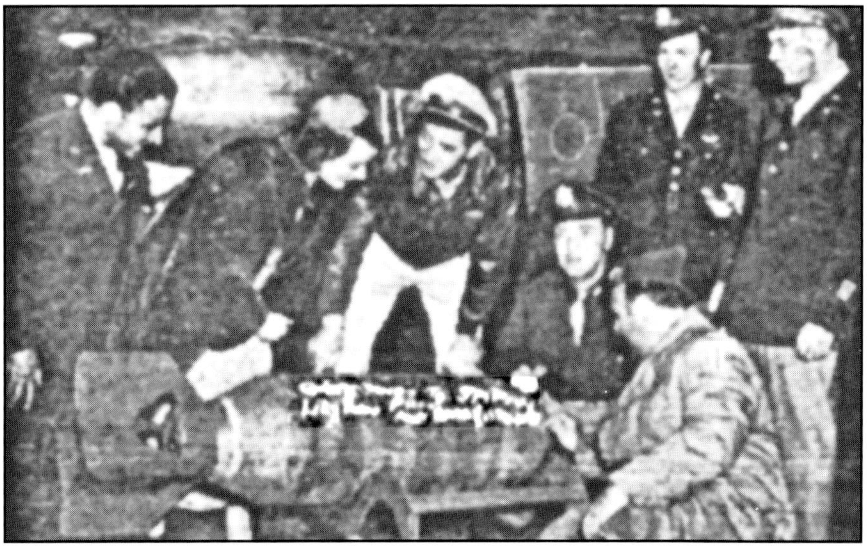

Before leaving an XX Bomber Command Base in India, Lily Pons and husband, Andre Kostelanetz, visited a B-29 being readied for a mission, and autographed the last bomb.

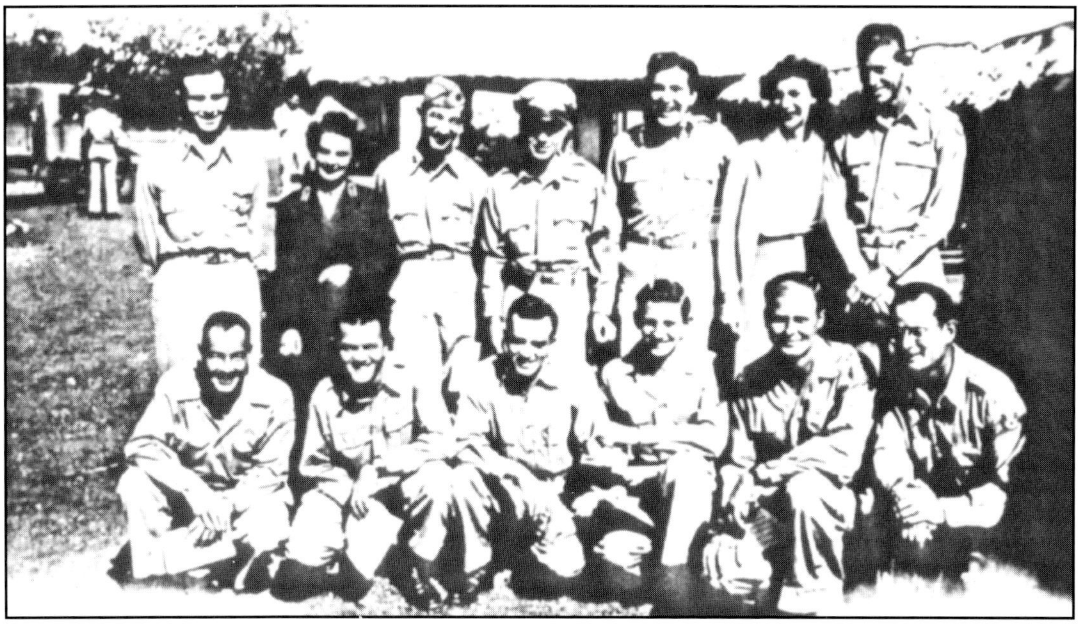

Some of Katie's choir

Unfortunately, a great catastrophe occurred in the afternoon. A plane, heavily loaded with bombs, exploded, setting off a series of explosions in other planes on the air strip. Casualties mounted close to a hundred, and volunteers were called into service to administer first aid and to assist the nurses. I was instructed on how to inject needles and perform a variety of emergency measures which under normal circumstances would have caused me to faint. I had never had a course in first aid and was rather squeamish about such things. Under these circumstances I had no time to think of myself and managed to give all the help of which I was capable. Because of this tragic event the musical performance had to be delayed, and Lily Pons had no choice but to be my roommate for two nights. I have a vivid memory of this great lady sitting on my rope bed, putting her hair up in my bobby pins. She was so petite and almost shy. She looked more like a young school girl than a famous diva. I told her about the number of times in New York that I had paid a "standing room only" fee to hear her sing. She was so modest; it seemed to me she blushed when I said words of praise.

Hours before the performance, Mr. Kostalanetz came to tell me Lily was suffering from a dry throat. This, of course, was not unusual in a climate with temperatures 100 degrees and up and with no means of cooling off. He said only pineapple juice would relieve this condition, and she had run out of the supply she had brought with her. I knew there was no such luxury on our kitchen shelves—shelves full of spam and C and K rations. Quickly I contacted our commanding officer. Communications started and finally a can of pineapple juice was located in Calcutta, about 200 miles from our base. Word traveled fast, and finally a plane took off, returning a short time before the performance - with this precious commodity. That had to be the most expensive can of pineapple juice in history, but it proved to be well worth it. Never had our spirits needed more to be lifted.

In her clear, bell-like voice, out in the open air, this great singer's notes soared to the heavens. She sang arias from light opera and popular songs from current shows. The men whistled and shouted, "More, more, Lily!" She gave several encores. They continued to shout for more. She was obviously very tired. Colonel Blanchard sensed this and came up on the stage to thank them. He placed a lei around her neck. She leaned up to give him a kiss to show her appreciation. She was so petite and Colonel Blanchard was so tall that she made several unsuccessful jumps. The boys shouted, "Bend over, Colonel, bend over!" She later remarked that never in her career had she sung before a more inspiring audience.

My chorus of singers gave such an exciting performance under the baton of the famous, beloved conductor that he begged to have them perform at other bases. This was, of course, impossible. They had to stay put and get the war over with. But possibly that goal was made a little easier after this performance, which raised the morale of the base to new heights.

The day they left, one of the crews, scheduled to take off on an important mission, asked Lily to sign one of the bombs, which she graciously did.

I walked beside Mr. Kostalanetz on the way to their plane. "Katie," he said.. "Do you realize how good this choir of yours is? Back home it would be impossible to gather together such a professional group of singers. They would be involved in opera, concerts or show business. To hear them perform here must give a lot of pleasure to a lot of people. I wish I could take them with us on our CBI tour."

"Thank you, Mr. Kostalanetz. I can tell you they give me a lot of pleasure. Sometimes I marvel at the sound they produce. But the best of all is the closeness that exists between the officers and enlisted men - the common bond of making music."

Perhaps we gave ample proof to this conductor and his famous wife that their unselfish, noble efforts were so worthwhile. Not too long ago a friend in California sent me a copy of Memoirs by Andre Kostalanetz, in which he singles out this particular performance, and graciously mentions my name as "the local conductor."

KASHMIR

Ever since I read *Arabian Nights* I dreamed of being transported one day on a magic carpet, floating through space to a world of eternal beauty and enchantment. The closest I came to that fantasy was when I lived for two weeks on a houseboat in Kashmir, a mecca situated in the magnificent snowcapped Himalaya Mountains.

After 18 months at our base in the jungles of India, another war-weary Red Cross worker, my friend Pat, and I met in Calcutta. We had worked together for about a year before she was transferred to a post in Burma. Many nights, sleepless because of the unrelenting jungle heat, we lay awake discussing the possibility of such a trip, and now it was becoming a reality.

Pat and I started out to cross the country, Kashmir bound, on a fairly hazardous journey and back again in the space of two weeks. Some people thought we were a bit insane to attempt it, but each moment of the trip made us even more sure we had made the right decision.

Travel in India, without a doubt, was a haphazard affair. Trains never ran on schedule; there were no reservations to be had; and information was totally unreliable.

We started out with nine pieces of baggage - two bedrolls, a makeshift container for use as an icebox, C and K rations, canned fruit juices, medical supplies, insect bombs, chlorinating equipment, etc. We drank only juices and saved our canteen water for teeth cleaning. Each of us carried a collapsible glass, which we cleaned with kleenex. It worked like a charm.

We boarded an old-fashioned, steam engine train without a central aisle, the entrance being gained only on either side of the car. We found our compartment with accommodations for twelve already filled with ten Indian men and women who eyed us with suspicion and misgiving. First, the Indians never were quite sure why the Americans became involved in the war, and in the second place, why we came to India.

We took a quick, cursory look around, and were thankful to find two free bunks, one over the other at the end of the compartment. There was little walking space and no curtains separating the bunks. Two naked 25-watt electric bulbs furnished the only evening light. We were thankful for our departure - only then, through the open windows, did we get relief from the stifling air of our quarters. This was to be home for the next four days while we traveled across the continent.

There was one lavatory, and every evening our bunk mates lined up to go in and prepare for the night. They washed (we hoped) and changed into pajamas. Since we were required to carry our own small washbowls, a canteen of chlorinated water for teeth cleaning, and a variety of disinfectants for use in all water, we decided to perform most of our "toilette" on the sides of our bunks. This caused a great deal of chattering among our neighbors as they crowded to witness this routine. It was a little unnerving at first, but was good for a laugh from these shy companions who spoke no English. Our Hindustani was only slightly better. We became accustomed to being watched, even when we prepared and ate our meals, which involved opening several cans of C rations, the Armed Services' survival kit. Pat, in her customary good humor, would say, "Let's start off tonight with a little caviar," and with a flair open our daily ration of spam. She made quite a ceremony in the preparation of our beverage, powdered milk and heavily chlorinated water with a few special safety pills thrown in. You might have thought it was an exotic, tropical drink.

We were not allowed to buy or eat Indian food because of the ever-present epidemics of disease. At station stops vendors sold food and tea through the open windows of the compartments. We could buy tea, but it had to be two cups. We had been instructed to buy one, swish it around to sterilize the cup, toss it out and pay for another to be poured into the same cup. We had been taught all sorts of safety measures by specially trained Air Force personnel. Bananas, the only fruit allowed, had to be peeled with cotton gloves.

Late one night during the trip there was an occasion which made our presence more welcome. A young woman screamed and our flashlight revealed a swarm of giant roaches coming from under her bunk. We quickly grabbed one of our magic bombs (part of basic gear) that killed the insects instantly. I was thankful for the open window, never quite sure what else that bomb might kill,

On the fourth morning, the train pulled into the end of the line. We had reached Rawalpindi, the last town this side of the mighty Himalayas. This was another world. It was cold! Through the early veil of light, we could distinguish men wrapped in heavy long robes, and women whose faces as well as their bodies were covered. Here there were sheep instead of the sickly, forlorn sacred cows of the South. The chill in the air and the tranquillity of the scene reminded me of Biblical pictures I had seen in my childhood at Sunday School. Many of those old pictures suddenly seemed to come to life. There were shepherds with sheep in the fields. It must have looked like that when Christ was born. Could this be part of the India we so recently left - temperatures sometimes 120 degrees, the monsoons, the famine, the poverty, disease, and the hopelessness of so many people?

When we arrived an unbelievable event occurred. Another ARC volunteer, who had been a shipmate of mine for the 28 day crossing, during which we had expressed to each other the hope of one day seeing Kashmir, had been waiting here for us for two days. I had written Sandy in Bombay, her base for the past year and a half, about our plans, giving an approximate date of our arrival here. Mail was a gamble in India; a letter might never leave for its destination nor ever arrive where it was supposed to, and the time it took was anybody's guess. We had a joyful reunion. One day to make final arrangements and we were on our way.

The only transportation available was an open touring car with makeshift isinglass windows. It looked like a 1920 vintage; a car that already had made too many trips over the mountains. A British officer, who had befriended us, felt uncomfortable about this driver and his jalopy. He tried to persuade us to wait until another car would be making the same trip so we could follow each other. Every hour was precious to us we explained to him. We just didn't have a day to spare. Unanimously we decided to go ahead.

We left at daybreak for the 14 hour hazardous journey, consoling ourselves by thinking nothing could be more scary than hitting the slit trenches when the Japs flew over our bases - three innocents abroad! Our Indian driver, a madman, spoke no English and had no intention of interpreting our sign language. The only time he slowed down was going uphill when the poor old jalopy slowed to a crawl, but once over the crest he growled and slammed his foot on the accelerator as if to get even with the tired old car. Hair pin curves were a challenge to him, and more than once we hovered dangerously on two wheels. Several times we stopped to have a cup of tea with the natives, simple mountain folk whose only contact with the outside world was seeing the few adventurous souls who came their way. Gradually it became very cold. We made bouillon from K-rations in a tin candy box, and ate chocolate to keep warm. We climbed higher and higher and discovered our fountain pens had begun to leak. Our hearing became faulty, but the scenery was more beautiful with every turn. A glance out the window revealed the exquisite beauty of these towering, snowcapped mountains. We felt happy to be alive.

It was Pat who spoke, "Well, the way this lunatic is driving we may never make it, but what a beautiful place to die!"

Around midnight we rounded a curve, and there, suddenly below us, was a small city with twinkling lights. It was surrounded by a lake which reflected moonbeams. The snow-covered mountains stood by in silence. All was peace and quiet. We were caught up in the magic spell. This is Kashmir, truly the land of enchantment and romance.

For security reasons we had been given permission to stay at only one particular hotel, operated by the British. The proprietor met us with bad news - not a vacant bed in the house. Aware of our predicament, he suggested we relax at the bar while he made arrangements to put up three cots in a hallway - just for one night. The only three seats left in the bar happened to be next to three attractive British officers. The magic spell of Kashmir was already at work!

We told them of our plight, and one of them replied, "The Air Force never forbade you to stay on a houseboat, did they?"

How clever are these British! "By chance a very beautiful one was vacated today." It just happened to be next to the houseboat of our newly-made friends, and truly was the most beautiful boat one could possibly imagine. We lost no time moving in.

The family who owned and operated it were included in the price. The father cooked, the mother cleaned, and the three sons were house bearers, similar to porters. Together they had constructed the houseboat, made of sweet-smelling sandalwood, and had made all the furniture as well. There was still more to come. Down a few steps outside was moored our private shikara, a small gondola-type boat fitted with exquisite Kashmir pillows and rugs. Two oarsmen awaited our wishes. This was the only means of transportation to the mainland.

We fell into bed that first night wondering when the bubble would burst. In the early morning we were awakened by one of the sons bringing us chodahazie, morning tea. "Memsahabs, it snowed during the night and the air is crisp. Would you enjoy breakfast by the fire?" Oh, heaven must be like this! It was Sandy who said, "Pinch me, I don't believe this is real."

Later in the day we decided to try out the shikara and explore the mainland. The eldest son, Karim, told us he would be our bodyguard, and a more conscientious one would be hard to find. From then on he followed us everywhere, warding off strangers, cautioning us where not to go and looking after our welfare in general.

The following morning, while we were luxuriating on our deck, the shikara of our British neighbors glided up to our mooring. The bearer presented us with a bouquet of flowers and a note, "Cocktails at six. Please come." This was the beginning of a ritual where we met at the same hour every evening for cocktails at either houseboat.

Our meals were some of the finest we had ever eaten. Dinner started with a small bowl of soup, never the same and always mysterious with delicious, exotic, unfamiliar flavorings. While having coffee by the fire in the evenings, the father appeared and Karim translated for him. "Father desires to know whether his dinner was pleasing to you."

One evening Karim asked us to

sign their guest book, Glancing through I was startled by the signature of a guest long ago. It read, "Neville Chamberlain, Lieutenant, British Army," - the man who later became Prime Minister of Great Britain. Another evening Karim proudly showed us a Bible written in his native language. Though I knew no Urdu, I remembered the first verse of the Bible and started to read, "In the beginning God.... "

"Excuse me, Memsahib," he said, "You are holding the book upside down."

One day Karim suggested a trip to the Shalimar Gardens.

Our British friends joined us for one of the most memorable days of my life, each couple rode in a shikara piled high with Kashmir pillows and rugs. Our caravan glided for several hours through canals and small lakes inhabited by swans and ducks and other exotic waterfowl. Finally, we arrived at the exquisitely beautiful gardens. Brilliantly colored flowers of every variety grew among the lush green shrubs and trees. History records that a Maharajah planned the gardens as the spot for reconciliation with a favorite of his harem with whom he had quarreled. In this atmosphere it wouldn't be hard to forgive anything. Karim had brought along tea and sandwiches, and spread out Persian rugs on which we sat. Early on we had decided not to mention the war, but it was not easy to forget that in a few days we would be headed back to our responsibilities. Farewells were difficult. Our newly-found friendship with the British neighbors had blossomed, and for Sandy even romance had found its beginnings. It ripened with time, survived the war, and eventually culminated in marriage. Karim and his simple, loving Mohammedan family stood on the steps as we waved good-bye; we took one last look at the sight which would remain forever indelible in our minds -the towering, snow-covered Himalayas standing majestic and serene.

THE RESTING PLACE

It took us a little less than a week to travel back to the plains, and a warm welcome awaited us. With all of its drawbacks, it somehow felt good to be back "home" with our old friends.

Some of the most meaningful, but heart-wrenching experiences, in which I shared a part, were the burials. They were of necessity very simple ceremonies. Any member of the military who died on the base, rather than on a mission, was buried there. There are no grave diggers in India; Hindus burn the bodies of their deceased loved ones and scatter the ashes on the sacred Ganges River. Early in the day one or two enlisted men assisted by several natives went to a designated area we called "The Resting Place" to prepare the ground for burial. Our chaplain drove an old truck and brought with him the men who had prepared the grave and the casket; it was a simple wooden box that contained the deceased and important, relevant information. There was no military fanfare. I rode in a jeep with those members of the choir who were not on a mission. We brought along an old, small pump organ, which they unloaded and placed beside the grave.

Father Adler, a beloved missionary priest attached to our base, usually presided. I would start out playing, 'Abide with Me', quietly hoping that the rickety old organ would do just that until the end of the service. The heat was unforgiving, Father Adler made his remarks brief. He suggested the choir members do a number, Jim Edmunds, the tail-gunner with a big smile and colorful disposition said, "Let's sing 'When the Saints Come Marching In'." we always sang it when Jim was there. Not only did he have a powerful voice, but he knew the words.

At one service, that took place during Holy Week, I sang "Were You There When They Crucified My Lord?" When I sang it again at the new Pentagon the first Good Friday after the war ended, I was there in body, but my spirit was back at "The Resting Place." At the end of the short service the keys of the organ were wet from dripping perspiration; my fingers slid off the keys. It was time to return. A benediction ended this moving service. There was an air of serenity about this place, far from the tension and turbulence of the runways.

After returning to the Red Cross Club, my thoughts generally lingered with the soldier we had just buried. I thought of his family and the inevitable shock and grief they would experience at the news of his death - formal, chilling words announced in a telegram or by an officer of the Armed Forces. Perhaps it might soften their grief a little to know there was a funeral service with a minister and music and some friends present. I decided to write to them. This proved to be a good, although not quite orthodox, decision. In some cases my letter arrived before the formal notification. The responses were warm and appreciative. Families yearned for more details which restrictions forbade me to tell. Most of the time I knew very little about the circumstances of the death. However, sometimes I had known the deceased in an association at the Red Cross Club. I was allowed to write about that, and I did. I kept up a correspondence with several of the families unti1 the end of the war, Actually their letters to me were especially welcome. They helped to ease the pain I felt at the loss of these young men. If anything was gained by these experiences, it was the knowledge that sharing tragedy makes it easier in the end to accept it.

The door opened and interrupted my reverie. Jim was whistling, "When The Saints Come Marching In." He gave me a pat on the back. "What are you thinking about, Katie?"

"Well, I was thinking it was great for us you weren't dropping bombs today."

INDISCRETIONS IN ICING

One day in early May a persistent rumor became a reality. The 20th Bomb Command was ordered to leave Chakulia, India for islands in the Pacific - Guam and Tinian. No one seemed to know exactly why, and certainly no one here anticipated the war would end in several months.

Headquarters in Washington refused to allow Red Cross workers to go to the islands. Colonel Blanchard, our commanding officer, tried several times to get them to change their minds, but they were adamant in their refusal. He gathered us. Connie spoke up. "It has to be something dramatic - something we'll all remember for the rest of our lives." She rose to her feet and paced up and down. "After all, we're saying farewell (she jestered with her arm) to these men we've lived with almost two years."

There was a short silence.

"I've got it!" Connie said. "Let's make a request to fly over the Taj Mahal on a night when the moon is full."

Without hesitation our wish was granted. The only difficulty was waiting for a full moon. Time was running short.

The next few weeks were exceptionally busy. Preparation for disassembling the base started while missions continued as usual. There was only one change in our routine.

Daily missions increased and consequently causalities. Morale was at a low point. We suggested, and were given official permission, to set up a table outside the building where interrogations were held following missions. Connie, May and I dressed in our seldom-worn dress uniforms and put on a little make-up and perfume, if we had any. We baked a large, chocolate sheet cake and served cokes. The crews were allowed to have cokes and cake and some casual conversation with us before being interrogated.

This plan worked out well. After a long mission it was heartwarming to see a smile on the tired, unshaven faces of the crew members as they relaxed a little - and made wisecracks about these "new" Red Cross girls.

One day I said to Connie, "How about my decorating the cake with something eye-catching?"

"Like what?"

"Well, I'll think of something."

"Good luck!"

I took some paper and folded it to make a funnel. Then I filled it with icing made from mixing sugar and water. I had had some lessons in drawing when I was in high school, On the first cake I drew a replica of "Hump-happy Baby." Another time there was a rickshaw and then a poor rendition of the Taj Mahal. One day I drew a B-29, from which bombs dropped. Below was written "Singapore."

I was called into the office of interrogation and given a thorough questioning. There was some explaining to do since Singapore had been the target that day. I was chagrined at my stupidity. Through my close relationship with one of the pilots, I often overheard classified information.

POEM TO MY CHOIR

Relationships were strained at the thought of separation and the unknown future. Everyone tried to put on a good front and act as though there was no concern for I remember the day not long ago,

Before the choir had started to grow.
We found a quartet that didn't sound bad,
At least those who sang seemed happy and glad,
So we ventured forth and got a few more.
Most were good - some few were poor.

We had started in fun and never thought
The day would come when we'd be sought.
But I've heard a CO often repeat
This choir of ours just can't be beat.

I heard a conductor of world renown
Say it was hard to beat that kind of sound.
It was rare and not on many occasions
Our songs suffered serious abrasions.

But the thing I like most of all
Is something I'll always like to recall.
Your spirit is high, your fellowship fine.
And I say this sincerely - it's not just a line.
It's guys like you that make it fun
For us to work in this goddamn sun.

MOONLIGHT AND THE TAJ MAHAL

At last the trip was scheduled. We were to see the Taj Mahal the night before the historic take-off for the Mariana Islands. The moon was out but not quite full. The powerful engines of the B-25 sounded like an explosion when we took off. We climbed quickly and then leveled off until we arrived in the vicinity of Agra, home of the Taj Mahal.

Our pilot descended as low as was safe for this powerful plane, and then we circled the magnificent Taj Mahal, even more exquisite at night. The rays of the moon cast eerie shadows on this masterpiece of marble and precious stones, the tomb of the favorite wife of a 17th century emperor.

With one last longing look, we returned to the base with heavy hearts, for the next day was the beginning of a new and uncertain chapter, not only in the war, but in our lives.

LAURA LOU

The GIs were leaving for the Marianna Islands.

Since I had difficulty recuperating from Dengue Fever, our doctors decided finally that I should have an examination at the General Hospital in Calcutta. It was a rewarding experience for me. One of my closest friends from Virginia, Laura Lou Lincoln, had been recently transferred there from New Caledonia. What a happy reunion we had.

Before she had left for her overseas assignment, we had concocted a secret code, whereby I would know where she was stationed. Different brands of cigarettes represented various countries, only we never thought to include New Caledonia.

"Come on with me, Katie," she said. "I was just planning to make the rounds in the wards."

As we entered one of them, I heard someone shout my name. I went to him and then recognized his face. He was a member of one of the crews from our base. His plane had crashed, but he and several of his crewmates had survived and been rescued. There were others from our base, recently released from the prison in Rangoon by an heroic English Wing Commander.

I shall never forget the profound joy I experienced with this reunion. It was as though they had come back from the dead. I wept and they wept.

Following my examination I was handed the diagnosis -"Must leave the Plains immediately."

Laura Lou was with me. She said she had accumulated some Leave Days.

"Let's go to Darjeeling. That's just a night and a day away and it's cool - around 8,000 feet high I think."

We were able to get the necessary travel papers the next day and took off that night. The train was small and antiquated. Columns of smoke rose from the smokestacks of its tiny engine. Tickets were collected before the train took off.

We shared our compartment with an English girl, Lila Brett. She told us her father was a colonel in the British army, and had been stationed in Darjeeling where she was born. She had lived there ever since. Lila often made the trip to Calcutta from Darjeeling.

"There are many things we need for our club that are available only in Calcutta. I make the trip often."

We locked the doors on either side, opened the windows and lay down on our bunks for the night. Some hours later I was awakened by something crawling on my hand. From the light of the small overhead bulb, it appeared to be long and black. I screamed. Lila turned on a brighter light and said, "It's a roach."

Laura Lou set off her mosquito bomb. It had absolutely no effect on this four-inch-long creature. In the meantime the mist from the bomb quickly filled the compartment and brought out more of these obnoxious bugs. They came in droves from under the bunks.

"Don't worry," said Lila. "I'll fix 'em." With her feet and bare hands she went after them while Laura Lou and I, perched on a bunk, watched in utter amazement. After Lila finished, the floor was full of these strange, dead insects.

"Don't worry," said Lila, "I'm used to these fellows. They live on the trains."

We made a pretty thorough search before we settled down once again for the night.

Early the next morning we were awakened by a knock on the window. An engineer told us in a half hour the train would stop. All passengers were expected to get off. Lila told us there were certain sections of the railroad track that had to cross very steep hills. The little engine couldn't make it unless sand was scattered on the tracks, and the cars were empty of the weight of the passengers. The engineers brought out sandbags and threw it by handfuls on the tracks. This occurred at intervals of several hours as we climbed higher and higher that day. We passengers were well acquainted with each other by the end of the trip.

We were spellbound by this view of the Himalayas. It was even more inspiring than Kashmir. The hotel where Laura Lou and I stayed rested on the top of a mountain overlooking the village. In front there was a terrace that stretched the length of the hotel. From there we had a sight unparalleled for beauty. The Himalayas surrounded us, and the clouds lay below. At rare intervals we could see in full view the snow capped Kenchenyunga Mountains, 28,000 feet high, the second highest range in the world. It stretched along the horizon as far as you could see in either direction. We had to strain our necks to see the tops.

As Laura Lou and I got settled in our room, we realized that we'd need a blanket at night and No Mosquito Netting. I felt better all ready.

India had been ruled by the British since before this century. This hill station, with its natural beauty and ideal climate was a great favorite of theirs. There were many soldiers stationed here. It was the preferred spot for British military recuperating from war casualties. There were many English clubs to which American soldiers and Red Cross staff were welcome. An informal atmosphere existed. Introductions were never necessary.

One day Laura Lou and I were having lunch with some GIs when a handsome Englishman approached and introduced himself.

"I'm John Saunders, Royal Air Force. We're having a party tomorrow night and we hope to do some singing." Looking at me, he said, "One of your boys at my table said you played the piano and sang. Will you come and join us? The rest of you are invited too."

A.L. Saunders (John) had the looks of Erol Flynn and the finesse of Charles Boyer. We all accepted.

The party was a lively affair, and to our surprise was given in honor of John. We had drinks and food accompanied by many toasts to this new war hero. However, it wasn't until the next day, when someone showed us an article in Time Magazine that we realized the extent of his heroism. Single-handedly, he had freed the prisoners from the notorious prison of Rangoon. He had been wounded and given a month's leave to recuperate.

Back at our hotel, some newly found friends were planning to take a five-day trek through the mountains. Laura Lou and I were asked to join them. There were seven of us, a British major and his wife, two young American officers - the inspector general and attorney general of the 40th Bomb Command (my outfit), and a former Ziegfield Follies middle-aged blond. Nine Tibetan coolies with three horses were to accompany us and carry supplies.

We planned to leave at five o'clock in the morning. When we gathered together everyone was given a canteen of water, a chocolate bar and a trail map which included the spot where we would gather for lunch. Confusion with last minute details held up our departure. The two American officers, Tom and Bob, and I decided to go ahead with one of the horses, saying, "If you don't catch up with us we'll meet you at the designated lunch stop."

We started off, climbing and taking turns on the horse. We ran into many landslides which forced us to alter our course. No one had warned us about them. One slide was so steep we had to force the horse to precede us. Then we crawled on our hands and knees as we cautiously made our way. We climbed and climbed, but never found the designated spot for lunch together. Obviously, we were hopelessly lost. All the water and chocolate we had brought with us had been consumed hours before. We were completely exhausted. The poor horse was panting and I could barely walk.

Suddenly we came upon a deserted-looking hut. On entering we saw some natives, crouched in the corner. Tom tried to explain to them our plight. There was no response, and they seemed terribly frightened. In the middle of the room a small fire flickered on the muddy ground. Bob said, "We must boil some water."

"Thank God, I always carry chlorination pills with me."

"Do we have anything we can give them?" I asked. "The only thing I have are pockets full of Kleenex. We're going to need them."

Tom pulled out of his pockets several rupees (money).

Finally we filled our canteens and gave the horse some water. Before leaving, Bob told them how grateful we were - they continued to look puzzled - and gave them his fountain pen, in lieu of money. Then he handed them the reins to the horse. We couldn't make the poor animal suffer anymore. We struggled along. Every step became more of an effort. We became actively ill. I wanted to lie down, but the boys wouldn't allow me. "You'll never get up if you stop."

After several more agonizing hours, one of the coolies found us and brought us to the little cabin where the rest of our group was waiting.

The three of us were sick all of that night and the following day. I, for the first time in almost two years, neglected to pay heed to the precautions pounded into us about sitting on wooden toilet holes. It was a price to pay - I contracted the dreaded, painful "jungle sores" which made it almost impossible for me to sit. This condition caused many embarrassing moments and lasted more than a week. I couldn't explain why I preferred to stand when a gentleman offered me his seat.

The remainder of the trek was, of course, called off. Bob had to be carried back to the hospital strapped to a horse. I went with him to the hospital fearing the worst about my condition. I never had the desire to climb again.

Laura Lou and I returned to Calcutta. She went back to the General Hospital and I to Red Cross Headquarters to await my new assignment. I was there four days before it was handed to me. When I opened the official letter, my face broke into smiles. I read "Darjeeling." What a place to fight the war!

The doctor who had examined me earlier explained to me my health would be severely jeopardized by remaining on the Plains. He said, "It's either Darjeeling or orders to return home." I took the funny little train the next day.

DARJEELING

The Red Cross Club and our living quarters were simple buildings with outhouses - a far cry from the luxurious accommodations at the hotel where I had stayed with Laura Lou the week before. The two other Red Cross girls, Midge and Gail, already stationed at the club in Darjeeling, and I decided to give the club a homey look. We went to town and bought curtains, a red and white checked tablecloth and a few plants. As we came out of the store, I came face to face with John Saunders.

"But I thought you had left," he said.

"Well, I guess I just missed you so much I had to come back," I said facetiously.

We both laughed, but our eyes

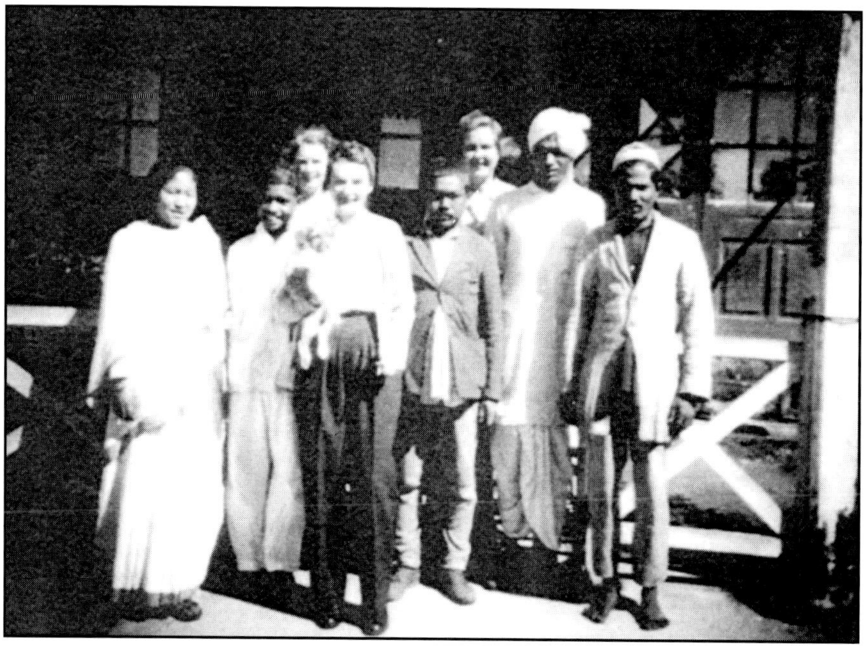

Katie, Cheenie and staff

met. I think this moment was the beginning of our future, deep relationship.

Life in Darjeeling and the new challenge at the Red Cross Club were as different from the B-29 Base in the jungle as spam is to filet mignon. Waking up in the morning with a cool breeze blowing across my face never ceased to be a surprise and delight.

Each morning I jumped out of bed and ran to the door to have another look at the Kanchenjunga. It was almost as though I wanted to make sure it was still there. I suppose, also, I wanted to drink in as much of its beauty as I could before the coming monsoon season. Then it would be visible only during brief periods.

I was amazingly ignorant of the war we were fighting - of its success or lack of it. The occasions were rare when we had news of the European Theater of War or the activity in the Pacific. It seemed I had followed a certain routine, as far as possible, with little thought of tomorrow. I think I even accepted tragedy, finally, as an inevitable part of that existence. And so, it was with surprise at my new assignment that I learned about General Stillwell and the Ledo Road.

The GIs visiting our Red Cross Club came from his outfit for a week or so to try to forget, temporarily, the extreme miseries encountered in the building of that road. Stillwell felt the road was necessary for the shipment of supplies to North Burma, still unconquered by the Japs.

The climate there was extremely hot and dry, except for the monsoon season which sometimes dropped as much as a foot or more of rain in 24 hours. Mud was everywhere. To build this road it was necessary to dynamite mountains, to build over torrential streams and to bypass canyons. Bulldozers were lost over banks and there were earth slides. The camps were infected by mosquitoes and a variety of insects. Malaria and typhus were constant threats. Frequently, supplies were delayed.

General Stillwell earned the title, "Vinegar Joe." He was a pretty tough master. However, it is said, he demanded as much from himself. He told the authorities at the Base Hospital as soon as any of his troops were able to get out of bed and stand up, they were to be dismissed and returned for work.

Our club was filled most of the time with these unhappy, thoroughly discouraged GIs. Often they would just sit and talk. A favorite pastime was watching the Red Cross mascot, Cheenie, our Himalayan half-dog half-jackal, perform tricks to commands in Hindustani. It was heartwarming to see them smile and once in a while even laugh.

One day we were all invited to one of the largest tea plantations, 25 hundred acres, to witness a tea-tasting session. It was quite an education. Five "tea experts" sat at a long table. In front of each were a row of cups and a large bowl. The judges took a mouthful from a cup, swiveled it around in their mouths, and with a faraway look in their eyes, spat it out in the bowl. They agreed on a winner after much debate. Elliot Mercer, our host, suggested several of the boys should give it a try. The reply was unanimous, "We'd rather have a beer."

Every time I see Darjeeling Tea advertised, I think of those "professional spitters."

Tom Deering turned to me and said, "Hey, look at this flat area." In Darjeeling, one rarely sees flat areas. "What a terrific baseball diamond this would make."

Elliot overheard him and responded quickly. "You get the equipment and we'll start playing. It will jolly well be the first baseball game in Darjeeling."

I called headquarters in Calcutta. "How soon can you get some baseball gear up here?"

"Are you going to try this on the side of a mountain?" was the reply.

The balls and the bats came quickly and the great day arrived. Elliot, our enthusiastic host, gave his tea-leaf pickers and factory workers - about 500 persons - holiday to watch the game.

At first, these workers were unresponsive. Then Elliot briefed them about the game in their native language. They quickly felt the spirit of the sport and responded by jumping up and down. The boys were happy and so was everyone else. It became a regular occasion - the most popular event of our activities.

We thanked Elliot - and he thanked us.

JOHN SAUNDERS

In my free time I had been seeing a good deal of John Saunders. He took me to fancy English clubs for dinner or dancing, and often both in the same evening. He was always recognized and "oh'd and ah'd" by the adoring English ladies.

"John," I said one day, "how about coming to the Club and telling the boys about your experience in Burma?"

He came and they were spellbound.

"I was on a reconnaissance mission in my trusty, little mosquito. As I circled that enormous, Japanese airfield, Mingaladon, I was startled to see it was completely empty -not a plane in sight. The Japs had fled. I circled several times and decided to land. I hit something on the runway -both my plane and I were slightly injured - nothing too serious."

Then he described to them how he went 12 miles by foot, ox cart and boat with the help of some natives until he reached the notorious Rangoon Prison. Fourteen hundred British, Americans and Indian prisoners were released.

After he finished he asked me to join him that night for dinner to meet a young Parsee couple, friends of his. Parsees, centuries ago, were driven out of Persia into India. They are generally intelligent, well-educated and cultured people. Agee was a graduate of Oxford University and also was a member of Parliament. Like all Indians, they were not allowed in English clubs. We had dinner in a restaurant. As I was saying "Good-bye" to Agee and Irin, they told me John was coming for a week-end with them. Could I come along?

I accepted, realizing time was running out for John and me to be together.

It was a "fairytale" week-end. Their apartment was palatial and luxurious. The furnishings had an air of elegance about them. There were overhead fans everywhere and many servants.

My hostess, Irin, suggested I might enjoy getting out of uniform and wearing the native garb. She opened a large trunk and said, "You select." She brought out exquisite gold and silver threaded saris, some studded with tiny pearls or semiprecious stones and others of fine, delicate, chiffon-type material.

This week-end stands out very especially in my memory, for various reasons. With all this beauty and luxury, I found it not only hard, but impossible, to enjoy fully. I could not erase from my memory the vision of the starving and sickly people so close by in the streets of Calcutta.

On the last day of our visit John and I spent some time alone. He told me that each "Wing" of the British Air Force was connected to one of the provinces of India. His was the area called Hyderabad, ruled by the Nizam, who at that time was reputed to be the wealthiest man in the world. Most of this wealth was in 24-karat gold, made into nuggets and buried in caves on his enormous estate.

John said he was always a welcome guest since his "Wing" was attached to the province of Hyderabad.

"Katie, dear, the Nizam has invited me to come for two weeks at Christmas time. He said I was welcome to bring a guest. Will you do me the honor to go with me?"

"Oh, John, I don't know what to say."

"Before you give me an answer, let me tell you what our visit will be like. As soon as we arrive a maid will be assigned to you - to unpack your suitcase, do your laundry, bring you tea, and to do whatever you desire of her. You will be asked to select a horse for riding. You know he has three hundred Arabian ponies. We will eat off gold plates, go tiger shooting, and have a car at our disposal. He's a nice chap. You'll like him, and when you leave, he'll give you a farewell gift of a gold nugget. You know, with all his gold, he could change the international gold standard if he wanted to. Now, how can you resist?"

"It sounds unbelievable, but, John, you know that is several months off. How do we know what will happen by then?"

He didn't answer, but asked me to close my eyes and put out my hand. I opened them to behold a beautiful ring he had put on my finger.

John said, "It's a topaz I bought in southern India. It is set in the Nizam's 24-karat gold."

"Oh, John, it's gorgeous!"

The hugh stone rolled over on its side.

"It's too large," he said. "I'll drop it by a jeweler I know. He'll make it smaller for you."

Quickly I held it tight under my finger. I didn't want to part with it

"I think it fits perfectly," I said.

John had told me before we left Darjeeling that he would not be returning with me. It was necessary for him to go back to Rangoon, and would leave from Calcutta, where his plane was.

"Here's the address of our quarters in Rangoon, but I'll be back in five days. I'll call as soon as I arrive."

"And I better get going. I have to be back at work tomorrow at 8:00 a.m."

I decided to surprise the girls. I didn't mention the ring when I arrived back at the club. Suddenly, Midge saw it and said, "What's that rock on your finger?"

"Oh, just something I picked up in a bazaar," I replied casually. Then I told her the whole story.

That night I decided to write John a note. I put it in the morning pick-up.

He didn't call on the fifth day, or the sixth, or the seventh. And then a letter arrived from Rangoon. It was from the second-in-command of John's "Wing."

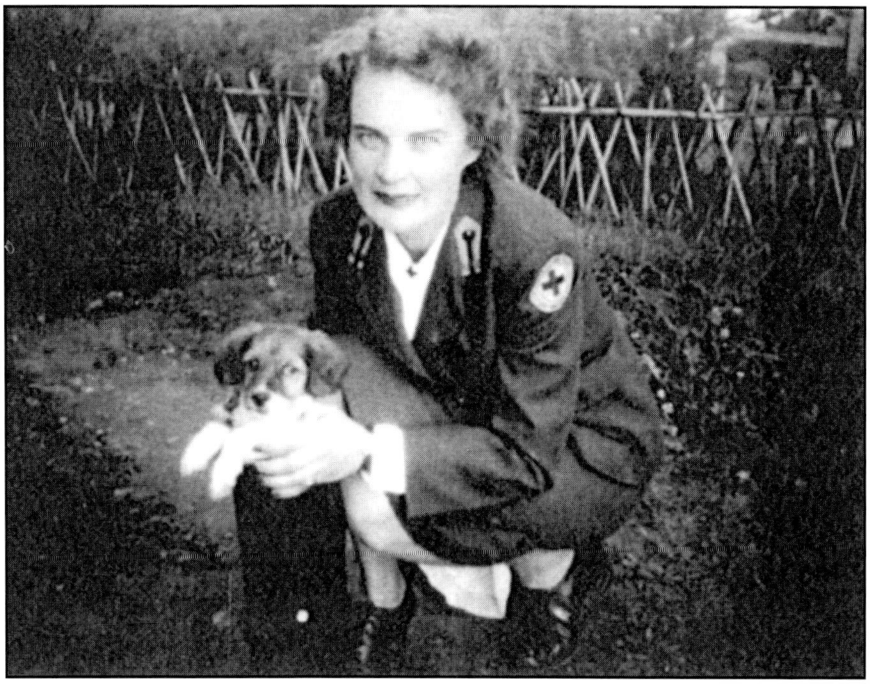

Katie and Cheenie

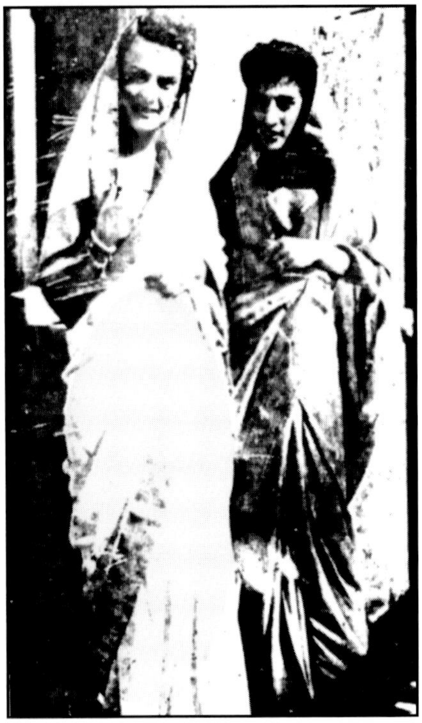

The Parsee Irin and Katie

S/LDR P.C. JOEL

110 (H) Squadron
RAF, SEAAF

4th August, 1945

Dear Miss Harris,

Your letter to W/Cdr. Saunders arrived here a few days ago and for reasons which I will explain it was necessary for me to open it.

Saunders left Calcutta on July 11 to return here by air, and the aircraft did not arrive at its destination and the crew and passengers have all been posted missing. We usually nominate a particular person to deal with all private mail in the event of casualty, and I felt it would be preferable to let you know in this case rather than for your letter to be returned unopened.

If I can be of any further assistance please do not hesitate to write.

Yours sincerely,
Peter Joel

I replied immediately, thanked him and asked if he would continue to keep in contact with me regarding any new information about John.

He replied and told me he personally had flown over the site where they had lost contact, but saw nothing. There was no trace of his plane. He said the area was in the Naga Hills in Northern Burma, where man-eating tribes lived.

This kind person kept in touch with me for the remainder of my time in India.

Irin wrote to me after a period of time. She said she had waited in the hopes that the initial news was not true. She and Agee were heartbroken at this sad news.

MOUNT EVEREST

My work in Darjeeling was of short duration - three months. World War II ended, and our first reaction was numbness. Is it true? Then we ran around hugging each other, we danced, and we cried. We all gathered under one roof and got drunk.

After the monsoon season the air was particularly clear. My desire to see Mt. Everest increased daily. I consulted an expert. "If you want to see the peak of Mount Everest, you must have perseverance," our Tibetan friend, Jaiwant, said. "It is rarely visible, and only for a few seconds at daybreak before a mist develops and covers its top. One may try many times before succeeding. It is an arduous climb during the night to reach the specific area in the lower Himalayas where Mount Everest can be seen, but a few have witnessed the fleeting sight of its summit."

Jaiwant introduced us - a fellow Red Cross worker, three British officers, two army nurses, and myself - to several Tibetan guides who consented to lead us on our trek the following morning.

We dressed in the warmest clothes we had and were ready to take off at 2:00 a.m. - the seven of us and three amiable guides. For the first hour or so we rode horseback. The horses were small, more like donkeys, and luckily seemed familiar with the treacherous terrain underfoot. The path was narrow and rocky. A cold breeze swept across my face. I pulled my scarf over my mouth and nose. After an hour or so, we were instructed to dismount and travel on foot. The trail was now too steep for the horses. I glanced back and saw Darjeeling drenched in flickering lights, It reminded me of Christmas.

Following our lead guide, we climbed in a zigzag pattern, which we were told, would make it easier to breathe in this rarefied air and cause less strain on our hearts. We made short stops to sip water from our canteens, or to eat chocolate for renewed energy. Finally we reached the designated area and spread blankets on the ground. We huddled together against the chill.

After a short time darkness began turning to gray. The guide told us to focus on one particular area. It was so high we had to bend our heads straight back. Gradually and imperceptibly, the darkness lessened. The sky became gray, then a shade lighter, then dawn. Suddenly, the jagged peak of Mount Everest stood out. It appeared like skeleton fingers reaching toward heaven. Hardly a minute later, the mist formed and eerily enshrouded this awesome sight.

There was nothing to say, but so much to feel. We had seen the topmost spot on earth. I said a silent prayer of gratitude for an experience that would remain fixed in my mind forever. Somehow, for a brief moment, we had been transported from earth. We embraced each other in silence, and slowly went back down the mountain.

LARRY

Our Liberty ship was slowly pushed out of the port of Calcutta. As I looked back at this country, my home for almost two years, I experienced mingled feelings. Certainly I had been enriched by exposure to one of the oldest cultures in the world. I had seen the exquisite beauty of its masterpieces in architecture, and the unexcelled beauty of its mountains. However, my overwhelming thoughts were concerned with India's billions of people - the caste system, which at birth forebodes one's future - the widespread poverty and resulting filth and disease. I could never erase from my mind the vision of starving humanity associated with this overpopulated country.

We rounded the Horn of India, crossed the Indian Ocean, and later entered the Red Sea.

This particular night was especially dark and the stars gave off brilliant luminescence. Lying on the deck of the USS *General Greeley*, I unconsciously raised my hand to touch them. I pulled the tarpaulin around me against a sudden breeze, infrequent in this hot, still climate. What a joy to feel it brush against my face! I lay awake this night as I had in other nights since leaving India, thanking God for the end of World War II and my return home.

There were several reasons why the Captain had assigned the eleven women on board - nurses and Red Cross workers -to this high, open gun turret on the troopship. It was ours alone and off limits to all males. The originally assigned cabin, on the lower deck was too small for the eleven of us, and it was unbearably hot. More important, a variety of reactions from the returning GIs to us, some very unpleasant, were responsible for this course of action.

The days were long and the heat overwhelming while we crossed the Indian Ocean and the Red Sea. I looked forward each day to sunset when I climbed the steps to our safe, little haven to remain until sunrise. Even though the war was officially over, our Captain declared the ship must be completely darkened during the night. Our guard, well equipped with a .45 and ammunition, counted heads and took his post at the bottom of the steps. He was obviously carried away with the importance of his responsibilities, and after he locked the gate to the turret, he reassured us, "Nothing to fear with old Joe in charge. Any guy so much as puts a foot on these steps is a dead duck. Got my orders straight from the boss."

He spoke the truth. More than once, over the loud speaker, the Captain threatened the thousands of troops crowded on the decks that he would tolerate no nonsense. "This ship is overloaded beyond capacity. We've all been at war too long, and it is my responsibility to get you home. I've heard of several unpleasant incidences directed towards the women on this ship, and this is my final warning: Shape up, treat the ladies with respect, or suffer the consequences - confinement in the brig for the remainder of the journey."

Lying awake and lulled by the gentle rolling of the ship and the monotonous whirring of the radar high above our heads, I thought about Larry. He was one of a number of GIs kept in solitary confinement in the bowels of the ship. They were referred to as "mental patients," because a terrible war experience had triggered an imbalance in their thinking process.

By accident I heard about these unfortunate soldiers. I learned there were no facilities on the ship for treatment. They were simply being guarded in cells until the ship reached New York, where they would be hospitalized. It bothered me to think of the fearful loneliness they were experiencing during this long journey. I asked permission to visit these boys. My first encounter was with Larry.

It was frightening when an armed guard led me to his cell and locked the door behind me. The room was small and bare; the air stale and stifling. The overcrowded decks above, with all the sun and heat, seemed like a paradise in comparison. Larry's frail body was clad only in pajama bottoms, and he sat on the floor in the corner. His head was framed by knotted curls, and large, hollow brown eyes looked at me impassively.

"Hi, Larry, I'm Katie," I said weakly, trying to conceal my nervousness.

There was silence. And then, "Sit down," he gestured to the floor.

More silence. Everything I had planned to say suddenly seemed wrong and inappropriate. I felt pity for him, for the injustice of his surroundings and for his returning home in such an inglorious fashion.

Suddenly, his eyes narrowed and he crossed his arms. I saw his fingers dig into his flesh. "And can you tell me why you are taking up the space of a soldier on this ship? Did you fight in the war?"

"Well, no, not exactly. I didn't fight in this war and I didn't ask to be sent home on this ship," I fumbled for words. "You know how the Army works. You take orders and don't ask why." I was glad to have thought of this hackneyed expression.

He half rose from the floor and said, "Now I'm giving orders - OUT!"

I stumbled to my feet and banged on the door, which opened quickly. It was all so futile. I burst into tears. As I left, I turned around and said, "Do you want me to come visit again?"

There was a long silence and then I heard a whisper, "Yes."

We became fast friends as the weeks went by, and my daily encounters with Larry gave me better insight into ways of helping other patients. I told him about life in the rest of the ship: how meals were scheduled around the clock in order to accommodate everyone; about the nights spent in the gun turret where improvisations was a constant challenge to weather conditions. Frequently he asked me to repeat the story of the night during a storm, when, in order not to roll overboard, we secured ourselves with ropes to the rails.

"I'm lucky," he said. "No danger of my going overboard."

Every day Larry inquired about our daily two hour show. "Do you mean you perform for a different audience every day? Are there really that many GIs up there? I'm glad I'm down here," he lied.

One day he asked me what I did in the show, and when I told him I sang, he said, "Prove it!" That was the beginning of my extra show every day.

I was able to have a farewell visit with Larry shortly before we landed.

I told him we were the first ship from the China-Burma-India theater to land in New York, and that we were being escorted by hundreds of gaily decorated, hornblowing boats, as well as official Army and Navy vessels.

"Oh, Larry, the church bells are ringing all over New York," I said. "The Statue of Liberty stands tall and more glorious than before. Her right arm reaches to the heavens, and the light of her torch is surely the symbol of new hope and peace in the world. At long last, Larry, we're home" Larry collapsed sobbing on my shoulder and we wept together.

HOMECOMING

It was just three months since World War II had ended and 23 days at sea when our troopship entered New York Harbor. We had slept little the night before. The decks were crowded with American soldiers and the few Red Cross volunteers and nurses. We were all eager for the familiar sights of the good old USA.

Standing on deck, as the ship prepared to dock, strange, haunting thoughts entered my mind. I began to wonder if my homeland, my family and friends had changed. At the beginning I had thought constantly about home and my loved ones. Then gradually that faded into the past, and my reality became the reality of the base. Letters from home took so long to arrive, and I found it increasingly difficult to write. With strict censorship there was little I could tell. My sister, who wrote to me so loyally about our family and the routine of home, got worried about me when my letters arrived with portions scissored out. How could anyone have guessed I was half way around the world at a secret B-29 base in India?

After a period of time I unconsciously developed a philosophy of living for each day with no thought of the future. That hurt too much.

An indescribable closeness was shared with my fellow workers as well as with the soldiers on our base. The association was akin to a family relationship, and this parting had not been easy.

A large flotilla of ships approached us with whistles blowing and flags waving and a large banner on a naval ship proclaimed, "Welcome Home - First troopship from the China-Burma-India Theater." Even the oil-slicked, littered harbor of New York was a welcome sight. As we docked we heard the ringing of church bells and saw crowds of people waving small American flags and shouting, "Welcome back! Welcome back!"

A group of Armed Forces and National Red Cross officials were waiting at the dock, and we, the Red Cross group, were taken to a hotel where the whole floor had been reserved. We were told it would be necessary to remain in New York several days for the purpose of interrogations, reorientation, physical examinations, and so on.

Since only New York knew of this momentous arrival, we were given permission to make a brief call home. My heart pounded as I gave the operator the number of my home in Baltimore. I was surprised I remembered it after this eternity.

My sister answered, "Hello?"

At the sound of her voice a lump in my throat delayed an answer.

She was impatient. "Hello ... hello?"

"I'm home - I mean New York." That wasn't what I had planned to say. I tried to be casual for fear of breaking down. "I've been in India - just back ... be released in several days... love to everybody, I'll call again... good-bye," and I hung up. It was more than I could handle at that moment.

After indulging in the amenities long forgotten: running water, a hot shower, flushing toilet, and best of all, a mattress on a real bed, I slept for 12 hours.

I was among the first to be called for a physical examination.

"Let's see," a pompous, but well-meaning, doctor said, reading my report. "It seems you've lost a considerable amount of weight in these two years. You experienced several, rather severe tropical illnesses, and you had some sort of accident from ... it says here 'home permanent set'." He snatched a quick glance above his glasses and noticed the burned, stubby ends of hair that covered my head. "Have you notified your family about these occurrences?"

"No, but they love me. They'll be glad to see me any way I am."

"Perhaps it would be advisable to call and prepare them - just indicate you're not quite the same person they said good-bye to a few years ago."

I didn't agree with him, but I called anyway and stammered through the routine he suggested. The response was loving and understanding. I later learned the welcoming party of family and friends they planned was then canceled. No more than senior members of the family would meet my train. They weren't quite sure what to expect.

The following morning I was awakened by an excited, jolly-faced official who told me she had contacted the Elizabeth Arden Salon and told them about the unfortunate accident that had happened to my hair. They had offered, as a contribution to the war effort, to call in experts to study the problem and determine the "proper action necessary to rectify this situation." She clapped her hands in gleeful expectation. "Get dressed and get over there fast. They are waiting for you."

I was given the red carpet treatment. I suppose I embodied every attendant's husband, brother, or lover who fought overseas. In addition to solving the hair problem, I was treated to a facial, massage, manicure, and a lunch so rich and different from the meager rations to which I had become accustomed that I promptly got sick. I walked out a very different person - head of curly, blonde ringlets, face renewed with the latest make-up, eyelashes extended, and a general look of well being.

I was issued a new uniform, white gloves, and a train ticket to Baltimore.

As I left my hotel room I passed a full length mirror, and I thought I was being followed by a very attractive person.

When the train pulled in, I saw the three anxious faces of my two brothers and sister. I couldn't resist - I fluttered my eyelashes, put out a white-gloved hand, and said, "What are you so worried about?"

CHEENIE

I had been home barely a month when it happened.

"A call from New York? For me? What was it about?"

"It came in last night while you were out... something about a dog with a letter attached to its collar, and it had your name and phone number on it. Doesn't make much sense, does it?" my nephew replied casually.

The word "dog" caused me to leap to my feet and race to the phone. I quickly put the call through, and shouted with delight, "It's Cheenie - she's here! Oh, thank you, God."

I lost no time in putting on my uniform, not forgetting to add the service stripes. Regulations forbid animals in train coaches, but since it was just three months since the end of the war, I would try to win the sympathy of the conductors. No time was lost getting to the station.

As the train bounced back and forth on the rails to New York, I relived the tearful farewell with my beloved dog. I never dreamed the complicated plans to smuggle her out of Darjeeling would ever materialize.

When I received my orders for the return trip home, my good English friend, Hugh Clark, was with me. He was stationed there with the British army in Darjeeling.

"Don't worry, Katie. I'll keep her in the barracks with me. The other chaps won't mind."

"Oh, Hugh, Thank you. " I was suddenly overwhelmed with tears. After returning to my room, I wrote to my sister telling her the good news of my impending departure and the heartbreak I felt leaving Cheenie behind.

After receiving my letter, she replied immediately. She wrote, "Your Cheenie sounds adorable. I wish you could bring her back with you. Elliot Roosefelt flew Blaze (White House Dog) back on a combat plane from Europe. The dog occupied a seat with returning troops. The event created quite a stir in the States. If he can get by with that, why don't you do something?"

"But how?" I thought.

I was the first one to receive my return orders and therefore, the first one to be given a farewell party. Midge presented me with a fancy, hand-embroidered, purple banner on which the Taj Mahal stood out in silver thread. Every guest added some sort of personal insignia which was attached to the farewell banner.

Among the guests was an attractive, American commander of a destroyer. It came to me like a bolt. This might be my only chance. I turned on the charm, all the charm of which I was capable. The next morning he told me he would take Cheenie back on his destroyer when it returned.

I was scheduled to leave in two days while the destroyer would be in dock for two weeks. The arrangements to get Cheenie to her final destination were formidable. Numerous friends were involved attending to the necessary details and getting her to the ship. Hugh Clark promised to care for her and see that she arrived in Calcutta by a certain date in September. Other friends offered to take care of inoculations. And finally she needed to be delivered by midnight to a specific spot on the Hoogly River outside of Calcutta. At this location she was to be picked up by a sailor from the destroyer. My close friend, had promised if she made it that far, he would bring her to the States. Once the ship had docked, he assured me, it would be simple to pretend she was the mascot and take her ashore for a walk. Sounds like a dream, doesn't it?

To think she had been a lost, three week old puppy when she was picked up by the military police patrolling the lower Himalayas Mountains. They had put her on my desk, and the first thing she did was to drink out of my inkwell. It had been such a challenge to keep her alive. She was so small she could nestle in the palm of my hand. To feed her, our hospital had given us a small bottle with a tiny opening. The boys had soldered a Red Cross pin to her collar for identification in the event she became lost and named her "Cheenie" - sugar in Hindustani.

"New York - all out for New York," the conductor called. It wasn't long before I was at the designated pet shop having the tearful reunion with a miserably thin, mangy, but happy dog. A note attached to her collar related the story of a long and stormy voyage that lasted about two months.

We hurried back to the station, down the steps, and faced a conductor standing by the train. "Can't take that on a coach - only in the baggage car."

"But, Sir, this is a dog - just returned from overseas. She did her share to win the war. She lived in a Red Cross Club, entertaining the troops with 10-day leaves from General Stillwell's Burma Road outfit. Those war-weary boys hadn't seen a dog since the beginning of the war, and she did more to raise morale than anything we could do." I made sure he saw my service stripes. "Oh, Sir, you wouldn't...."

"Take her on, and by the way, make sure she gets a seat."

The trains were filled with troops returning from overseas, and it wasn't long before I decided to see if Cheenie remembered her performing acts. To commands in Hindustani, the dog turned somersaults, jumped over shoulders, replied to questions with the correct number of barks, and danced up and down the aisles. It was quite a show, and I couldn't conceal my pride.

Later on that day, several soldiers suggested going to the diner. I hesitated, and they said, "Awe, come on. We'll buy Cheenie a beer."

The head waiter took one look at us and said, "How did that animal get on this train? - strictly against regulations - take it away."

When he heard her history, considerably embellished by the GIs, he softened, and told us about his youngest son stationed with the army in England.

"Let me show you to a table, and be sure your little hero gets something to eat. That dog deserves the best."

I was nibbling on a cheese sandwich when suddenly the head waiter appeared with a large plate piled high with hunks of meat. With a flourish he placed it in front of Cheenie and said, "For distinguished services overseas."

The train pulled into Baltimore, and we two travelers, tired and sleepy, found a taxi whose driver hesitated to allow the dog in his cab, then consented only if it remained on the floor. Since cars, and cabs in particular, were scarce because of the war, it was necessary to have a full capacity of passengers before leaving for a destination. After a long wait, and a subsequent lengthy journey, I realized we were the last riders. It was then that I told the driver my story. He was so fascinated he proposed a free ride if I would put the dog through her tricks in front of his headlights. "I can't wait to tell my kids," he said.

It was past midnight when I arrived home, but the show went on - that is until a neighbor raised his window and shouted, "What in the hell is going on at this time of night? I'm going to call the police!"

I thought to myself, I'll tell him the story - tomorrow - or the next day - or the next. We're going to be home for a long time.

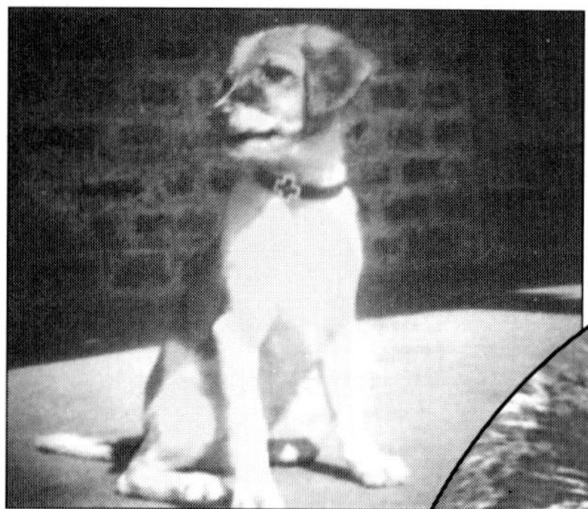

Cheenie

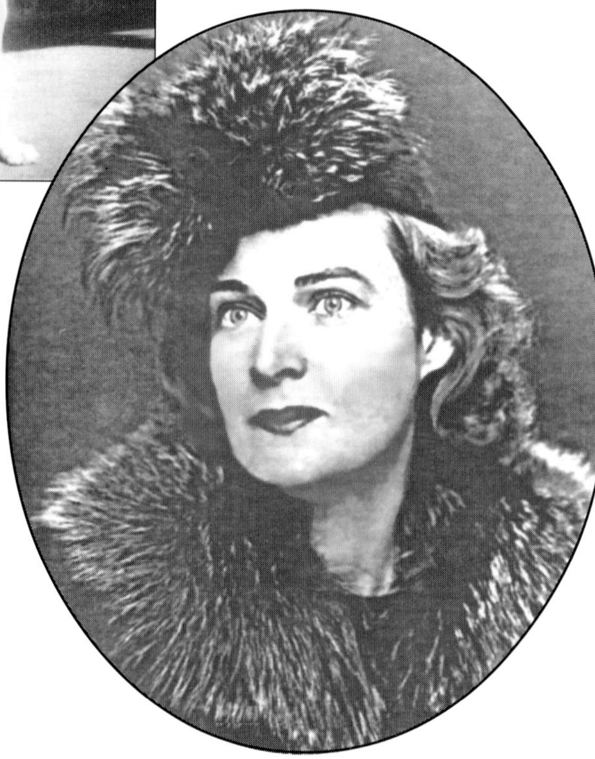

Katie out of uniform

Hollywood Celebrities and the Cherry Blossom Dance

by Margaret Truitt Joyal

Some of my clearest memories are the visits of Hollywood celebrities to entertain and amuse patients. Walter Reed Army Hospital received visits from such celebrities as Marlene Dietrich, Bob Hope and Linda Darnell. At the Forest Glen Section of Walter Reed, I escorted Bill Cosby whose humor had ambulatory patients literally rolling in the aisles. The most memorable visit was from Joan Crawford to the US Army Hospital at Ft. Dix, NJ. She arrived in a pale yellow satin dress with matching pill box hat. She visited one of the wards where patients had put up signs welcoming her. Afterward, the commanding officer brought her to the "Rec" hall where a lovely feast had been prepared. Miss Crawford declined the refreshments and proceeded to the television set where she settled into a chair, kicked off her shoes and said, "I'm taking my own daughter's place in today's soap opera, and I want to see if I performed all right." With that, all the patients, nurses and staff sat quietly until the end of the program whereupon Miss Crawford got up, waved good-bye to everybody and, left without another word. The staff was stunned! Needless to say the commanding officer, who had had to sit quietly by and watch Miss Crawford's TV performance, had few good words to say about her visit — only expletives!

As the recreation worker at the US Air Force Hospital in Nagoya, Japan, I had the pleasure of working with the Japanese liaison official, a good friend, who brought programs to the hospital to entertain the patients. Among these were large groups of children dressed in beautiful kimonos who danced and sang and brought gifts. Mr. Fukuoka

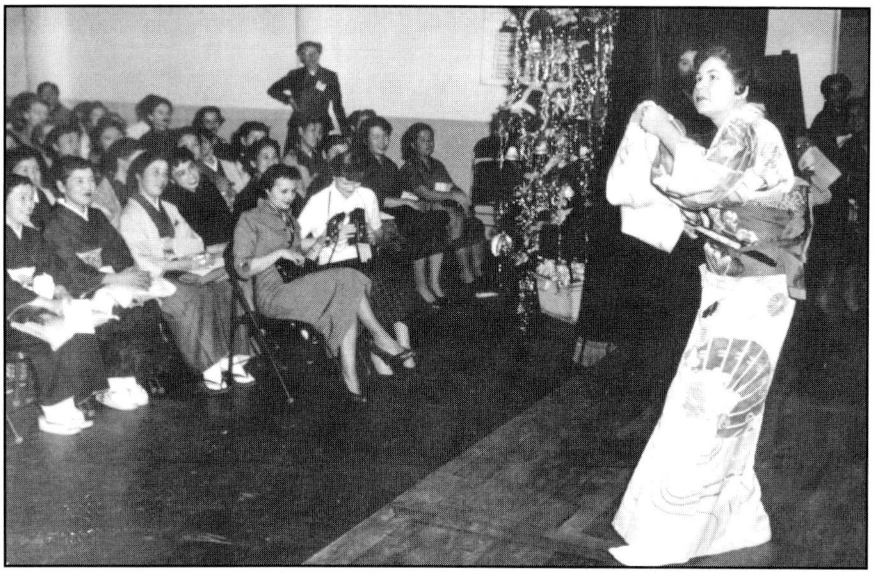

Margaret Joyal and members of the Japanese/American Cultural Association in Nagoya, Japan, ca. 1955

also brought cultural activities such as tea ceremonies, Koto players and others. As a form of personal recreation, I tried learning the children's "Cherry Blossom Dance." As a result, I was asked to perform this dance before the members of a joint Japanese-American Women's Cultural Club, which I tried to do dressed in my own Japanese kimono. My efforts were rewarded with flowers, a picture in the newspaper and a brief flash on the local movie news. I had truly tried to show appreciation in return for the many kindnesses that our Japanese friends had done for our patients.

Hospital Ship

by Phoebe Steffey

One of the most memorable experiences of my Red Cross career occurred when I was Red Cross representative on an US Army Hospital ship. At the invasion of Southern France the ship served essentially as a field hospital taking aboard the wounded servicemen directly from the battlefields of the invasion. My job was to be on hand as the men were boarded to assist in offering them cool drinks and to provide needed comfort supplies. (Red Cross chapters had made individual kits of toilet articles that had been placed on board ship in the USA.) The men's courage was deeply moving.

On each assignment aboard ship a most significant aspect of the job of the Red Cross staff member(s) was to make referrals to the appropriate local Red Cross of individuals who needed assistance or supporting in coping with some aspect of arrival in the US.

In the case of the hospital ship, most referrals were to the SMH field director at the military hospital to which the servicemen would be transferred.

The Brideship Operation brought to New York the faraway wives (and some children) of servicemen. The men had been urged not to come to New York to meet their wives, but to await their arrival in their new hometown. Many men did not follow this advice, to the delight of their wives. And to the wives of those men who did obey it came the troubling question: didn't their husbands care enough to come? To be reassuring was a principal role of Red Cross staff, including that of the New York Chapter who made arrangements for telephone calls and assisted in

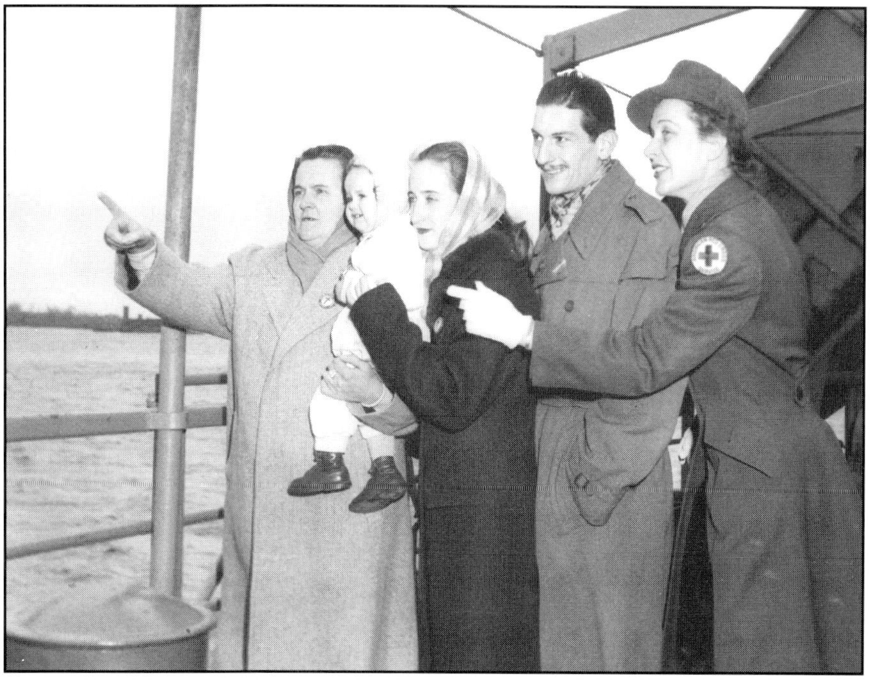

A Hungarian refugee family, gets its first look at the United States as Navy Transport Eltinge steams toward a landing at the Brooklyn docks. Pointing out the skyline is Red Cross Worker Phoebe Steffey. Left to right, Ozv Hornyak Balane, Frigyes, Amaryll, and Fribyesene Szhertnere. The family fled from Budapest.

making arrangements for expeditious travel to places all over the USA.

On the SS *Elbinge* a 14-year-old boy had managed to come aboard without disclosing that he had no connection to any adult on board. This fact came to light on arrival in New York when his fears about "What now?" became apparent. The New York Red Cross made arrangements for his temporary placement and the development of a longer range plan for him — a very moving situation.

Recreation

by Esther H. Smith

When stationed at the USAF hospital in Tachikawa, Japan, the colonel of the hospital and I met the crew of a B-52 Bomber, which had been shot down in China. The crew was brought to the hospital for physicals and surprisingly the member attracting the most attention by the press was a young man whose wife, believing him dead, had remarried. By international telephone arrangement each crew member was allowed a five minute conversation with his family by the Red Cross. It worked like clockwork. The crew member whose wife had remarried was closely guarded by government agents and with the help of veterans organizations in her home town, we heard that the reunion took place.

While at the hospital, the Gray Ladies shopped for all the men and accompanied them around the hospital. The crew leader was the one who had been tortured the most and needed the greatest medical care.

I learned they all arrived back in the States safely and one sergeant whose girl had waited for him, was soon married to her.

When stationed on Guam (1954), the captain of an Avon Moore ship fell 36 feet down the hold of his ship. It seems he had just passed over it, but someone had opened it as he returned and he plunged down it, breaking almost all the bones in one side of his body.

Our naval hospital was the nearest medical facility, so he was brought there. The surgeon who had wired his bones together asked me as the person having the nearest to an English accent, to keep talking to the unconscious man to try to get some response from him. As I had lived in England, I spoke of his homeland and talked about my life there. After a few weeks he began to talk and I became a steady visitor when he was moved to the ward surrounded by young patients. He participated in crafts (still a bed patient), then when he started to use crutches, the doctor asked me to try to get him out to functions, so I wheeled him to the Officers' Club, and then to a Brown, Pacific Maxim construction company cookout. A contact was made with the Qantas Air Lines manager who visited him, and took him for rides around the Island.

After three months, he was airlifted to Hong Kong where he was taken over by his steamship line, arriving in England before Christmas.

The steamship line wrote a delightful letter of appreciation to the volunteers of the Red Cross at the naval hospital, and we were glad he was safely home.

In 1944-45, I was assigned in England (Erlestoke Park) near Devises, in a 1,000 bed hospital. Our unit was visited by the chaplain and a few officers from the 10th Armored Division stationed at Warminster, who said their group had a lot of talented men who would like to entertain our patients.

We discussed time and the need for ward shows as well as recreation hall shows for the ambulatory. When a group of musicians and vocalists came within a few weeks, the talented men wowed the entire base with great music. Every few weeks, a group came. One night as the show was to begin, all the lights went out. Not to be deterred, the men went to their trucks, returning with flares placed on tin plates, which they lighted, casting a soft glow over the hall. The show went on and an Irish tenor sang too-ra-loo-ra-loo-ra to an audience of wounded men lulled by the beauty of the presentation. When the 10th Armored left to fight in the "Battle of the Bulge," we were saddened to think of our benefactors in the midst of danger and for weeks afterwards we tried to learn as much as we could about their welfare.

Midway Kansas Chapter

by Gayle Anderson-Savage

In 1974 the Midway Kansas Chapter of the American Red Cross, "headquartered" in Wichita, Kansas, responded to the need for a local agency to sponsor a senior nutrition program by contract with the local Area Agency on Aging, and funded primarily through the Older Americans Act. The program was set up in Sedgwick, Harvey and Butler counties, the counties that comprised the Central Plains Area Agency on Aging.

A committee of the chapter board was formed to oversee the program, and a director, program coordinator and secretary were hired. The program began operating 12 meal sites during January and February, with a catering firm providing food to the Wichita sites and restaurants in outlying towns providing space and meals for the seniors. According to Older Americans Act guidelines, meals were served five days a week at noon to participants who came to the sites, and were delivered to those temporarily homebound. All meals were on a contribution basis. Within less than a year and a half the program grew to 16 meal sites.

On July 1, 1975 I was hired by Tom Irving, then chapter manager, to be director of what was named the Good Neighbor Nutrition Program. Previously, I had worked 10 years for the Wichita YWCA, helping to develop and direct a preschool program in a minority neighborhood, and later directing program in the downtown YWCA. In this work I had known Tom Irving through interagency committees, and I was delighted to be offered this position in what I knew to be a wonderful Red Cross Chapter.

I served as GNNP director for 16 years, until my retirement in October 1991. During those years the number of meal sites grew to 36, as a result of increased funding from federal and local sources, and of the strong support of Midway Kansas Chapter, and of the great number of volunteers. The staff increased from three to nine, and many supportive services were added, including outreach, nutrition education, transportation and information provided to participants on a wide variety of subjects to increase their quality of life.

A transportation service at the chapter was enlarged to a full department by the manager and the board, and rides were provided to and from the meal sites and to special events. The meal sites were operated primarily by volunteers supervised by a site manager who worked two and one-half hours a day. All transportation drivers were volunteers, and most were seniors themselves. This service was essential to the operation of the program. Because of sponsorship of the nutrition program by the Red Cross, GNNP was able to provide more support services than many such programs across the nation that were sponsored by other agencies and institutions. It is to the credit of Tom Irving, subsequent managers and CEO's George Hutchins and Bill Hamelau, and an outstanding chapter board that this important service to seniors was initiated, supported, and is still operating in Wichita and surrounding areas. It was my good fortune to have been a part of an exciting and unique service by the American Red Cross, and I enjoyed and treasure the memories of my 16 years at Midway Kansas Chapter.

Can't You Tell Time?

by Melbern Robinson

The first sergeant of D Company, 2nd Rifle Battalion, was a friend of mine and told me of his search for a Company runner. The infrastructure of post-war Germany still had some way to go before practical telephone service could be established all the way down to Company level, therefore there was need for a runner.

My friend selected one promising young man from the hills of Tennessee who demonstrated an excellent memory. This private could repeat back the longest message the first sergeant would give him, if not with ease, then at least with a higher degree of accuracy than any of the other soldiers in the unit. Unfortunately, every time the first sergeant sent the private up to Battalion, he wouldn't be back for hours. After several "chew-out" sessions, the private finally confessed that he could not tell time. The first sergeant was flabbergasted, but bought a large alarm clock from the Post Exchange and taught the private to tell time.

For a month, the private carried the clock around, practicing. Emboldened by his success, he went to the Post Exchange and bought a watch, and returned the alarm clock to the first sergeant. Sure enough, the very first time he got sent to Battalion with a message, he was an hour late in returning.

The first sergeant asked him, "What's wrong with you. I know you can tell time, and I know you have a watch. What's the problem?"

"Top," the soldier responded, "This here watch they-uns at the PX sold me, it's broke. Durned thing don't work right. I can't read it." He extended his wrist out to the NCO to show him the face. The watch was working, the hour and minute hands were in the right place for that time of day, and the second hand was sweeping dutifully in its' circle. But then it dawned on the first sergeant. The private had bought a watch with Roman numerals!

A Memorable Red Cross Experience

by John R. Russell

In my 37 years with Red Cross, I was exposed to a wide variety of experiences, some pleasant, some not so pleasant, but all were stimulating, learning situations. The most unusual or unique was the following: In 1954 a hurricane pushed up the Rio Grande Valley in Texas. The accompanying heavy rains produced major flooding in such towns as Ozona, Eagle Pass and Laredo. I was sent down to serve as the Red Cross operational director, opening a headquarters office in Del Rio, and regional offices in the towns named previously.

The staff assigned were experienced, some speaking Spanish. One whom we were particularly fortunate to have with us was Carlos Patterne, Director of Disaster Relief in San Juan, Puerto Rico. As will be told later, his contribution to the successful operation was profound.

On the second day in Del Rio, I received a phone call from Ray Shaeffer, National Director of Disaster Services. Ray reported that his office had received word of heavy flood losses and many deaths on the Mexican side of the valley. The US State Department had made contact with the Mexican Government through the Mexican Embassy, offering assistance. The Mexican Government declined, not wishing to appear dependent on the "Big Brother" to the north. However, in the conversation, it was learned that "assistance" from the American people through the American Red Cross would be acceptable. This position was relayed from the State Department to Red Cross National Headquarters.

In his call, Ray gave me instructions on how to proceed under the circumstances. First, the next day, I was to go to Nueva Laredo to meet with Mr. Chavez, Mexican Secretary of Hydraulic Resources, (similar to our Secretary of the Interior) and negotiate the plan for assisting. Second, I would be guided to the meeting place by the American Consul in Nueva Laredo, but that he would not be involved in the meeting. Third, I should go in as much style as I could muster, thus giving face to the importance of the meeting. Fourth, I should take an interpreter along, since it was not known in which language the conversations would be held. Fifth, I should avoid the use of US Military Forces in giving assistance. Otherwise I had a "blank check to use as needed." Sixth, all food was to be purchased in Mexico, using US currency. Last, I should proceed with all haste, so as to be there promptly at 10:00 a.m. the next morning.

Contact with the USAF at Lackland Air Base was made to arrange for a plane to fly the 10 miles or so from Laredo to Nueva Laredo. (Thus the right "face" was being placed on the approach.) I contacted our office in Laredo to have Carlos Patterne ready to accompany me. He was to be my interpreter and advisor. The 200 mile drive from Del Rio to Laredo gave me a chance to collect my thoughts.

The next morning, our flight to Nueva Laredo took about 20 minutes. We were met by the American Consul, who took us to the meeting place in the town Plaza. He said that he had been told to get us there, but to stay away from the meeting.

When we entered the second floor meeting room, we were greeted by Secretary Chavez and an assistant. Chavez was dressed in a military uniform. We were told by the Secretary's assistant that the language of the meeting would be Spanish. However, I felt certain that Chavez spoke English.

Not knowing how to proceed otherwise, I quickly and bluntly asked Mr. Chavez what was needed from us. He as quickly replied "beginning tomorrow morning, to feed 8,000 refugees in the Nueva Laredo area and continue feeding for three weeks. After that, the Mexican Army will take over." We also learned that the refugees were housed in various school buildings in the area. I agreed that we would meet his request, although I was certain that to do so would require the involvement of US Troops.

Chavez' assistant indicated that the scene for the meeting would shift. We were to go to the airport, get in a Mexican Army transport to fly to Piedras Negras (across from Eagle Pass) for a meeting there. The group, plus two Mexican soldiers as "helpers," boarded the Mexican plane.

We landed on a flat strip in the desert and were greeted by the governor of the State, Mr. Cepeda. Folding chairs and bottles of water were brought out of the plane by the two "helpers" and set up in the shadow of the plane wings. In 10 minutes or less, Governor Cepeda made known his needs: medicine, vaccines, antibiotics, bandages, etc. Again, I immediately agreed and stated that we would have the supplies there in 24 hours.

Governor Cepeda, speaking on behalf of the town of Ciudad Acuna, asked if we could feed 3,000 people there for three weeks. The town was now isolated because the bridges and roads were washed away. I agreed to his request, but knew that it would take an airlift by a US helicopter to deliver the food.

Our visit was completed, and we flew back to Nueva Laredo. There we parted company with Mr. Chavez, without a word of thanks or gratitude from him. He was formal and very abrupt. So was I. I did tell the American Consul of our agreements.

When I called Mr. Shaeffer, he understood the situation and agreed that the help of the US Army was required. Further he advised that he would arrange for it with the State Department and the Pentagon. As a result, by dusk that day, a CO-54 with 108 men and full cooking equipment landed in Nueva Laredo, and breakfast was prepared the next morning for the refugees. Mexican women pitched in to help.

The requests from Governor Cepeda were fulfilled including setting up a helicopter airlift to Ciudad Acuna.

My last action was to ask Carlos Patterne to move over to Nueva Laredo for the next several weeks, do all of the food buying as ordered by the army, and pay all expenditures in US currency. Our temporary accounting office in Del Rio received a full and proper accounting from Patterne.

World War II In India And Germany

by Carla Ross

In the summer of 1944, the Red Cross sent me to the China-India-Burma Theater headquarters in Calcutta, India. My assignment was to set up a program to teach the troops for the invasion of Japan. They had to be able to swim with everything they wore and carried. We built swimming pools where ships unloaded, Calcutta and Karachi. We taught the Breast Stroke only, since that was easy to do with full combat gear, the GI boots were good with the frog kick. We had the program going good when the atom bomb ended the necessity of an invasion.

In September of 1945, I was sent from India to Europe. My headquarters were in Munich, Bavaria. My job there was to provide First Aid training for the military forces who were to be the constabulary police force of Europe.

The US. military had taken over Hitler's winter sports area at Garmish-Partenkirchen and hired 22 Swiss-German and German ski instructors to patrol and teach the US military who used the area as a Rest & Recreation center. The Germans didn't know First Aid since in Europe (unlike the US) skiers aren't allowed on the slopes until they are very experienced. We taught the instructors American National Ski Patrol Technique in two weeks.

I was able to get a ticket to the Nuremburg Military Tribunal. It was quite an experience. The room was long and narrow with the court sitting against one long wall and the prisoners against the other facing the court. The spectator gallery was along the end of the room. I was seated close to Gerhing. If I had leaned forward I could have touched him.

Field Director in Phu Bai, Vietnam

by Melvin Fredericksen

Phu Bai, Vietnam: Rakkasan, Bastogne, Veghal and Tomahawk are their names. There are others like them.

All are rugged hilltop fire bases in defoliated jungle about 40 miles from the DMZ. Soldiers of the Army's 101st Airborne Division man these embattled enclaves.

Charlie is very much around. Tomahawk recently was forced to move to more strategic higher ground after NVA regulars overran the base.

Conditions are very primitive and there are few creature comforts. American Red Cross Field Director, Melvin Fredericksen, cannot do much about the Viet Cong or North Vietnamese but he is trying to help make things a little easier for the American men at these remote outposts.

Flying out by helicopter from 101st Headquarters at Phu Bai. Frederickson and his assistant Field Director Raymond Kohlman in a recent trip visited some of those fire bases. They carried with them boxes filled with various comfort items: stationary, pens, playing cards, combs, nail clippers, bar soap and heavy, vinyl bags to protect belongings from the damp weather. All are gifts of the American people through the Red Cross.

When their Huey helicopter put down at Fire Base Bastogne, the landing zone was afire with dusty sunlight. Few of the men inhabiting this heavily bunkered hill were moving in the dazzling midday heat.

A sergeant emerged to talk with them and men were dispatched to unload the chopper and carry the boxes into the bunkers.

The men came out to chat with Frederickson and Kohlman, "It's great you could come," someone said. "Be glad to have the Red Cross come here more often. The men appreciate these things."

Fredericksen, from Lawton, Oklahoma, and Kohlman, from Newport, Rhode Island, thinks theme visits are important. "Naturally they are glad to see us." Fredericksen said. "It lets them know someone is interested in them, and that the people back home have not forgotten about them."

Kohlman added, "These guys will make good use of everything we bring. It isn't really enough for everyone, but the message of someone caring gets through. That's important for morale, especially in a war we say we are no longer trying to win and which many people do not support."

They had traveled to four bases that day when hostile action in the

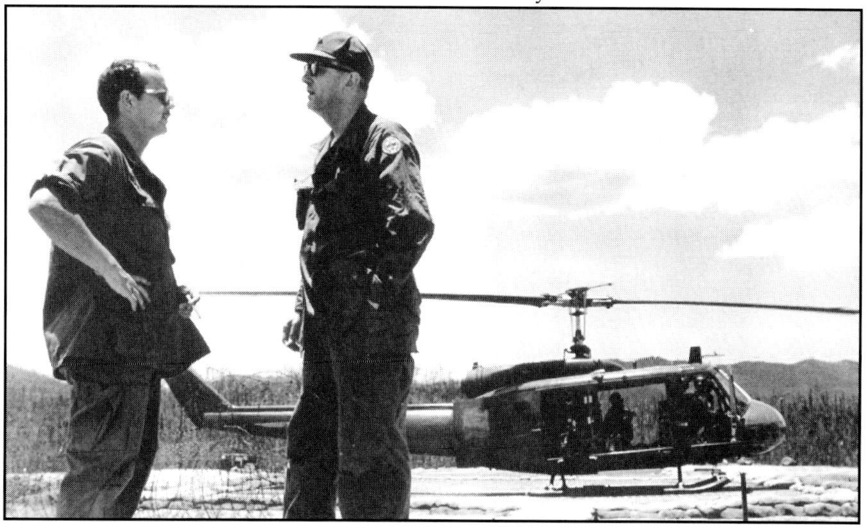

At Bastogne, Fredricksen confers with Sgt. Steve R. Swanson concerning comfort articles for GIs at the firebase.

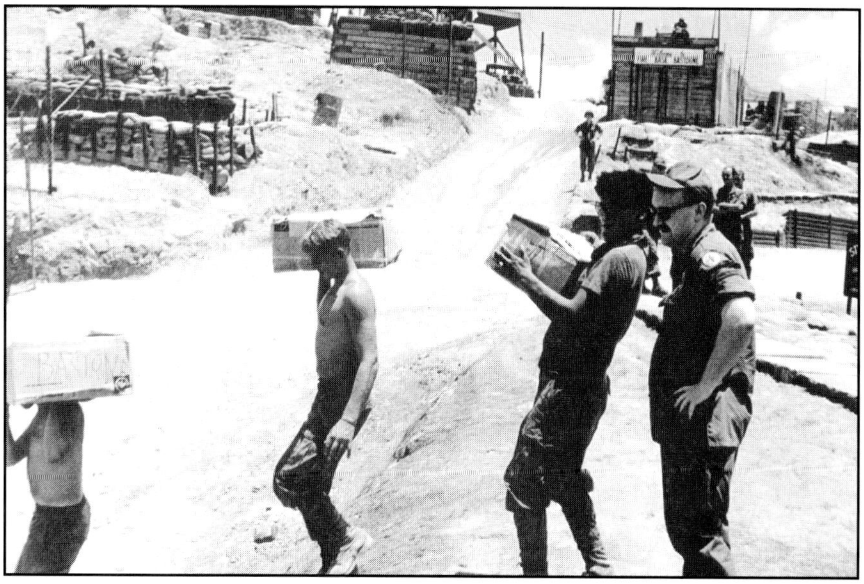

At Bastogne, Kohlman watches GIs carrying boxes of comfort articles from the chopper.

area forced an early return to Phu Bai. The Red Cross men had to wait for another day to continue their visits.

There are approximately 150 Red Cross workers serving at military installations throughout Vietnam handling emergency communications and health and welfare inquiries from servicemen's families back in the States. They counsel servicemen with personal problems, assist with requests for emergency leave, as well as help and advise servicemen to obtain government benefits to which they are entitled.

Frederickson is no stranger to the military, he has spent 21 years in the US Army and is a retired 1st sergeant. After retiring, he taught high school for a year before taking the post as city manager for Burnet, Texas. He joined the Red Cross in 1965 and has served at Fort Sill, Oklahoma, Korea, Japan, Fort Leavenworth, Kansas and now in Vietnam.

"I felt that in the Red Cross I could accomplish something worthwhile and be especially effective because of my familiarity with the military," Fredericksen explained. "I know I could help these men and with my Army background could better understand their problems." Regular visits to the 101st far flung fire bases are important because "lots of guys have problems and can't get in to see us and our visiting them is the only way to make contact." He said.

While Frederickson, who is married and has two grown children, brings paternal interest and military experience to his Red Cross job, 25-year-old Kohlman feels he brings the advantage of youth and a college degree in psychology and theology. The combination makes him well qualified to understand servicemen and their problems.

A graduate of Barrington College in Barrington, Rhode Island, Kohlman is the son of Mrs. Eleanor Harriet Kohlman who lives in Lewiston, Maine. His wife Kathleen lives in Newport, Rhode Island with their 2-year-old son.

His greatest satisfaction, he said, is when "some GI comes to me with a problem and I'm able to solve that problem, and watch him walk away happy." He particularly likes the Red Cross work because "for the most part I'm my own boss. The responsibility is on my shoulders."

Nearly Trapped By Big German Push

submitted by Joseph Willicombe Jr.

PARIS, DEC. 30 - (INS) - A young American Red Cross heroine of the US First Army front, beautiful, blonde Margaret "Peggy" Henry, came back to Paris tonight with a dramatic story of her breath-taking escape through the German lines in Luxembourg. Twenty-four-year-old Peggy, from Columbus, Ohio, whose vivacious smile, gay wit, doughnuts and coffee have brought joy to GIs from the Normandy beaches to the German frontier, told this correspondent of her experience - one of the epic narratives of the war.

Known as "the last rose of no man's land," Peggy was stationed within 1,000 yards of the German lines when Marshal von Rundstedt launched his desperation drive against the First Army.

This young beauty had been sent there to operate the recreation club of an army division rest center because her record had shown a brilliant mind and a steady, cheerful disposition. She had served with distinction in England and Normandy for 15 months.

"This place was supposed to be a rest center for the American First Army troops," explained Peggy, who holds BA, BS and MA degrees from Ohio State University and taught English in the Main-Montrose Junior High School in Columbus four years before she joined the Red Cross.

"I had been there six weeks during which things were very quiet. There was nothing to indicate that the Germans were going to launch any offensive in that sector.

"The first definite indication I had of what the Nazis were up to was early in the morning of December 16. I was asleep in Headquarters of the Rest Center Hotel when I was awakened by explosions. I figured they must be enemy shells so I got up, put on my house coat and went downstairs. On the way, I knocked at the door of the colonel, commanding officer of the rest center, and asked him if the explosions were from enemy shells. He said they undoubtedly were and were undoubtedly aimed at us. The shells kept getting closer and closer, so we all went down in the basement and stayed there a couple of hours. Then the shelling stopped for a while. I had breakfast and went back to bed for about an hour, when the shelling started all over again.

"I got up once more and decided this time to stay up. The second period of shelling lasted about an hour and when it stopped the colonel said he was going to send me away until things quieted down. But we received word that the roads leading out of town were under fire, so I couldn't leave. All of us at the rest center were 'alerted' and restricted to the hotel."

Peggy, who was the only American woman in the town, continued:

"When everything was quiet for a while again we believed it had all blown over, so I opened my club and put up a big brave sign on the door: 'Of course, we are open.'

"All the boys came in and told me I should be wearing a Combat Infantry badge because I had earned it by then. There was a movie for the troops, but that afternoon the Nazis started shelling again. From then on, we were all under an 'alert' and as the situation became increasingly serious. we all stayed in the lobby of the hotel where runners from various platoons came in and brought news during the evening that our town was definitely an objective of the German offensive and that tanks were on their way.

"We also heard there were some

reinforcements on their way but that they probably could not reach us in time. I was scared when I heard that, but I couldn't show it. After a while, I put a blanket down on the floor, and tried to get some more sleep thinking it might be the last I'd get for some time."

The pretty Red Cross worker said she could not really sleep very much under the circumstances and finally got up only to learn that the Germans were then only four miles away.

"There was increasing small arms fire around us, and continuous shelling from mortars somewhere in the hills behind the hotel," she continued.

"The firing kept getting closer and closer and then we could actually hear the approaching rumble of the German tanks. My job was to continue serving coffee and cigarettes to the patrons that came in and the runners and others who were going to and from the combat zones. We all kidded about it to keep up our spirits but at the same time we felt our situation was rapidly becoming pretty hopeless. I was told it would probably be impossible to escape, and it was suggested that I throw away all divisional insignia and anything that might in any way jeopardize me in case of capture.

"During the afternoon, we were ordered into the basement, because it was getting so hot and so close it was dangerous to remain in the lobby of the hotel. Soldiers took up positions on the stairway of the basement and in front of me while I tried to keep five civilian women quiet so German patrols would not hear us. We stood there for 15 minutes not knowing when we would see the first Nazi troops.

"As I threw my insignia away, an officer remarked, 'Peggy, if you are lucky you'll be captured.' I just prayed I wouldn't and hoped for the best.

"Suddenly the telephone rang. Lt. Col. Trapani answered it and received orders suggesting that we move to cover which was situated about 30 minutes away on the top of a hill. By that time, however, the Germans had already moved into the town and it was necessary to get through their lines before the designated destination could be reached.

"First of all, we had to cross the street in front of the hotel which was now under direct machine-gun fire. Our colonel went first. We didn't expect him to get across. But he did, firing at the Germans en route. Then I followed, then the others, one at a time. Altogether, there-were eight of us, including three civilian girls. The Germans fired at us constantly as we crept along the walls of old buildings.

"As we crept along, the colonel and a lieutenant endangered their own lives trying to protect me. I tried to hug the walls so closely that I might look like one of the stone slabs.

"The Germans used searchlights now that it was dark and whenever they came near we froze there while they shot away in our direction, and then went on.

"Finally, we reached the road leading to our place of cover. Shells were continually whistling by us. We lost our way after a bit and had to cut, uphill and cross country before we finally approached the building that was our destination. The colonel went ahead to tell the American guards there not to fire on us. Then when we got the signal we went on and rushed into the building. The three civilian girls, whom the Army feared the Nazis might kill if they were captured, and I were quickly assigned to a truck convoy which was making a desperate effort to get out of the area over a back road.

"The shelling continued more fiercely than ever. Five guards on our truck jumped off to protect us each time we were challenged by sentries along the roads. On one occasion I had to take the girls off and get them into a ditch when shells exploded close by our truck.

"An hour later, we met some infantry marching up to reinforce the garrison of the town we had just left. That was the first time I really realized that infantrymen had to walk, and single file too. We kept moving as fast as we could and as we got further away I could see shells in the distance and it was hard to believe we had really gotten away from the Germans.

"An hour or two later, we reached Bastogne. I got an hour of sleep there when suddenly we were alerted all over again. There were other mobile club workers in Bastogne and all of us were again ordered to evacuate at once. All night long the Luftwaffe was strafing the town and the main road was under heavy fire. Finally, we were moved along a circuitous route and managed to make our way back to Mezieres and safety.

"I could still hear the sounds of battle Christmas morning when we managed to move back 30 more miles. We had our Christmas dinner with troops on the run — a small can of C-ration hash, one piece of bread and a cup of coffee.

"From that time on, everything happened so fast it was hard to keep track of all that was going on, but I learned later that the brave boys who got me to Bastogne on the truck convoy rushed back to the front to help stem the German drive.

"I'll never forget how those soldiers in the heat of combat still found time to help us escape."

Custody Assistance

by Doye Fannin

Searching my memory for a special story, I found it very difficult to select just one. Over the many years of my service, to military installations, I encountered hundreds of special situations.

In the story chosen, a divorced mother died suddenly, leaving her young daughter (age 6), with no parent in the home. The situation came to the attention of my office in Germany, by a message from a hometown chapter of the American Red Cross. The chapter directed the message to my office, requesting contact of the child's father (Army

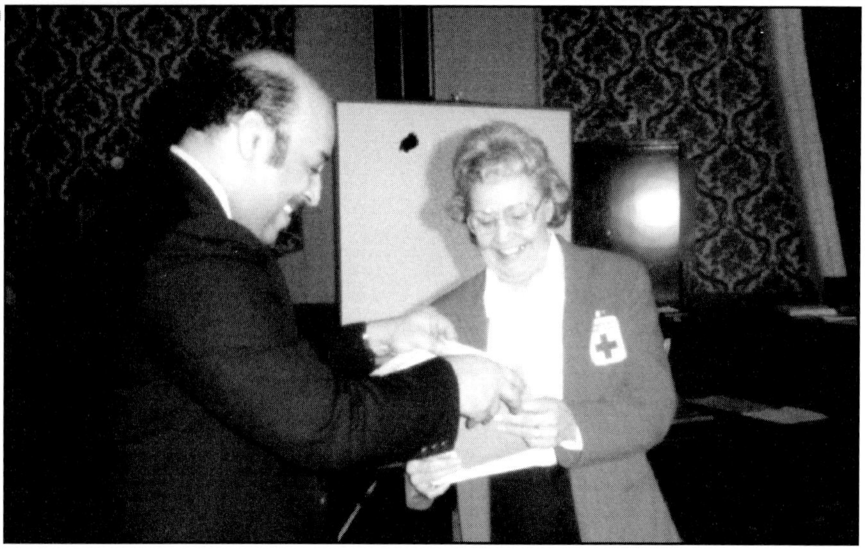

Winter 1983. Red Cross District Director presents 25-year Service Pin and certificate to Doye Fannin, SD, at Grafenwoehr, Germany.

Sergeant), stationed on the military base that I served.

Getting the child's father home became problematic, because the sergeant had no accrued leave time. However, after bringing the little girl's plight to the attention of the sergeant's unit commander, he granted advance leave against the time remaining on the sergeant's enlistment.

When the girl's father arrived in the US, another complicating situation confronted him. The child's grandparents (ex-wife's parents) brought action in the court to gain custody of the child. They claimed that his military service and his status as a single parent, prevented the father from providing a proper home and supervision for his daughter. The judge issued an order enjoining the father from taking custody of his daughter, pending adjudication of the case. After being informed that disposition of the case could take weeks, if not months, the father had no recourse but to return to Germany, without his daughter.

Soon after the sergeant returned to his duty station in Germany, he came to my office to thank Red Cross for the assistance given him. When asked about the status of his daughter's custody, he advised me of the suit by the child's grandparents. He stated that the Court appointed an attorney for him and that he gave a deposition before he left. He also left a copy of his former wife's will, in which she indicated she wanted him to have custody of their daughter. He said his court appointed attorney (a former JAG officer) advised him to seek assistance from the military, to document that he could provide proper care and supervision of his daughter.

I asked the sergeant if he had taken any action to secure the documents. He indicated that he was not sure how to proceed, and that he felt reluctant to make further requests of his commanding officer for help. Asked if he would like me to contact his unit commander, he stated that he would very much appreciate my assistance.

I contacted his first sergeant and apprised him of the sergeant's need to provide evidence, for his attorney, and the court, to support the sergeant's claim for custody of his daughter.

The commanding officer took swift action, to provide the sergeant with family quarters, located near his place of duty. The nature of the sergeant's duty permitted flexible hours, so that he could escort his daughter to and from school, and allow him to be with her at all times, during evening hours. The sergeant, having no leave time accrued, was unable to take leave without being placed in a "no pay due" status. To avoid having the sergeant lose income, the Military Transportation Office made arrangements to have the sergeant's daughter travel to Germany in the company of a military family being assigned to that station. To assure a smooth adjustment for the sergeant and his daughter, the commanding officer provided for special counseling.

After finalizing all the arrangements, the commanding officer gathered all the documents and forwarded them, with his own letter, to the sergeant's attorney and the court. Within two months of this action, the court released the sergeant's daughter to his custody and she joined him in Germany.

Serving Troops In Greece And Turkey

by Byron W. Evans

In the mid-50s, the need for American Red Cross service to troops in Greece and Turkey manifested itself. European headquarters in Stuttgart, Germany selected me as the field director in charge of that operation.

Because the military command at Athens, Greece had invited the Red Cross to establish offices in Athens, it was decided to make this the base of operations for Greece and Turkey. The United States Air Force maintained an air base in Athens, thus a resource for regular visits to units in Turkey by Red Cross personnel.

As a routine, the American Express was used as the banking resource for all Red Cross offices in Europe. These banks accepted checks issued by the Red Cross for American dollars, an important factor. Military personnel purchased food and other needs from the commissary or post exchange, both of which required US dollars for purchases. It was anticipated the same program could be instituted in Greece.

Such was not the case. Greek money was legal tender for

American Express. Once American Express checks were cashed, the recipient could exchange Greek money for American dollars for a fee. This was unacceptable because recipients of financial assistance often interpreted this charge as a fee for Red Cross service. In addition it was cumbersome.

Turkey presented another problem. Checks written on American Express in Greece were not honored. Hence, Red Cross was unable to render financial assistance to military personnel and their families through the use of existing banking facilities.

It became apparent the only solution was to establish an account in a bank in the United States for the Athens office. When this solution was reviewed by the European headquarters, it was met with disbelief. In all Europe it had never occurred. My supervisor, assigned the task of solving the problem, reported that the suggested solution was the only viable one. It was then that an account on a US bank was opened for the Athens office. Checks written on this account were cashed by military finance offices.

Another problem occurred, tangential to the one described above. Service to troops in Turkey was limited, because I visited military units routinely, but irregularly. This was particularly difficult for personnel and their families facing emergency financial needs. I finally solved it by issuing revolving funds to military chaplains located in three central locations in Turkey. They were given the authority to advance funds to military personnel to meet emergency needs. This plan, inaugurated with the approval of the military, solved a difficult situation, and permitted me to discharge obligations to service personnel and their families in an effective, efficient and timely manner.

Again, personnel at European headquarters voiced consternation and disapproval of this arrangement. Subsequent review by supervisory staff approved the arrangement, expressing gratification at the plan's uniqueness.

Had the solutions not occurred it would have been impossible to provide traditional Red Cross services to members of armed forces. Personnel in emergency situations would have been without the means to meet them—funds for family emergencies, funds to finance emergency leaves, and other situations requiring money in the form of loans or grants. The problem and solution described, affected countless numbers of military personnel and their families located in far flung foreign areas.

How I Lent President Kennedy My Hands

by Neal T. English

Why did President Kennedy appear with my hands attached to his body when his annual Red Cross Month appeal appeared on the three television networks? After Kennedy's death, why did President Johnson lose his cool doing the same type of appeal for the Red Cross?

One situation was a very interesting video combining of anatomies. The other a somewhat frightening and eye-opening experience. This was especially true for one who had lived a very sheltered life in Loveland, Ohio. One from that a small town does not expect to encounter two presidents under such circumstances, if any. But as National Director of the Office of Public Information for the American National Red Cross, in Washington, DC, I experienced these events across the street at the White House.

Regarding the hands situation, I was amazed at how lax security was at the White House at that time. I walked from ANRC Headquarters across 17th Street to the White House gate. I had a bulging briefcase. There were no hand-held metal detectors, or standing ones, as we now see in many locations. No one asked to look into the briefcase. A simple, "I'm Neal English from the Red Cross and have an appointment with the President," was all that was needed to gain entrance through the gate. Passing security at the White House door was the same.

I was especially aware of this lack of security. At an earlier date, I had seen President Kennedy lingering and waving to tourists at the side entrance to the Daughters of the American Revolution, opposite my office window.

At that time, anyone could enter the three ANRC buildings without being stopped and go to any floor, office or the roof. The President's schedule was published daily in the *Washington Post*.

Arriving in the White House Cabinet Room for the Kennedy filming, I found the NBC-TV crew setting up lights and cameras. I introduced myself and asked how I could help. I was asked to put a Red Cross symbol on the desk if I had one. Naturally, one of the items in the briefcase was a cardboard, fold-up emblem I had anticipated would be helpful for ANRC identity as a cut-a-way from the President during the appeal.

At the appointed time, the door opened and President Kennedy breezed in, smiled and greeted everyone. He sat at the desk and quickly delivered the Red Cross message. "I think I can do better on that. Let's do it again," he said. After that, he thanked the crew and left. As the door closed, the NBC director said, "We didn't get the shot with his hands on the desk near the Red Cross emblem. We need it to provide some pace to the message and for the emblem identity." He then said, "We cannot ask him to come back. Who has a blue pinstripe suit like he was wearing?" Suddenly everyone was looking at me. So the NBC director said, "Just sit down, in the President's chair, locate your arms and hands exactly as he had his near the emblem." I did, and those are the hands seen, apparently as those of the President, in prime time on CBS-TV,

ABC-TV and NBC-TV that year. That film was later requested by the Kennedy Library, and Red Gross gave them a copy.

Prior to President Johnson's first meeting with the Cabinet in the White House, after JFK's death, the filming of the Red Cross Month appeal had been scheduled. Since the crew was filming in the same room, for all three networks, chaos resulted.

The NBC-TV crew had just started unpacking equipment prior to the appointed time, when the door flew open, and there was LBJ huffing and puffing: "Aren't you ready yet? Get moving," he yelled. "I've got a Cabinet meeting to do." He later returned, spoke to no one, sat down at the desk and then said, "Are you ready?" He rushed through the message, jumped up and departed. There were sighs of relief through the room. A couple minutes later, the door flew open. There he was again, yelling wildly, "Look at this mess. Get those lights, wires and equipment out of here. Get those chairs back where they belong." He was fuming. He departed slamming the door. NBC-TV crew members were shocked. (Probably wished they had gotten that performance on film.) I was, too. They grabbed everything in sight without bothering to roll up cords, fold lights or pack cases and dashed for the hall. I ran around moving the heavy chairs back in place around the Cabinet Room table, hoping the door would not open before I could get out of there.

At the next election, I did not vote for LBJ. Most other people did. Later when I was National Public Relations and Advertising Director for the American Institute of Architects, I conducted a press conference in Portland, Oregon for Lady Bird Johnson and was invited to a dinner she held for a number of people at a ski lodge on Mt. Hood. Earlier, and still, I have been impressed with the fantastic job she did beautifying Washington, DC, and the nation. I was even more impressed in finding her to be such a gentle, polite, considerate lady.

The press in Portland felt the same way for her convention speech and press conference for the American Institute of Architects resulted in an 8-column wide headline on page 1 in the daily *Oregonian*. I never had that happen for any other press conference including those for convention speakers such as Princess Grace, Adalai Stevenson, Lorne Greene and others. They say opposites attract in marriage. It was certainly true for the Johnsons.

VJ Night In Manila, PI

by Elizabeth Reed Denman

It was late in August 1945. I was stationed as a recreation worker at a 1500 bed general hospital in Manila, PI, which was set up in the grandstand of a horse racing track called The Jockey Club. Almost all 1500 beds were occupied.

On this night, I met my date at the hospital gate and we went to a small club run by the officers of an amphibious engineer unit for dinner. After dinner we were dancing and enjoying the conversation of the group when we noticed a sudden absence of voices at the bar. We too fell silent as a friend came toward us. In a low voice he told us that the radio had just carried a brief announcement that an immense bombing raid had hit a city in Japan, thought to be Hiroshima, and it was thought the war would end soon. There were no details. No one knew where the statement originated. We too became speechless for a time. We couldn't believe it—were afraid to believe it. Where was Hiroshima?

Our sources of news were the Armed Forces Radio, *Stars and Stripes* newspaper, and Tokyo Rose. The first two carried almost no news of the combat situation and the latter, of course, was totally unreliable.

Every man in the room, every man in the Far East knew his assignment for the invasion of the Japanese main islands which was expected to take place very soon. They knew that this would be the hardest, bloodiest, and most dangerous campaign of a most terrible war. Many of those present probably would not survive it. Everyone was psyched up to do what had to be done and was trying not to think about the planned invasion. Now, could it be possible they wouldn't have to do it? Nobody knew any way to find out. We were all stunned. Everybody sat talking in hushed tones, listening for further information from the radio at the bar which never came. What a cruel thing to have their defenses weakened if the report were not true!

After an hour or so, the other woman and I decided that we should return to the hospital in case there was something we could do there to ease the situation for the patients.

As our escorts drove us to the hospital, close to midnight (curfew time), the streets were even more quiet than usual. When we reached the hospital, we found that nearly everyone there had a similar reaction to ours. Almost all off duty personnel and ambulatory patients were aimlessly wandering around outside the buildings hardly talking at all and when they did, it was in whispers. This went on most of the night.

It was several days until we got enough news from "solid" sources so that we could believe that the raids had taken place and that the surrender was genuine.

THEN THE CELEBRATIONS BEGAN!

Clubmobile Days At 1st Cavalry, Korea

by Lucie Davidson

On the 18 February 1960 our class picture was taken at the ARC National Headquarters in Washington, DC. There were seven of us standing tall and proud and smiling nervously as we wore our Class-A Red Cross uniform for the first time. We had just completed two weeks of training in DC to learn all

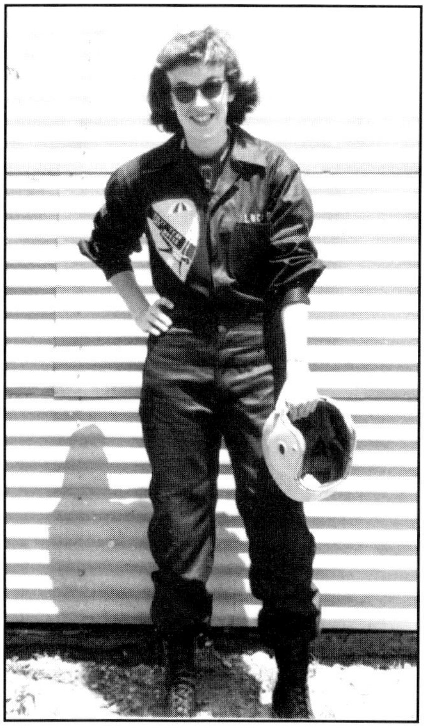

Lucie Davidson in front of the 1st Cav. Skydivers Clubhouse at CC#4 near Mun San Nee, Korea

about the Red Cross, to learn a little about the military, to get to know our classmates, to get to know our clubmobile leaders and most important, to learn just an inkling of what our job was to be for the next 12 months. We were ready and raring to go to Korea, we were the March 1960 class of Clubmobile girls.

An inkling of our job was all that was possible during those early training days as this assignment and job turned out to be like no other in the world! I remember feeling very confused and just a little bit scared—or was it terrified? I also remember the feeling that we were all in for something quite out of the ordinary, something most unusual and something that I already felt proud to be a part of.

I remember the cross country flight to California. I think it was at Fort Mason where we got our fatigues, finger printed, ID carded and dog tagged. I remember the long flight across the Pacific on a military airplane with stops at Guam and Midway Island and finally arriving at Tachikawa AFB, Japan. We were one of the last classes to have another full week of training at Camp Zama, Japan before arriving in Korea.

Finally we were off to the "land of the morning calm" and would soon arrive at what was to be our home for the next year. We did not know where we were going until that last morning in Japan. There were five SRAO units in Korea at that time: 1st Cavalry (Camp Pelham), ASCOM (HQ, 20th Gen. Sup. Gp.), 7th Division (Camp Casey), HQ I Corps (Camp Red Cloud) and I Corps (Gp) Artillery at Camp St. Barbara. I was lucky as another girl in our class (Cindy) and I were assigned to the same unit, the biggest and, I might add, the best unit in Korea—the 1st Cavalry.

Cindy and I climbed into a helicopter and off we went. Home for us turned out to be Cavelle Hall, 19th Field Artillery. We each had our own small room in a cement block

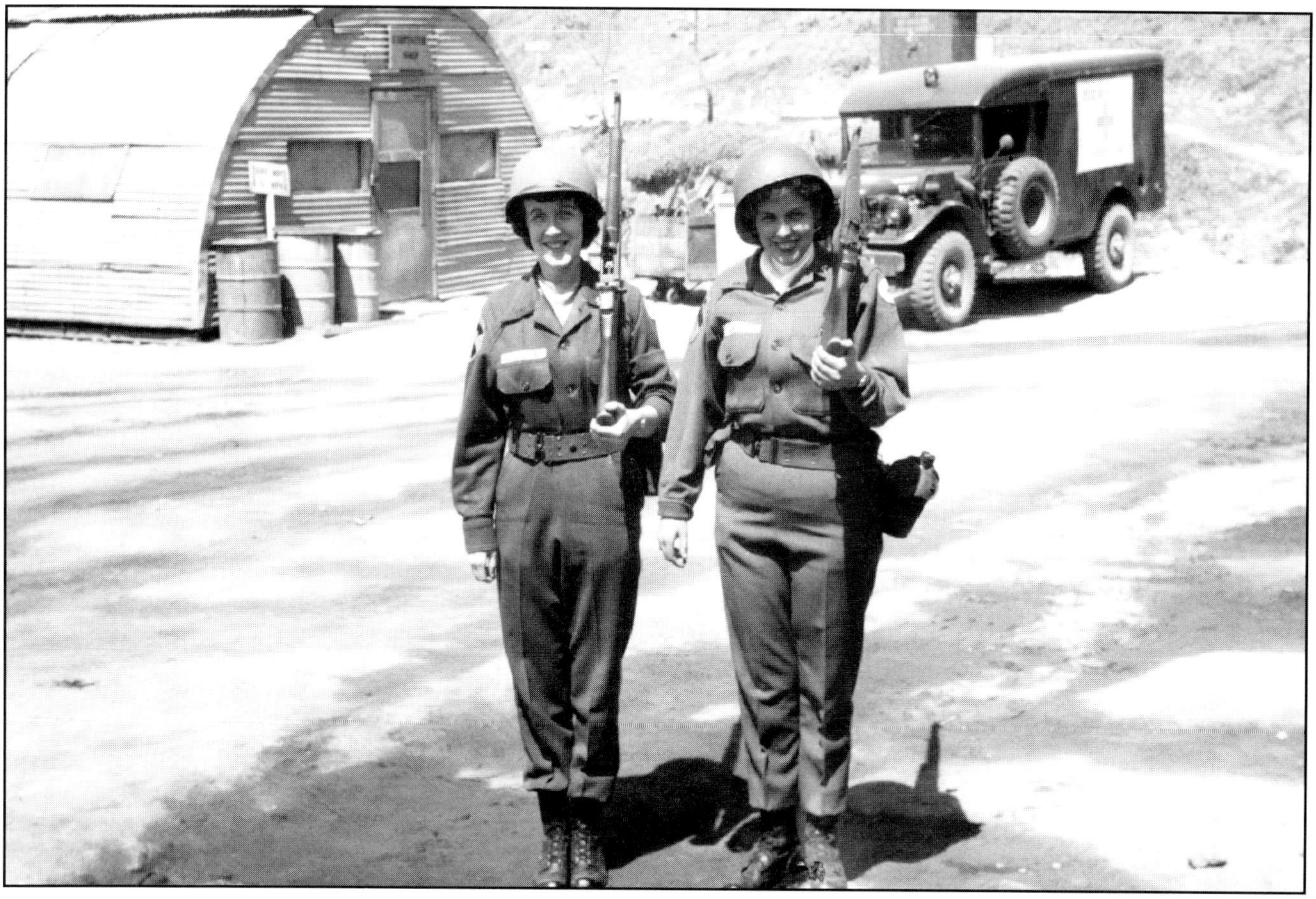

Lucie Davidson and Cindy (Oliphant) Meadows participating in a practice alert at 1st Cav

building. There was a very large Quonset hut crossing one end of the building complete with a stone fireplace, this was our lounge. We did have indoor facilities and showers with hot and cold running water (most of the time) and electricity (most of the time). Flowers, snacks, cokes and Welcome Books had been placed in our rooms to make us feel at home. (I still have my Welcome Books from Cavalry and ASCOM.)

I remember we only had the week-end to be the "new girls in the unit." Monday morning, hobbling along in fatigues, combat boots and field jackets (under the protective wing of an old timer in the unit) we were introduced to the joys of programming to the troops. I remember being very scared and I remember that I survived, what happened between these two memories, I have no idea!

Though I could not remember programming that first day, it did not take very long before many memories started to accumulate. I remember walking into the office at 0700 hours and being greeted by the marvelous odor of baking donuts. The coffee was always ready and waiting for us thanks to the great Korean bakers who started their day at 0500 hrs. It was a nice touch on a cold and frosty morning. I remember the bare, pink hills surrounding our home. I remember the dust and the mud, the snow, the rain and the frozen rice paddies. (It should be noted that I had skated professionally and frequently had my ice skates in the truck. Upon occasion, weather permitting, we would stop for a quick skate through the rice shoots.)

My greatest memory from my 1st Cavalry assignment had to do with seeing war movies as a kid. I always thought that someday I would like to make a parachute jump. Imagine my surprise when I discovered a Sky Diving Club just down the road from 1st Cavalry at CC4. Cindy and I were welcomed, once the men knew we were serious in learning the sport, and from then on most of our spare time was spent at the Club House. Red Cross would only let the Clubmobile girls fly on official business and for some reason skydiving was not on the list as official business. Though we were both fully trained, we respected the rule and did not jump in Korea. The skydivers really appreciated us because we could run the drop zone as well as any one of them, therefore, they could all jump every time they got a plane and did not have to leave a ground crew behind. These men were our good friends, we had many fun and unusual adventures with them, both in Seoul and in the DMZ, 'nuff said! I ran into many of them through the years as I stayed working for and with the military. Now and then they helped me present a program on skydiving to the troops in Turkey, France and Vietnam. After I returned to the States and was doing ARC Hospital recreation work in El Paso, Texas, I finally had my chance to make several jumps. It was worth the long wait!

I spent 18 months in Korea and after my six months at 1st Cavalry I was transferred to ASCOM for about seven months and ended my tour at the new unit in Taegu. Being a "Donut Dolly" in Korea was the greatest experience of my life. I thank the Red Cross for organizing such a program, the American people for supporting such a program and most of all the troops who welcomed us week after week and seemed to have a good time relaxing and enjoying themselves as they participated in our program presentations.

The Commodore

by Gaylord W. Colle

A huge man sat at a luncheon table at a well known eating establishment in George Town

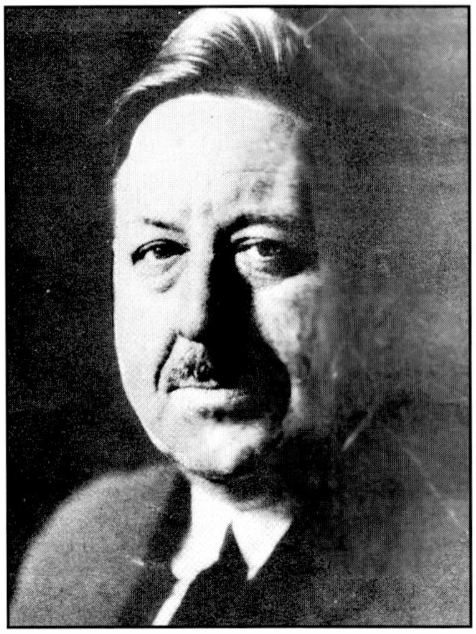

Commodore Wilbert E. Longfellow, d. 1947. Established Water Safety and Life Savings Corps

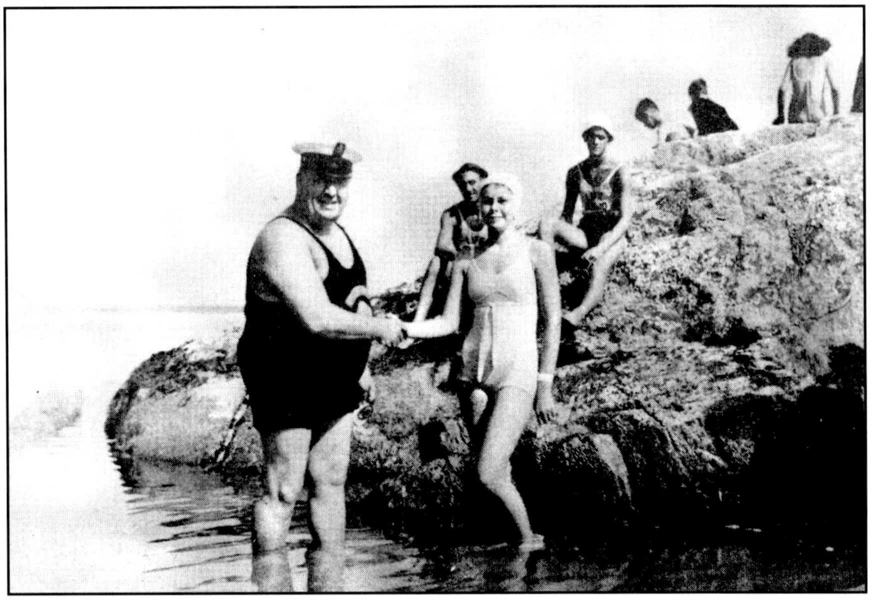

Commodore awarding the Millionth Life saving Certificate

Maryland. With his napkin tucked under his shirt collar, he dined with great gusto. His three companions, sharing with him the mid-day repast, were nonplused as well known Washingtonians stopped to pay their respects to Wilbert E. "Commodore" Longfellow their companion.

The three men dining with the "Commodore" were Robert "Bob" Duncan, Director of First Aid, Water Safety and Accident Prevention Services for the Washington DC Chapter of the American Red Cross, John "Johnny" Gates, his assistant, and Gaylord Colle, staff member.

The four had joined for lunch shortly after the Pearl Harbor bombing and entry of the United States into World War II. All branches of government were, understandably, under great pressure to gain preparedness for self protection and self reliance. There was fear that the capitol itself might be subject to attack.

Longfellow was director of National Red Cross Water Safety. The three chapter men, along with the National organization, foresaw an upcoming massive effort to meet an expected demand for first aid training.

Through Harold E. "Skipper" Enlows, Director of First Aid, Water Safety and Accident Prevention's Office of the National Organization, "Commodore" had been assigned to assist the Chapter in the gigantic effort.

According to the plan the four "brainstormed," at that fateful luncheon, there would be three stages of action for the operation. One of the three men would accompany the "Commodore" to top echelon planning meetings of the government offices during phase one.

In Phase Two, selected staff members of that office would be chosen as candidates for instructor training. The training would consist of instruction in standard and advanced First Aid as a requirement for the instructor course. The standard and advanced courses were often by chapter volunteers. Government offices that were close to each other merged classes.

Bob, John and Gaylord would meet the brunt of most of the instructor presentations. As the amount of demand developed, it was necessary to bring in from the eastern area of the Red Cross other professional staff for instructor courses. During all this, the three chapter men employed two more staff. Even with five local instructors, there were at times other National's in Washington teaching these Government and citizen members.

During the late 1941 period through 1942 there were more first aiders taught than in all previous approximate 35 years' history of the organization. From less than 200 qualified instructors the number increased to nearly 3,000.

"Commodore" Longfellow's engaging personality "carried the day" in those first visits to heads of departments. He was already nationally known in his efforts to "water proof" America. Another long narration could be written about his remarkable career.

"Johnny" Gates drove an old fashioned touring car. On one trip to a government office he was chauffeuring "Commodore." The seats to this vehicle were secured by bolts through the wooden floor. "Commodore" settled his tremendous girth into the front passenger seat. As he leaned back against the upright seat he was startled when the bolts tore up through the floor boards. Needless to say "Johnny" was dumbfounded and embarrassed. He helped 'Commodore" from the predicament to the back seat where "Commodore" finished the trip "in style!"

Gaylord had met "Commodore" four years earlier in the Wichita Kansas Red Cross Chapter. At that time Gaylord was a volunteer. Later he was to have further experiences with Longfellow. Gaylord was to become Director of First Aid, Water Safety and Accident Prevention Services for the Kansas City Missouri Chapter of the Red Cross.

Mabel Boardman

by Gaylord W. Colle

Gaylord was stooped over the rear door of an ambulance-type vehicle. The vehicle was one of several owned by the Washington DC Chapter of the Red Cross during the World War II era.

"Young man I want to introduce myself to you," exclaimed a strong female voice behind him. When Gaylord straightened up and turned around, he was confronted by a rather tall lady with a "ram rod" back.

"I am Mabel Boardman," the strong voiced woman exclaimed. Gaylord had just been "on the job" at the First Aid, Water Safety, and Accident Prevention Services of the DC Chapter a few days.

When Gaylord had reported for work, or soon after, either Bob D. or John G. had told him about Ms. Boardman. She was the National Chairman Of Women Volunteers of the American Red Cross. As Red Cross historians may know, the late Clara Barton had been the founder of the organization. On Ms. Barton's demise, Ms. Boardman had been Clara's successor.

It was said Ms. Barton the nurse-humanitarian, although founder of the American Red Cross, was not a business minded type of person. So it was reported Ms. Boardman was the one who put the organization on a professional foundation. She was the one who finalized it with the United States Congress, Ms. Barton's request for a Congressional Charter to the American National Red Cross. Ms. Boardman's lobbying of members in Congress resulted in such a Government Charter to the organization.

Such designation to a volunteer organization is rare. The charter strictly stipulates, by law, the American Red Cross must perform in three major functions. One is international relations within the organization. Two is that the organization must perform services for natural disaster victims and third that it serve military families and individuals for emergency assistance. Further, though Government designated, the Red Cross does not receive government financial assistance in any way.

Ms. Boardman had heard of Gaylord's appointment to the chapter staff and had crossed the garden from the National office to meet the neophyte member. After preliminary greetings, Ms. Boardman sternly stated "Young man we have a project I want to see carried on successfully by your Chapter office!"

The project Ms. Boardman had designed and instigated was called "The Truck Ambulance Corps." The program was designed to support medical transportation facilities in times of major disasters or war casualties.

A basic unit, as Ms. Boardman had designed, was a box like frame made up of galvanized piping. With two sizes of pipes it could be shortened, lengthened, widened or adjusted with butterfly nuts to fit various sizes of delivery trucks or vans. At the center of the four upright legs was welded a metal hook. At the center of the two crossmember pipes was hung four web straps with metal rings. These hooks and rings were designed to fit the handles of military type litter-stretchers. Placed inside the truck unit the pipe frame converted the vehicle into an emergency ambulance capable of carrying four litter bound casualties.

Company owners of medium size enclosed trucks and vans would be asked to make their vehicles available in times of mass disaster or war time situations. To complete the plan, for the company participation, the company drivers would be needed as volunteers to drive and man the equipment.

The drivers would receive first aid and litter bearing training. The company vehicles would have available quickly applied Red Cross identification. The drivers would keep available Red Cross identification materials such arm bands, bump helmets, etc.

Gaylord was to learn from Ms. Boardman and Bob Duncand that the Washington DC Chapter First Aid Service already owned 10 of these units. In other words, the department had four of the box-pipe frames in storage along with 40 Army type litters. Already first aid litter bearing training was underway for several companies and their drivers. The large department store Hechts was participating in the effort.

Leper Colony

by Lucile Allen

In Palawan, Lucile had a most interesting experience. She had, while in the USA, read a book called *Who Walk Alone* by Perry Burgess. It was the story of the Culion Leper Colony near Palawan and Lucile was very eager to visit there. With four other ARC staff members she obtained permission from ARC Headquarters to go for one day. They flew from Palawan, a short trip, and saw, from the plane, many of the same views pictured in Mr. Burgess' book.

Still living in Culion at that time was an American veteran of the Spanish-American War. The five Red Cross women were told that they were the first Americans to offer help since the Japanese troops left, taking most of the medical personnel with them. Remaining were some French nuns who had been on Culion for several years and who stayed to help the people there.

The Mission Service Center

The Red Cross Mission Service Center was established in September 1971. The estimated population it serves is about 162,000 consisting of approximately 6,700 Blacks; 10,000 Asians, Chinese, Samoans and Philippines; and 100,000 Whites, mostly Latins from Central American countries.

The Center organized an Advisory Committee composed of 11 members to provide community leadership for implementing Red Cross services, providing publicity, recruiting of volunteers instructors, recruiting class participants, and recommending possible innovative activities.

The Mission Service Center has been for more than 10 years providing basic Red Cross programs: social services, safety classes, blood pressure screening, vital English and citizenship classes, legal screening and information and referrals on community resources.

In addition to these activities, the Mission Service Center has been working with senior citizens providing bilingual services for senior citizens who need information and help in obtaining SSI, housing, Medicare and social security benefits.

American Red Cross Community Support

by Eloise B. Waite

As the crisis in Vietnam accelerated in 1975, service to military families (SMF) at Red Cross national headquarters was deluged by inquiries asking for help in locating missing persons and reuniting families. These inquiries came not just from chapters and individuals in the United States, but from around the world. This task was beyond the capacity of the national staff that was working overtime to handle daily routine business prompted by the Vietnam crisis and of Red Cross chapters to respond to requests for service that were essential to community support of the Red Cross.

I discussed the need for staff reinforcement with Mr. Foley, the Vice President, to whom SMF reported. I had submitted a detailed estimate of staff and dollars needed and of additional office space. Mr. Foley was not optimistic about possibilities of obtaining the funding and I told him that if it could not be provided promptly, I would bring the inquiries in bushel baskets and put them on his desk. The next day, Mr. Foley called with the welcome news that funding had been approved and that SMF might proceed with staffing.

Since I didn't know one thing about selecting bilingual staff for such an assignment, I pressed into service a Vietnamese friend whom I had met on a seven hour taxi ride from Kuala Lumpur to Peneng, Malaysia. We kept in touch and when Vietnam fell, Thoa Nguyen arrived on my door step as a refugee. We later found him a job at Sears Roebuck as a tailor and an apartment down the street.

I persuaded Thoa to leave Sears and come to the Red Cross for a job in the Refugee Locator Unit, (RLU). We agreed that he would take care of hiring and of managing the RLU and I would be responsible for funding and logistics. This arrangement worked splendidly. RLU staff, fresh off the boat from Vietnam, could not believe that they had full time jobs and regular salaries in the Red Cross, an organization which they regarded so highly in their own country. In the mornings when the regular national headquarters staff arrived at 8:30 am, the RLU staff was already assembled in the lobbey waiting for work to begin.

The pleasure they experienced in their work was delightful. When clapping or cheering resounded over office partitions, we knew that a family had been reunited.

The RLU flourishes and since its origin has been expanded to serve refugees worldwide. On the several occasions that we have had RLU reunions, I have been impressed with the numbers who express what this experience has meant to their careers and to their lives in the United States. Many have gone from Red Cross to important and lucrative jobs. Frequent is the comments that if one has worked for the Red Cross, references need not be checked.

I Remember

by Elaine M. Sweet

In the early 1960's, the American Red Cross Blood Center in our Chapter, in cooperation with major hospitals in our state, became involved in a new and exciting life-saving procedure — Open Heart surgery. At that time, this new medical development, attempted by only a few top surgeons, required a very personal relationship between the patient due to undergo surgery and the local Red Cross office.

In this early stage of development, only blood drawn on the day of actual surgery was acceptable. When the surgeon determined that this operation was to be performed on his patient, the hospital notified the Red Cross Blood Center with specific information on blood needs. In turn, the Red Cross Chapter in which the patient resided was contacted. An initial contact was made with the patient to explain the role of Red Cross in providing blood for the surgery and to determine if any family members were possible blood donors. The next step was to explore donor files, contact prospective donors of the required blood type and ask if they would be willing to be 'typed' for this special surgical procedure. Approximately 15 donors were needed, more if enough compatible donors were not found on the first testing. When the necessary number were selected and the surgery date confirmed plans were made to assure everyone would be present at the hospital early on the morning of the operation.

Vividly recalled is a cold, snowy morning, opening the Red Cross office at 5:00 a.m. to welcome the donors with a hot cup of coffee, and see them all, 12 very wonderful individuals, on their way. They were due at the hospital by 6:45 a.m. with drawings to begin at 7:00 a.m.. When our near-by hospital was the location there was little problem however this surgery was to be performed at a hospital 45 miles away. There were many concerns on this very stormy morning. Because of the very personal nature of this process a feeling of close relationship with the patient was formed. Donors frequently phoned the Red Cross office days after the surgery to inquire about the progress of "their patient".

One particular patient stands out in memory, a six year old girl who, in 1963 was an open heart patient. As a special Welcome Home, I thought it might be nice to present her with something to remind her of all her new friends. Quickly assembled was a doll dressed in a red and white dress and parasol, several changes of costume, all in a carrying case made from a hat box (remember them?). On the parasol were printed the names of the 12 donors selected for Linda's surgery. The under skirt of the dress held the names of the over 40 donors who donated in Linda's name at a blood drive. Christened 'Rosie Red Cross', the package was delivered to Linda and her mother in the hope that it would give the little girl something to play with during the many weeks she would be recouperating.

NOTE: It was not until many years later that I learned that Linda had kept Rosie and how much it meant to her. We were able to meet and share continued to share a friendship until her untimely death.

Working With Military Families

by Gladys L. Longoria

Very soon after Japan surrendered to the United States (August 1945, World War II) I was asked to apply to the Laredo, Texas Chapter as caseworker. I was hired on the spot and for my training, I was to "read the Handbook".

Working with military families in the Laredo area, to include many living in Nuevo Laredo, Mexico whose sons/husbands had joined the U. S. Forces, became very interesting and challenging. Soon many of those on active duty became veterans. Long hours were spent in helping them file claims for benefits made available through the Veterans Administration.

Nearly two years later we moved to Austin, Texas where I applied to this chapter. I continued in that position until 1952 when I was made Director of Service to Military Families and Veterans. Challenges and experiences broadened in working with volunteers and numerous community social agencies. The Korean and Vietnam Wars brought expanded needs to help new generations to adjustments to family separations and problems arising through these periods.

In 1970 our chapter became one of the division headquarters named by National ARC. We became Capital Area Division and covered 29 counties. Thus, being Division Director of SMF & V I thoroughly enjoyed visiting those chapters with a large percent handled by volunteers.

After my retirement in June, 1978, 1 became a National Disaster Reserve worker until late 1983. 1 volunteered with the local chapter from my retirement until July, 1996.

Over the years I had a husband, four children and much roundthe-clock emergency duty. An extra minute of time was very important to me. I feel honored and grateful to have been associated with the American Red Cross for fifty-one years. The entire time was filled with exciting, personal experiences.

From Disaster Exercise to Genuine Disaster

by Helen L. Ettlin

It was the thing to do in the days when I was Safety Services Director of the Tacoma-Pierce County Chapter, Tacoma, Washington, We were holding another disaster exercise to test the readiness of chapter volunteers in both First Aid and Disaster. The First Aid Chainnan had designed the exercise: a downed aircraft which hadjust taken off from Sea-Tac. We were using an abandoned air strip on the outskirts of town and were counting ourselves extremely lucky to have men from nearby Fort Lewis do the "injuries on about forty high school students from Bethel High School. My daughter, Karen, was among those students.

Volunteers from Tacoma, from Fort Lewis, from McChord Air Base and Madigan Army Hospital were participating along with local firefighters and law enforcement personnel, Local hospitals and ambulance companies were involved. It was a full-scale exercise and was going with precision.

Suddenly there was an announcement that a Red Cross worker had had injured by the rear rotor blade on one of the hospital helicopters. The volunteer had been assisting an "injured" victim and had gotten too close to the rear of the 'copter. As a registered nurse, I rushed to help, and was immediately restrained by the county sheriff. It was then I learned the volunteer had indeed been killed.

Our mock disaster turned into a real one. I had a number of hysterical high school students on my hands, and my daughter was terrified when she heard that a "Red Cross nurse" had been killed. She thought it was me that was killed! Trauma was the name of the day.

The exercise was cancelled and I spent the rest of the day rounding up students who had already been dispatched to local participating hospitals. We waited for school buses to return at the end of the aftemoon.

It was a long time before I could hear a helicopter without reliving that day.

A Red Cross Career

by John R. Russell

My Red Cross career began June 14, 1943, when I reported as a new hiree to the Eastern Area Office in Alexandria, VA. I had applied for a position as Assistant Field Director in Services to the Armed Forces and had gone through the interviewing/selection process some weeks before.

The first assignment I received was to report to American University for training. During that first week, our group listened to speeches designed to orient us to Red Cross history and development. They were impressive, and served to get us identified with the purposes of the organization. It was exciting and gratifying to become part of an organization so big and involved in world events.

Adding to the excitement of that first week was the selection and purchase of uniforms. We were given credit slips at specific stores for specific items. The outfits we were alloted were standard army officers uniforms, winter and summer, on to which we fastened Red Cross insignia. We were a proud bunch in those clothes and felt more a part of Red Cross.

After the week in Washington, we were assigned to training units in various military installations across the country. I went to Camp Claiborne, LA, a large encampment in the western middle of that state. It was a raw place of tar paper buildings. For two weeks under the supervision of a training supervisor, we dealt with the variety of problems brought to Red Cross by soldiers in the camp. There was a wide variety of problems, but the most common was the verification of need for an emergency furlough because of a critical situation in the family at home. Also, the man usually needed funds to meet transportation costs, so a grant or loan would be involved.

The needs were so simple and basic that we trainees quickly became effective at handling the "cases". Hometown Red Cross Chapters, replying by telegraph or telephone, verified the family emergency, while the commanding officer identified the financial need of the soldier. Emergency furloughs were granted by the Commander, using the information supplied.

From Camp Claiborne, I went to

my first "permanent" assignment.. Camp Campbell, (now Fort Campbell) KY. For the next six months, I served as an Assistant Field Director in a staff of about twelve, handling "cases" pretty much as at Camp Claiborne.There was one unusual difference in the work. Because of my pre-Red Cross work background in prisons, I was assigned to service the sizeable German Prisoner of War group at Camp Campbell. The primary activity was to clarify procedures for handling communications from the prisoners to families at home. Also each man could write to a designated person in this country. That fact led to an unusual experience. Most of the German prisoners were members of the Africa Corps. One fellow, a tall handsome blond who spoke good English, had been corresponding with an American girl whom he had met pre-war while he was in the United States. She worked at a well-known eastern women's college. After receiving letters from the young prisoner, she became concerned that she might be accused of spying if the correspondence continued, so she contacted the local Red Cross chapter and asked if the prisoner could be contacted and told to stop writing. It became my job to inform the German. The company Commander was an American Captain who lived in the same B.O.Q. as I. Arrangements were made for me to meet the prisoner at the Captain's office in the camp. The orderly room was next door. When the prisoner came into the room, two other Germans continued to work in the adjoining room. I explained the request to the German and he quickly asked who might suspect the young lady of spying. I wasn't sure how to answer.' I said, "Probably the FBI." He in turn asked "What's the FBI?" Again, at a loss to immediately explain, I blurted out, "Like the Gestapo." The German snapped to attention. The two men in the adjoining room did likewise and he replied "I understand fully. There will be no more letters." The local Red Cross chapter was notified.

After six months at Camp Campbell, I was assigned as Field Director at Northern Field, Tullahoma, TN. My wife Dorothy and two year old son Mike joined me there. We stayed for three months as I closed down the office. We lived in what had been the W.A.C. officers quarters, complete with coal fired cooking stove and wooden bunk beds .... enough said!

From Northern Field I was assigned to Esler Field, LA near Alexandria, LA. Dorothy went back home to Terre Haute to await word of my locating suitable housing. I did locate a nice unfurnished apartment. For six months, our furniture consisted of a card table, two camp chairs, a mattress and springs and a baby bed for Mike.

The Red Cross office at Esler was in a tar paper covered building, open to the outside by a double door and a window on each side of the single room. We had a lone damaged eight-inch fan and no water cooler. The area office, at my request, granted $10 to purchase a water cooler which I found at a local store — a 10 gallon wooden keg with a spout. Each day I got ice from the mess hall across the street. Day after day, the little thermometer on the office wall registered 108 degrees in mid-afternoon.

Added to the physical discomfort was the job demand that I be at the Alexandria railroad station at 2:00 a.m. almost every night to write loans or grants to soldiers leaving on the North bound train. All in all, it was the most physically demanding job I had in my 37 years with Red Cross.

After six months at Esler and a variety of other unique experiences, I was reassigned, this time to the Southeastern Area Office in Atlanta as Assistant Director of Training. Thus began a stretch of 35 years of wonderfully gratifying experiences in general administration and disaster relief.

For the next twelve years I served first in the Training office, followed by Chapter Service, then Assistant Director of Disaster Relief, and finally, in 1950 to Director of Disaster Relief for the Southeast.

In those twelve years, I directed relief operations following tornadoes, floods, hurricanes or fires in Florida, South Carolina, Illinois, Louisiana, Mississippi, Georgia, North Carolina, Alabama, Tennessee and Texas. These assignments provided a wide variety of experiences, too numerous to relay here. Those serve to highlight the fact that Red Cross had to adjust to and work through a wide range of situations, some pleasant and some not so pleasant, to carry out its relief mission.

A fact I must point out is that I was fortunate to be working in these situations with resourceful, intelligent, dedicated staff and volunteers. Red Cross can and must be proud of them.

In 1955 I was assigned to National Headquarters in Washington, as Deputy National Director of Disaster Service. The experiences in Washington were a mixed bag, some pleasant, some frustrating. All in all I was too far from the satisfaction of direct action, which work in the field provided. I did have an interesting oportunity in 1957 to direct the flood relief operation in Appalachia. It was the biggest single relief activity of my life.... 18,000 families affected with 600 relief workers assigned. It was the first Disaster Relief experience for the then new President of Red Cross, General Alfred Gruenther. I was pleased to have a chance to visit the flood area by helicopter with the General, and Kentucky Governor, "Happy" Chandler. One exciting episode came for all of us when the General's helicopter got lost. To finally orient themselves in the Kentucky Hills, they landed in a cornfield behind a gasoline station, and asked the assembled group which way to go. It was hilarious to hear General Gruenther say that each person there pointed in a different direction.

In 1958, I became assistant area manager in Eastern Area. Disaster Relief, First Aid and Water Safety, Public Relations, Junior Red Cross and Office of Volunteers reported to my desk. The challenges were numerous and demanding but still a long way from the field of direct action.

In 1960, when I was offered the position of manager in the Hartford, Connecticut Chapter, I jumped at it. It offered endless opportunity ... administrative responsibility for a magnificent state-wide blood program, a new chapter building, a chapter operation in need of a complete overhaul and a community backed by the vast wealth and leadership of the insurance industry. The eight years in Hartford were a particularly satisfying period in my Red Cross career. We rebuilt the chapter from the ground up and blended the blood program operation with the chapter so that they were mutually supportive. The blood program grew to be the fourth largest in the country. Further, the Hartford community offered the unusual opportunity and need to create a United Fund. Largely through Red Cross efforts, the Community Chest and Red Cross Chapter joined forces to establish the Community Chest/ Red Cross Fund Campaign. Separately, the two organizations had been only moderately successful in fund raising, but combined, and with community support, the campaign was very successful. In addition, the Red Cross Chapter received some generous legacies. The finances were on solid ground. Programs were strengthened and internal operations polished. The chapter moved into a much more effective position in the community. Its image was improved and its place in Community affairs solidified.

In the summer of 1968, word came that the Chapter Executive Director's position in Indianapolis would be open as the incumbent was retiring. Dorothy and I had always wanted to return to Indiana. It was home to both of us, and our families were still there. Thus, I filed an application for the job and made such supportive contacts as I could. In September, after interviews I received notice that I was hired. It was the best move I made in my Red Cross career. It built the backdrop for retirement in 1980.

We quickly entered into community life in Indianapolis, thanks to old friends and a helpful Chapter Board of Directors. For the next twelve years, until retirement at the end of 1980, work effort was focused on strengthening the staff, raising morale and increasing program output. The efforts were rewarded by success in all areas. When it came time to go, the Chapter was in the strongest financial position of its history. That fact added to the glow of satisfaction in leaving after thirtyseven happy rewarding years.

Pianist in Vietnam

by M. Victoria Bain

My tour of duty in Vietnam often presented opportunities for service outside my usual 10-hour day duty as FOA in the HQ III MAF American Red Cross office. As a somewhat amateur pianist, I was pressed into playing piano at our chapel both at III MAF and MAG-16 when some of the chaplains found out I could do a passable job of playing four-part harmony, which meant I could play most Protestant hymns. I was very happy to do this.

In April 1969, a fire which started on the Vietnamese side of the river at a garbage dump had flamed out of control resulting in a conflagration which spread to the nearby ammo dump. This resulted in $80 million of ordnance going up in a spectacular fire and explosion which reverberated all over the area of Da Nang, complete with all the pyrotechnics. It was like a dozen Fourth of Julys combined into one gigantic fireworks display. The Sunday after this catastrophe, the III MAF compound was trying to proceed as usual, including chapel services, even though there were several windows broken in the buildings including the plastic "stained glass" windows in the chapel. Neon lights dangled from the ceiling and pieces of windows lay strewn everywhere. However the chapel was still habitable. I came to chapel services as usual and was asked to play for the service as the duty Navy lieutenant organist was unable to get there from Camp Tien Sha. It was Communion Sunday and as I sat down to play the opening hymns, I have never felt such a sense of awe at being in the right place at the right time to do what I was meant to do. During communion, I played many of the passion hymns familiar to any Protestant from my childhood to adulthood. The chapel was well-attended and the whole scene was so meaningful. Through flood, fire, wars and turmoil, the certainty and permanence of one's spiritual beliefs shone through. I have had many memorable experiences during my Red Cross service, but nothing stands out in my mind quite like that day.

Emergency Loans and Alleged Emergencies at Home

by Wilber Daniel Conn

One of my most memorable experiences with the RC occurred while working at the Charleston AFB, SC field dir. office, they made many emergency loans to military personnel arriving from overseas locations. Many of these same personnel would return to our base upon completion of their emergency leave for return travel overseas. One airman, who had received one of these emergency leave loans, walked into the RC office upon his return and announced that he would "like to reopen his account."

While on field maneuvers near New Orleans with an army unit, a CO said a SVCMN's wife had been bugging him day and night regarding alleged emergencies at home. He asked us to verify any emergency need for the soldier's presence. I phoned the New Orleans Chapter and asked their assistance. The Chapter worker called back to advise that the wife's doctor said the wife was "nuts." I asked if that meant she had psychological problems. "No," the Chapter worker replied, "The doctor says the wife 'is just nuts.'" The CO gave up and approved the emergency leave.

Blood Bank

By Ruth Furse

The Red Cross Mobile Blood Unit collected blood in northeastern Ohio, traveling in Cleveland and surrounding areas. At one factory we were in, a young man came into my unit, saying, "I can't do this. I can't give blood!" My response was, "Then why are you here? You don't have to give blood." He replied, "I want to be a part of our Blood Bank." The reason I finally learned was that his wife was pregnant. We got a good unit of blood and before he left his remark of thanks was, "You sure talked me through that." This, I feel demonstrates our deepest desires: to love, to be loved and to help others.

Japanese Brides

submitted by Mary Minamoto

Japanese brides of US servicemen are invited into homes of Red Cross volunteers in Japan as part of the Brides' School training. In Yokohama, Mrs. Mildred (right in photo), a staff aide, coaches Mrs. Kyoko Sanders (seated in photo) in "tea ceremony" western style. Miss Mary Minamoto (center in photo), a Nisei from Portland, Oregon, interprets to Mrs. Sanders and other brides who are being trained in western ways by Red Cross.

Below: *Bride's School training, Yokohama*

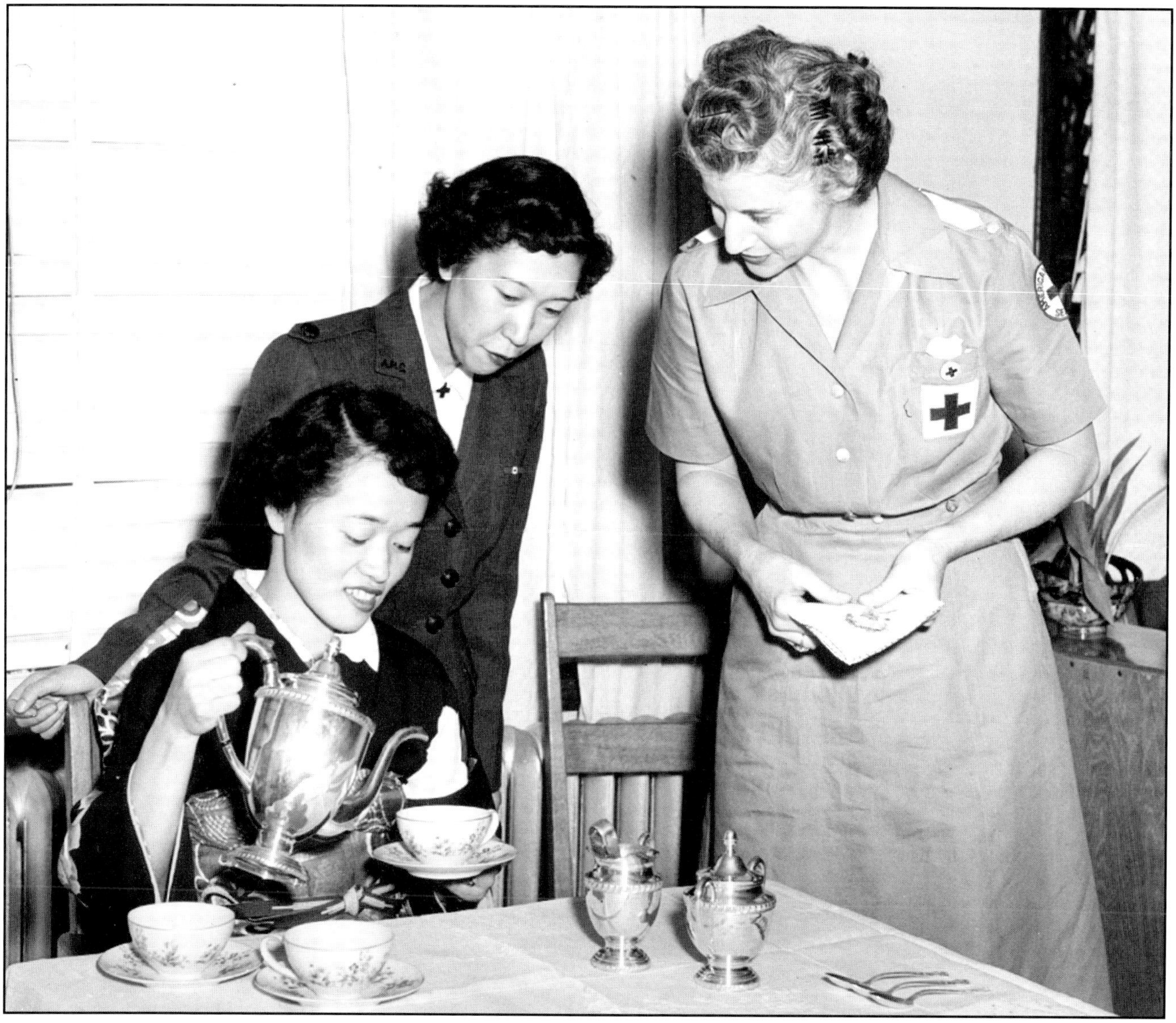

Flower Children

submitted by Marge Klass and Helen M. Grandcolas

In the history of the Midwestern Area office, in St. Louis, Missouri, there are two staff award ceremonies we would like to remember.

During the administration of Philip Schenkenberg, area manager, the first such event occurred in 1969. Phil Gaddis, then assistant director of Public Information, conceived the idea and planned the hilarious show featuring Phil Schenkenberg as "Uncle Sam" and Helen Grandcolas, director of personnel, as "Statue of Liberty." The following quote from "Crossroades," the staff publication of MWA says it all. "From the moment Uncle Sam was introduced by Chet Elick, chairman of the staff council, there were no holds barred. Most of the jibes went to Miss Liberty, unforgettably dressed in a couch cover and missing a "spoke." Incidentally, there were 19 awards made that day ranging from five years to thirty years to staff in the area office.

The other occasion was a similar event in 1971 entitled "The Happening," with reference to the looks and activities of the youth of the 60s. Phil Schenkenberg portrayed a guru, Helen Grandcolas and Marge Klass, chairman of the staff council, dressed as "flower children," presided over the ceremony. A number of other staff members appropriately dressed for the occasion participated in the entertainment.

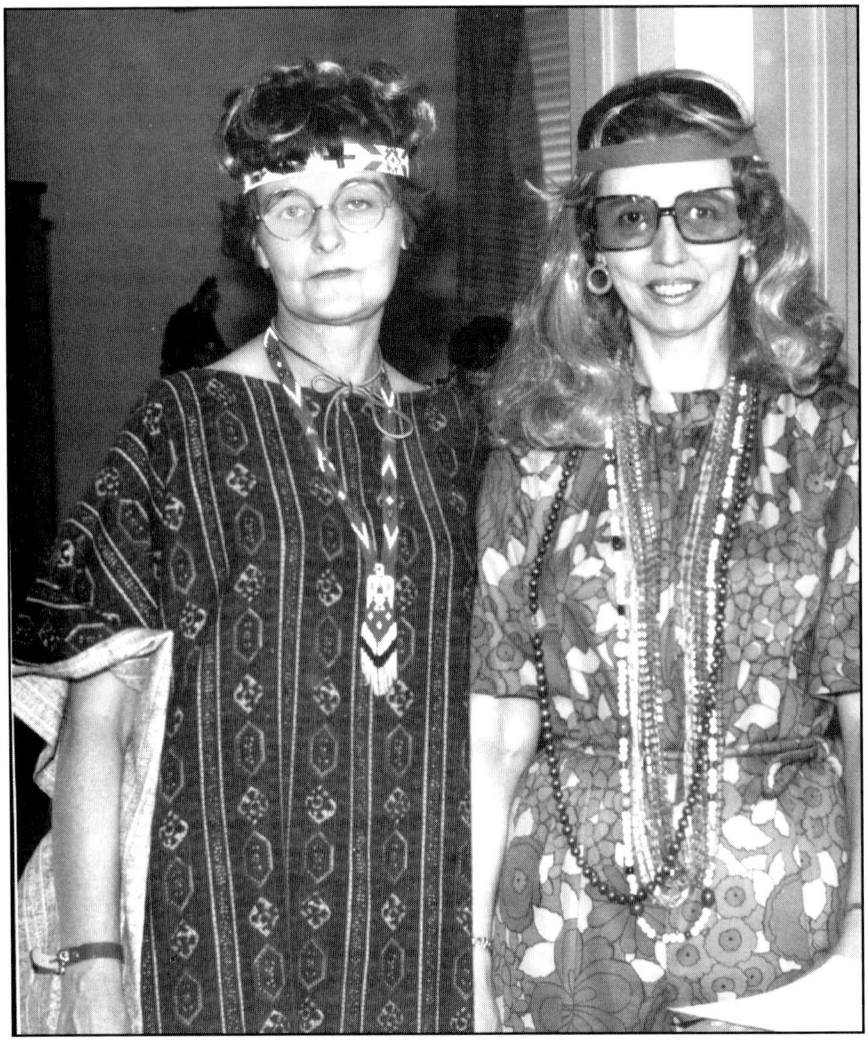

Helen and Marge as flower children

The Bradshaws' Release

submitted by Lucile Allen

Dr. and Mrs. Homer Bradshaw, missionaries to China, were held prisoners by the Chinese Reds for nearly five years. Following is a letter written by Miss Lucille Allen of the Red Cross to Mrs. Robert L. Lewis concerning the services rendered by the American Red Cross to the Bradshaws upon their arrival from China and Hong Kong in 1955:

Dec. 23 Friday
Dearest Dort and all,

Thought I would write you about the Bradshaws. If you ever receive a box I sent with the diary kept in HK you'll see where I wrote that Mrs. Bradshaw was expected to come out then while I was in HK. She refused to come out tho unless Dr. Homer Bradshaw her husband also was released. I knew this in November when Mr. Tomlin told me that the Communists wanted to release her.

Well, you probably have read in the papers about their release together. On Friday, 16 Dec. Mr. Tomlin wired from HK to me that Mrs. B would come out on 20 Dec. and that I should ask if our hospital would take her as a patient. That is because the military hospital doesn't ordinarily take civilians. He also asked that I see if the hospital would send a doctor and a nurse and a plane and that indications were that she was mentally sick as well as physically ill. The C.O. said he'd take her and that he'd send a doctor, nurse and a corpsman.

They all flew up Tues. and returned Wed. About an hour before they arrived at Clark, they send a message in that they also had Dr. Bradshaw!! I don't know yet the details or why the Reds let him out. The day before there was an article in the paper saying he'd die before he signed any confessions.

Much excitement here and on Wed. a.m. 7:30 the doctor phoned me to come and see Dr. Bradshaw as they wanted Red Cross to take care of some clothing for him. Mary Waldrop and I went right over ... Before I knew Dr. B was coming I'd bought (with Red Cross money) some things for her [Mrs. Bradshaw]. I got the

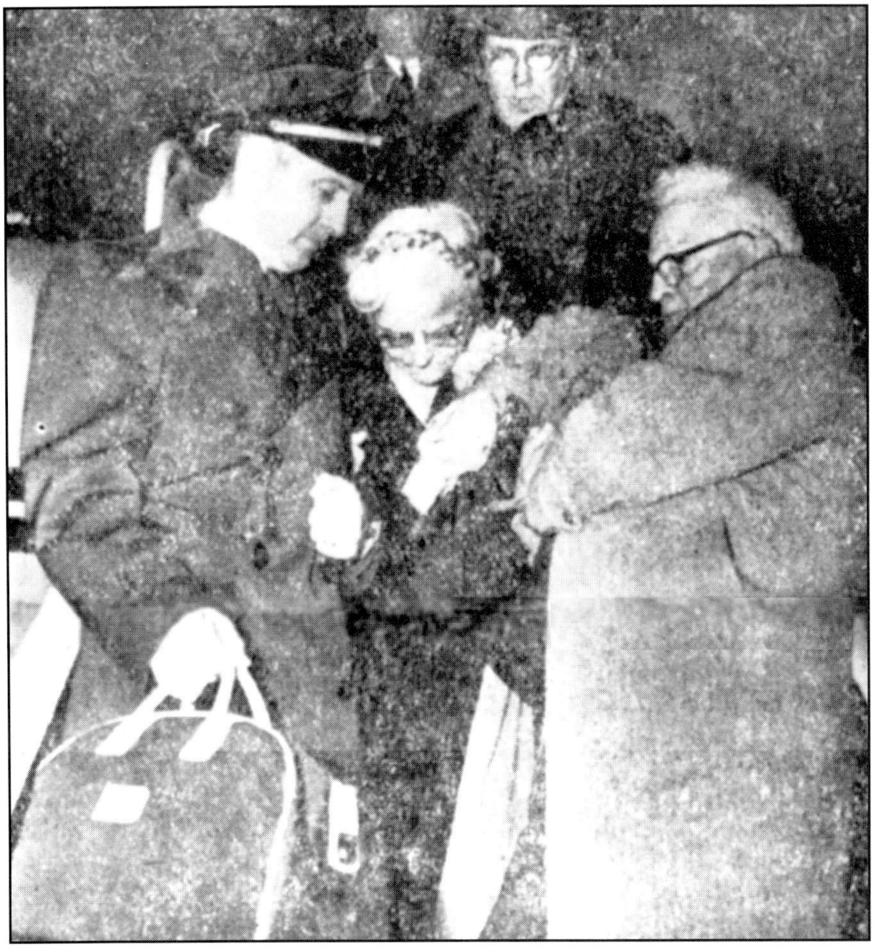

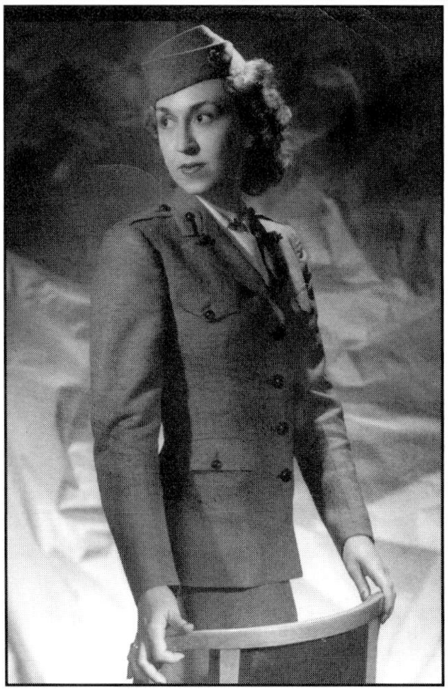

Above: Lucile Allen

Left: Mrs. Homer Bradshaw, held prisoner by the Chinese for nearly five years, arrives home.

nicest smelling things I could in plastic containers. I'd heard she was quite unmanageable from Mr. Tomlin who got the word from Mrs. Laura Lou an American woman married to a Chinese missionary. He is in prison, but she was released and sent to the U.S. three weeks ago ... I thought that plastic best in case she threw them on the floor. Got name brands of things in case she would recognize U.S. things. This is a good plug for an ad, eh? Ipana toothpaste, Propholactyc brush, a comb (blue), blue soap case, and nail brush, Yardley's lavendar soap, E. Arden deodorant, Rubenstein talcum, Kleenex, 3 wash cloths, bobbie pins.

Well, Mary and I went on to the ward to see him. They had adjoining rooms — very small and cell like with high windows, typical military hospital style and uninviting. They are moving them in 2-3 days to a sunporch on another ward where they can see out.

Well, his doctor, Dr. E. Cooper, a Negro, an internist, knocked on the door. Doctor was very nervous for some reason. Dr. Bradshaw opened the door. Small emaciated man with gray longish hair in a hassle on top of head, glasses ... he stood quavering in a hospital cotton robe like one I clean house in. Dr. Cooper introduced us. I offered to shake hands and we did so. I said I was so glad to have the honor of meeting him and so glad he and Mrs. B had returned. He thanked me and I introduced Mary. He cupped an ear, "What's your name again?"

Then I said I'd heard he wanted to send some clothes to a cleaner and could I help him. He tried to pull a suitcase from under bed. I peered under and when I offered to help, our doctor caught on and pulled them out. Dr. B said he had new luggage. They got it for him yesterday in HK. Wonderingly he said it was taken in a luggage shop and the owner said., "Hello, Dr. Bradshaw." He said, "I guess he saw my picture in paper." I said, I guess everyone knew about him now.

He began to pull out his clothes, trying to do it neatly and not untie the ribbons of suitcase. He smelled of each thing as he took it out, so I did, too. He said he could tell if things were dirty that way. I said they smelled mildewed and asked if they had been stored. He said some were in HK in storage someplace. He had 4 cheap suits from Bond Co. and an extra pair trousers with each one, several worn white shirts, 2 horrible sweaters — that is they were not holey or tattered, but cheap — a white pullover which he said, "I wore that in the cage they put me in," I smelled of it and said it smelled OK and he said someone washed it last week. Another khaki pullover — also clean but both shrunk, a khaki scarf — wool — a terribly soiled bloody, rusty appearing suit of long underwear. Absolutely unwashed. Neither of us smelled of this. Then a sleeveless undersuit of his wife's. He sent a nurse in her room to see if she wanted it washed. Answer: yes. He smelled of the only pair sox — red. I said, "Let me get you a pair." "These are all right. " he said. I said, "How are your shoes?" He showed me brown low-cut oxfords. Heels were chewed off and run over, thread all rotted. This stuff has been stored since they were kidnapped 3/51. I said, "I'll get these fixed." He asks me if I'll see about his watch, too. It is engraved:

Homer V. Bradshaw, MD
street address
Grove City, PA

Finally, we had the load, and he said jokingly, "That's the works."

We have had it all cleaned, etc. And today when I took it back he was out being questioned but Mrs. B was in her room, sitting by bed, weighs 80 lbs., snow white hair, dark eyes and black eyebrows ... extremely fearful of everyone. Refuses to let anyone take her clothes to be washed. Refuses to open her box from us. I told nurse to open and place things around on night table. She hardly speaks. She is very bad shape. But she won her freedom by refusing to eat. Scared the communists and they put her under house arrest, but she still refused.

Dr. B has sent this note to the American Red Cross which he wrote in prison when he thought his wife would get out and before he knew he'd be released. I copied it:

The Local Representatives
Prison No. I
of the American Red Cross Hong Kong
Canton, Kwangtung
December 18, 1955

Yesterday, I was informed by a local representation of the Chinese Red Cross that on Dec. 19, 1955 one of them is to take Mrs. Bradshaw (Wilda H. Bradshaw) to the border town between Hong Kong and China and about noon on Dec. 20, 1955 a representative of the American Red Cross will meet her there and take care of her. I assume you will take her to the PMH ... and she will be given into the care of the APM (American Presbyterian Mission). Whether they decide to have someone take her on home now or have her remain in HK for treatment of her present condition, I am unable to say. Whatever they decide is best for Mrs. Bradshaw is of course ok with me. It would be wonderful for us to fly home TOGETHER next March after my release, but whether it is best for her to remain in HK for treatment or be taken home for it, I leave for our APM friends to decide. In any case, Mrs. Bradshaw's parents should be notified of her arrival in HK...

I would like very much if it is possible in HK to have a COMPLETE vitamin analysis done on Mrs. Bradshaw as soon as possible. She knows and is known by Dr. Gordon King and Dr. Samuel Moore...Either would know if such a test is possible in HK and could arrange for it if it is possible. Any expense involved would be paid by the APM ... and be charged to our account with them.

If Mrs. Bradshaw is to remain in HK for treatment, I would greatly appreciate it if the American Red Cross would let me know fortnightly Mrs. Bradshaw's condition. This information could be sent to me... c/o The Chinese Red Cross, Canton...and they will pass on to me any reports from you until and including March 2, 1956. If she is to be taken home now, then please let me know as soon as possible the date she left (or is to leave) and with whom.

May I take this opportunity to thank the American Red Cross from the bottom of my heart for this kindness to me as well as Mrs. Bradshaw for your meeting her on Dec. 20, 1955 and any other kindnesses to her.

May I also thank the American Red Cross for receiving from them via the Chinese Red Cross the gift parcels I have been receiving since the first one 7/26/55 and the 14th one but recently. These "Homeside" things are SURE much appreciated.

Again thanking you for all these courtesies I remain, most gratefully yours,

Dr. H.V. Bradshaw, M.D.

Then on another little slip he entered an account of the dates he received the American Red Cross gift parcels. These were first given in May but his never came until July...

I saw them both tonight. He's on ward in a suit I had cleaned, looking very chipper, in wheelchair, but pushing hnnself around. Had seen movie on ward. Wife still sitting by bed but did stagger out to listen to part of a Christmas carol. The Officers' Wives Choral Group came on ward to sing.

We are all ready for Christmas ... I work this weekend...

Lots of love and Merry Christmas,

L.

LETTER FROM DR. BRADSHAW TO MR. NICHOLSON OF THE RED CROSS:

Presbyterian Hospital
Pittsburgh, PA
January 25, 19,56

Mr. James T. Nicholson
The American National Red Cross
Washington, DC

Dear Mr. Nicholson:

Yesterday I read and today reread your letter of January 18, 1956 to my oldest brother, Dr. Wm. A. Bradshaw, and the enclosed detailed report of the services rendered to Mrs. Bradshaw and me. It is the report of a task well done in a most efficient and kindly manner. Being one of the recipient of these services, I know whereof I speak.

May I take this opportunity to express in so far as mere words can do so my personal heartfelt appreciation and that of Mrs. Bradshaw, of these services rendered to both of us (who were so badly in need of help), by the American National Red Cross. Our sincere gratitude is extended to the entire organization for what you have done for us, but particularly to "Dick" Tomlin, Miss Allen, Miss Waldrop and the rest of his most efficicnt staff there at Clark Field, P.I, and also to the other Red Cross groups along our route of travel from Clark Field to and including Pittsburgh via Guam, Kwajalein, Honolulu and

Travis, Cal. Our thanks would be incomplete indeed if we did not include the kindness and services of that also grand group — the Gray Ladies. I salute you all. Last but not least, also the Red Cross group here in the U.S.A. who kept our relatives and friends "posted" as to our progress both physical and geographical.

To say the gift parcels, of which I received 14 from 7/26 through 12/16/55, were life savers for me is putting it mildly. In so far as it is possible for words to do so, I again express my grateful thanks for each and every one of them.

Trusting you will pass these thanks along to those who were so kind and helpful to us I remain, an eternal debtor to the American National Red Cross.

Homer V. Bradshaw, M.D.
c/o Dr. Wm. A. Bradshaw
1315 Beechwood Blvd.
Pittsburgh, Pa.

REPLY:

January 27, 1956

Dear Dr. Bradshaw:

It was more than thoughtful of you to write me as of January 25th and to be so generous in your expression of appreciation of what the American National Red Cross endeavored to do for the welfare of Mrs. Bradshaw and you. You may assured that we only wish we might have done a lot more. In any case, what we did was the least that we could do, considering the aims and purposes of the Red Cross.

It is very much our hope that Mrs. Bradshaw and you are making a rapid recovery from the effects of the hardships and suffering you both experienced in the People's Republic of China. A number of us have had you both very much in our hearts and do hope that from now on, life may recompense you for all that you have gone through. If at any, time you should be in Washington, I would appreciate very much the privilege of meeting you.

With our every good wish,

Sincerely yours,

James T. Nicholson
Executive Vice President

Dr. Homer V. Bradshaw
Care of Dr. William A. Bradshaw
1315 Beechwood Boulevard
Pittsburgh, Pennsylvania

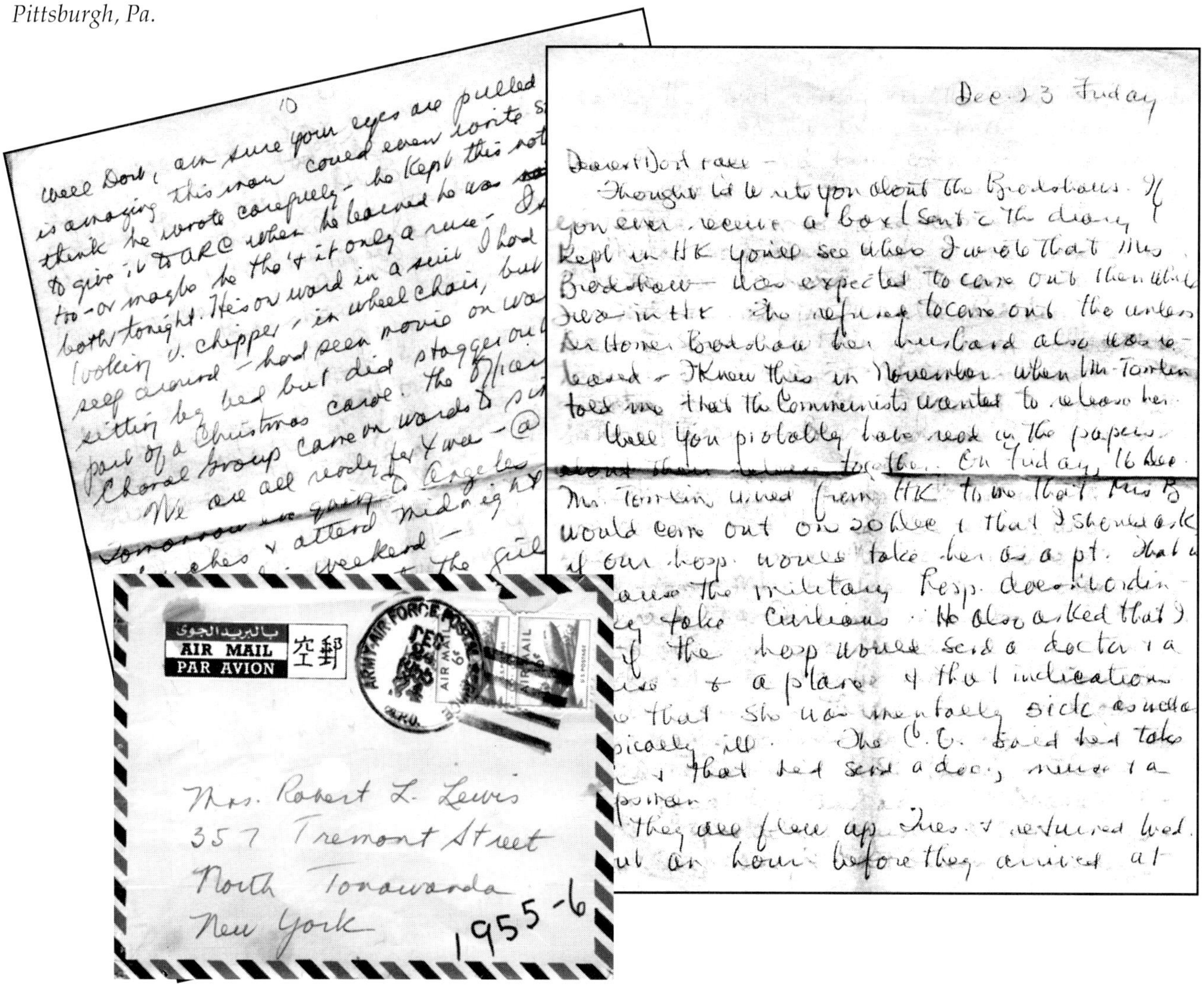

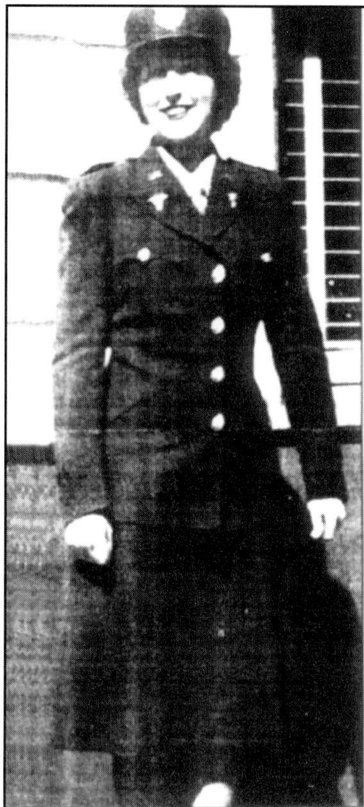

Lou Ferenz as a Flight Nurse in 1943—

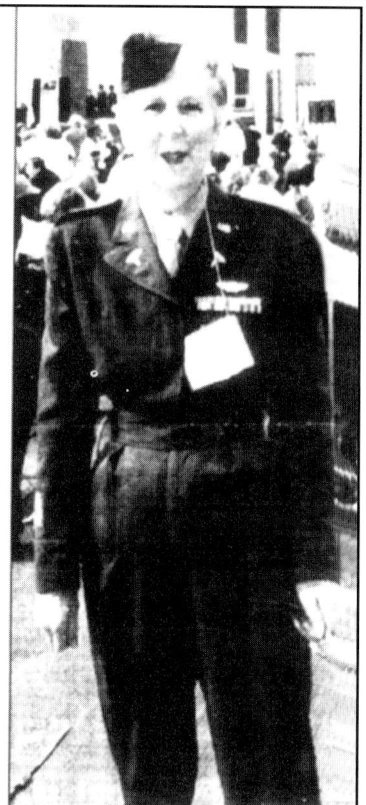

Lou Ferenz Rice, ~~last year~~ Oct 1997. The lady is still full of vim, vigor and vitality.

She still fits into her World War II uniform

by Lloyd Cory

Villager Ludmilla "Lou" Ferenz Rice, unlike about 99.44% of World War II vets, can still wear her uniform, which is over half a century old.

Lou had aimed at becoming an airline stewardess. In those days a stewardess also had to be a nurse. So she went into nurse's training at New York's St. Luke's Hospital.

But before graduation the Japanese attacked Pearl Harbor. The government froze nurses out of becoming stewardesses because they were greatly needed for the war effort.

So Lou, at 22, joined the Air Corps part of the U.S. Army Nurse Corps. She underwent basic training at Mitchell Field air base in New York. She wasn't gung ho about digging foxholes, sleeping outdoors, wearing gas masks and other tough duties, but she gamely endured them.

She got her commission as a second lieutenant. (Later she got upped to first lieutenant.) At first she served in Stockton, CA and Kearney, NJ.

Then the coveted gold wings were pinned on her uniform and she flew to Hickham air field, her new home base, in Hawaii. From there Lou and other medical people island-hopped, picking up seriously wounded men from Guam, Saipan, Johnston, Kwajalein, Luzon and Leyte and Manila, Luzon in the Philippines and later Japan.

Lou says she is the only nurse who still has her flight log, showing all stops, times, mileages, names of pilots, number of patients carried and dropped off. She also kept all her military records. She says she was a "memento collector;" her husband says she is a "pack rat."

In the states she flew in C-47s. Overseas she flew in C-54s, which were larger and carried 40 litters.

As she flew she cared for shell-shocked cases and men with multiple wounds. She talked one of the former out of opening a door and jumping out of a plane in flight.

Once Gen. Douglas MacArthur took her 30th Squadron's planes to evacuate folk who had been Japanese POWs for years.

A chapter on Lou Frenz appears in *Women in America's Wars*. The book's author was a former patient of Lou's.

Last year a World War II Flight Nurses' Reunion was held in Tulsa. Old friends could only fit into their old caps. When they saw Lou wearing her old uniform some claimed that they hated her.

In October 1997 Lou went to the "Women in Military Service to America" dedication and memorial at Arlington Cemetery, Washington, D.C. It was a quality program, featuring Al and Tipper Gore, Janet Reno, Kenny Rogers, heads of the military services, Loretta Swit and Connie Stevens. They honored women in the military today.

Next year's reunion may be held at the Air Force Academy, Colorado Springs.

Lou was a widow for years. For 20 years she worked as a nurse in Whittier, CA. Then she became a Red Cross nurse in charge of Bloodmobiles, which job she held from '74 to '85.

Then she met Banner Rice in the Civil Air Patrol in Van Nuys. (The CAP performs many search and rescue operations.) They married in '87.

They read about HSV in *Modern Maturity*, which named it as one of the 10 best places to retire. They bought a lot in '91 and moved to the Village in '92. They love it here.

Banner had his basic training at Camp Roberts, CA went to OCS school in Ft. Benning, GA and served at Camp Croft, SC and Camp Robinson, AR. Then he joined a heavy weapons unit of the 80th Division, in Germany. He came out of the Army as a captain, then later retired from the reserves as a full colonel, after becoming a licensed pilot before his 60th birthday.

The Rices have served their country well.

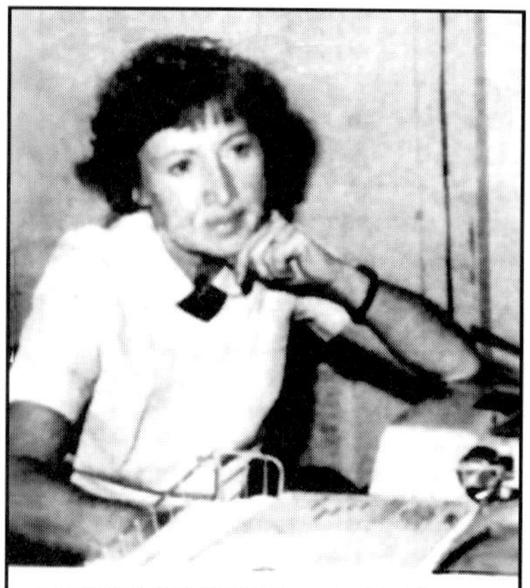

A UNIQUE CHRISTMAS was had by Erna Guy, Red Cross Field Director here, in Vietnam. She describes her holiday, "When I was serving with the Red Cross in 1969, I was stationed at Tan-Son-Nhut, a Saigon Air Base. We received a surprise at 4 p.m. on Christmas Eve ... a shipment of Christmas trees, donated by a businessman in Oregon. As we hurriedly distributed the trees to the troops, one of the men commented, 'Now I can throw away that bottle and celebrate without it.' We decorated the trees with what we had. IBM cards, sprayed with glitter that was mixed with insect repellent, cut up socks for bows, roses which were abundant there and paper snowflakes made for a very different look. We promised the servicemen a 'white Christmas,' and came through with the promise in a substitute way ... by having the Navy men in their Dress Whites around the tree! The youngest soldier present received the traditional stocking goodies in one of my high heeled shoes, since the climate was not condusive to ever wearing stockings. A traditional Christmas dinner was at least the right color, we called it our red and green meal, which consisted of beets and creme de mint. It was all we had that Christmas, but the spirit was there."

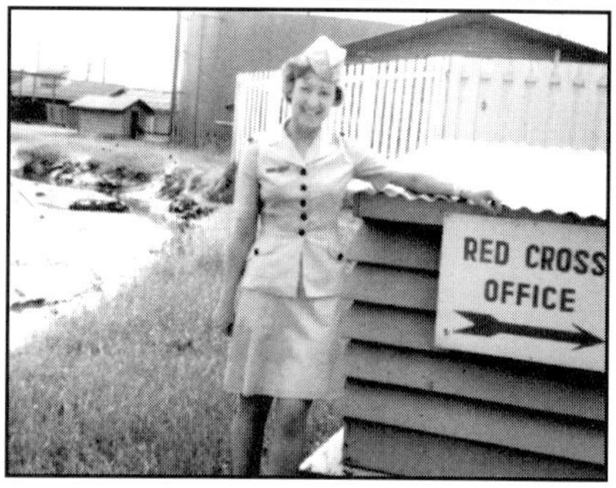

Above: *Erna M. Guy on South-East Asia tour, Tan-Son-Nhut AB, 1970-1971.* ***Below:*** *Erna M. Guy giving out candy after the medicine.*

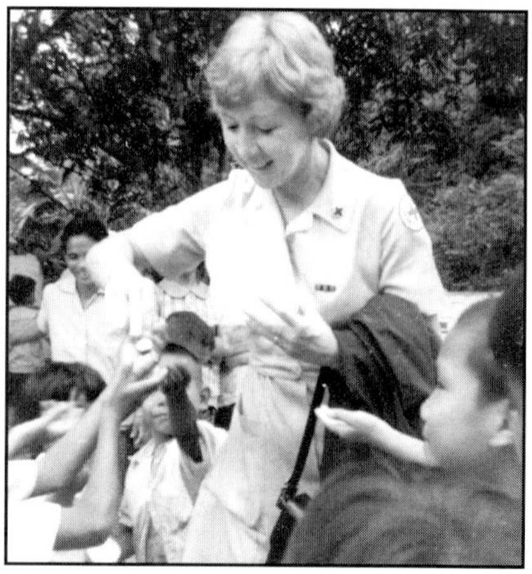

Red Cross field dir. commended for work

After more than two years of service to Marines, sailors and their dependents at The Combat Center, Mrs. Erna Guy, field director for the American Red Cross here, will be leaving for her new assignment in Germany, January 26.

Mrs. Guy was honored at a farewell luncheon, January 16, at the home of Mrs. Rene Tilley, chairman of volunteers for the American Red Cross here. The luncheon was given by eight members of the Red Cross Board of Volunteers and was attended by Mrs. Carol Glasgow, honorary chairman for the Red Cross here, Mrs. Joyce McHenry and Lieutenant Colonel John P. Caynak.

Prior to the luncheon, Mrs. Guy was presented with a Certificate of Commendation by LtCol Caynak for her exemplary performance of duty while assigned as the American Red Cross Field Director at The Combat Center. She was also presented with a ceramic statue of a roadrunner by the members of the Red Cross Board of Volunteers.

Following the presentations, Mrs. Guy gave the Board of Volunteers an original volume of **The Red Cross**, written by Clara Barton, founder of the American Red Cross, and published in 1898. The book is a collection of Clara Barton's memoirs and letters during the founding period of the Red Cross.

Mrs. Guy was appointed an American Red Cross professional staff member in June, 1966, after more than 10 years of volunteer service. She has served with the Armed Forces in Georgia, Florida, Vietnam and Thailand before her arrival at The Combat Center in September, 1978.

Her next assignment will take her to the United States Army's Third Infantry Division Headquarters in Wuerzburg, Germany for three years. "I've already told them that I want to come back to The Combat Center," said Mrs. Guy. "I'm just a real desert lover at heart and I love working with the Marines."

Mrs. Guy is a native of Munich, Germany and a citizen of the United States since 1951. She has two daughters, one a student at the University of California at Los Angeles and the other a journalist in Honolulu, Hawaii.

At this time, Mrs. Guy's replacement has not been appointed. Mrs. Mary Alcaraz, currently the assistant field director, will be the acting Field Director until a permanent replacement arrives at The Combat Center, probably in February or March, according to Mrs. Guy.

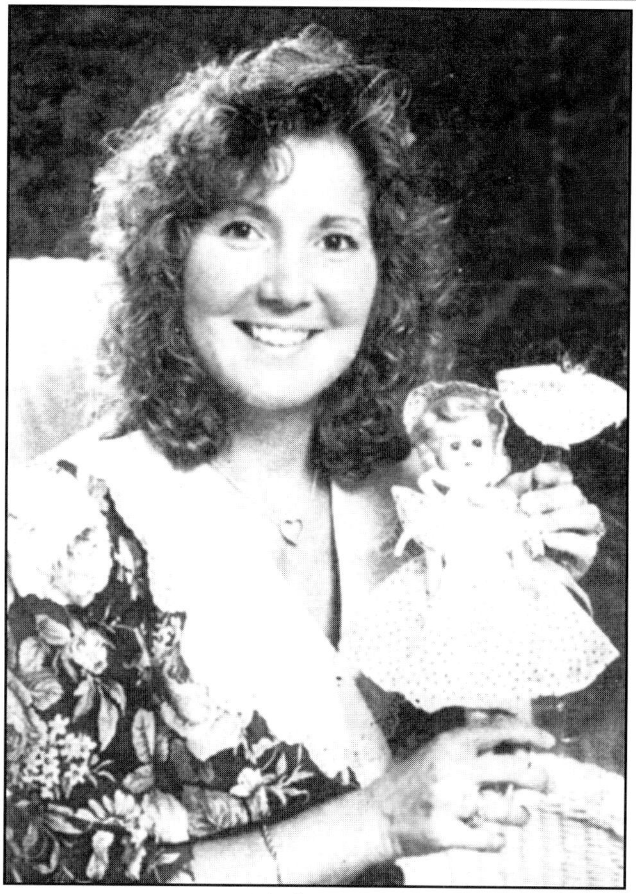

Linda Jones

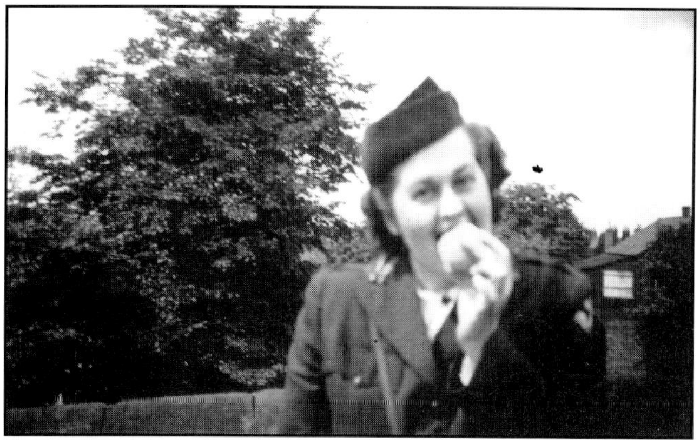

Mae Culler, England, 1944.

"People carry a lot of care in their hearts."

Linda Hayes, now Jones, of Willimantic was born with two heart defects, first identified when she was only four months old. In 1963 she had the first of what would be three open heart surgeries. She was seven years old.

In those days the blood was drawn on the actual day of the surgery. The Red Cross arranged rides for 12 donors with matching blood types to donate for Linda. Not only did she get her donors but she also received a doll she named Rosie.

Over the years, the doll remains a symbol of profound joy in Linda's life. It symbolizes the care that people carry in their hearts every time they donate blood.

Father, Son Serve in Viet

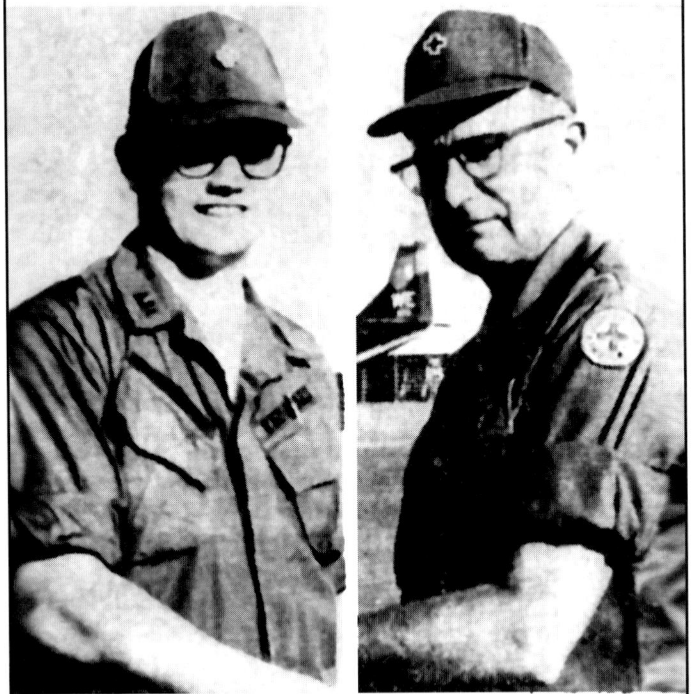

IT WASN'T "home for the holidays" but perhaps the next best thing for Neil M. Clark Sr., right, of Boise and San Francisco, was when his son, Neil M. Clark Jr., left, arrived in late November for a one-year tour of duty in Vietnam with the American Red Cross in which the elder Clark also serves. Clark Senior's parents are Mr. and Mrs. Clifford H. Clark, 5712 Castle Drive, and his wife is the daughter of Col. and Mrs. Clarence Boggs, 2422 West State.

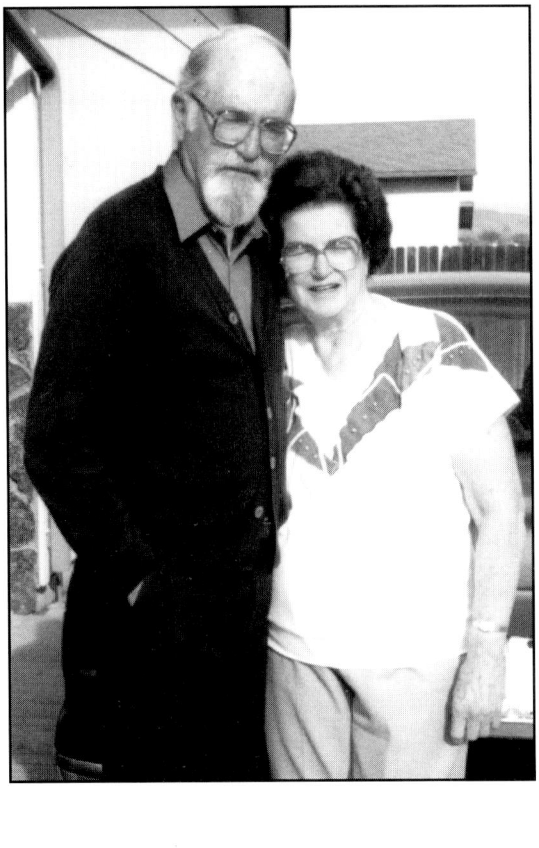

Mr. and Mrs. Clark, today

Red Cross on Berlin Duty Since Last War

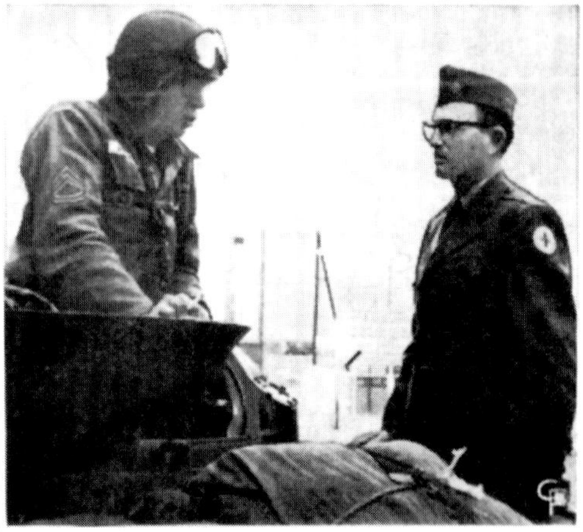

Sgt. Glenn Hedrick of Mead, Wash., chats with Neil M. Clark, an American Red Cross field director, just a few yards from the barrier on the Wilhelmstrasse, Berlin, which separates West from East.

By Central Press Association

BERLIN, Germany — The 1,500 U. S. Army men who were rushed here in mid-August to bolster the American garrison force had to leave their homes in West Germany on just a few hours' notice.

The men, however, found the American Red Cross on the job here, ready to help them solve family and personal problems that the sudden move had accented.

Neil M. Clark, ARC field director, and Miss Mary Moffatt, his assistant, are the latest of a long series of Red Cross staff people who have been on duty in West Berlin since the end of World War II.

* * *

ARRIVAL of the new contingent of U. S. servicemen actually may cause a relatively moderate increase in their total workload, Clark and Miss Moffatt explained. Dependents of the latest group of American troopers now are being allowed three-day visits to West Berlin, and many of the families will be able to solve their own problems as they develop.

"The East-West tension that brought about the present crisis had already increased our workload by half since last June," Clark said. "The 110-mile corridor through East Germany that leads to Berlin from the West creates many communication and travel difficulties for the U. S. troops stationed here.

"And the German-born wives of many American soldiers stationed all around the world are asking the American Red Cross for welfare reports on relatives who still live in either half of Berlin."

* * *

CLARK CITED one recent case that points up the problems involved in living in an "island city" where normal travel is restricted.

The 10-year-old son of a Berlin-based sergeant was attending summer camp in Frankfurt, 400 miles west of here. He became homesick, and camp officials called the father to advise him to come for his son immeditaely. Because of travel restrictions and the time and expense involved, the soldier called on Clark for help.

The Red Cross man notified the ARC field director in Frankfurt, and the latter purchased a plane ticket for the boy and put him aboard the plane. The next day, homesickness forgotten, the boy ran happily off the plane at Templehof Airfield in West Berlin where he was met by his parents.

* * *

ANOTHER recent case involved a search for the German father-in-law of an American serviceman in France. The wife had learned her father was planning to leave the East Zone through Berlin, and the couple asked the American Red Cross to help locate him.

With her German secretary to do the interpreting, Miss Moffatt went to the main West German Red Cross refugee camp of Marienfelde in Berlin. Officials there had no record of the father-in-law, but said he might try to come through later.

Other refugee camps in Europe have been alerted to watch for the man and tell him he could get in touch with his daughter through the American Red Cross. "We and the family haven't given up hope," Miss Moffatt said.

* * *

IN ADDITION to the two career staff members here, the American Red Cross has a volunteer staff of Gray Ladies and staff aides serving in the U. S. military hospital. Wives of both enlisted men and officers, they work together to help the patients — serving coffee and snacks, playing the piano, singing, playing cards, checkers and chess — providing a touch of home to men far from home.

Anticipating that the Red Cross job in Berlin will continue to increase, the organization is adding a hospital field director to the staff in Berlin. This will free Clark and Miss Moffatt to work exclusively with the able-bodied members of the American armed forces and their dependents living here with them.

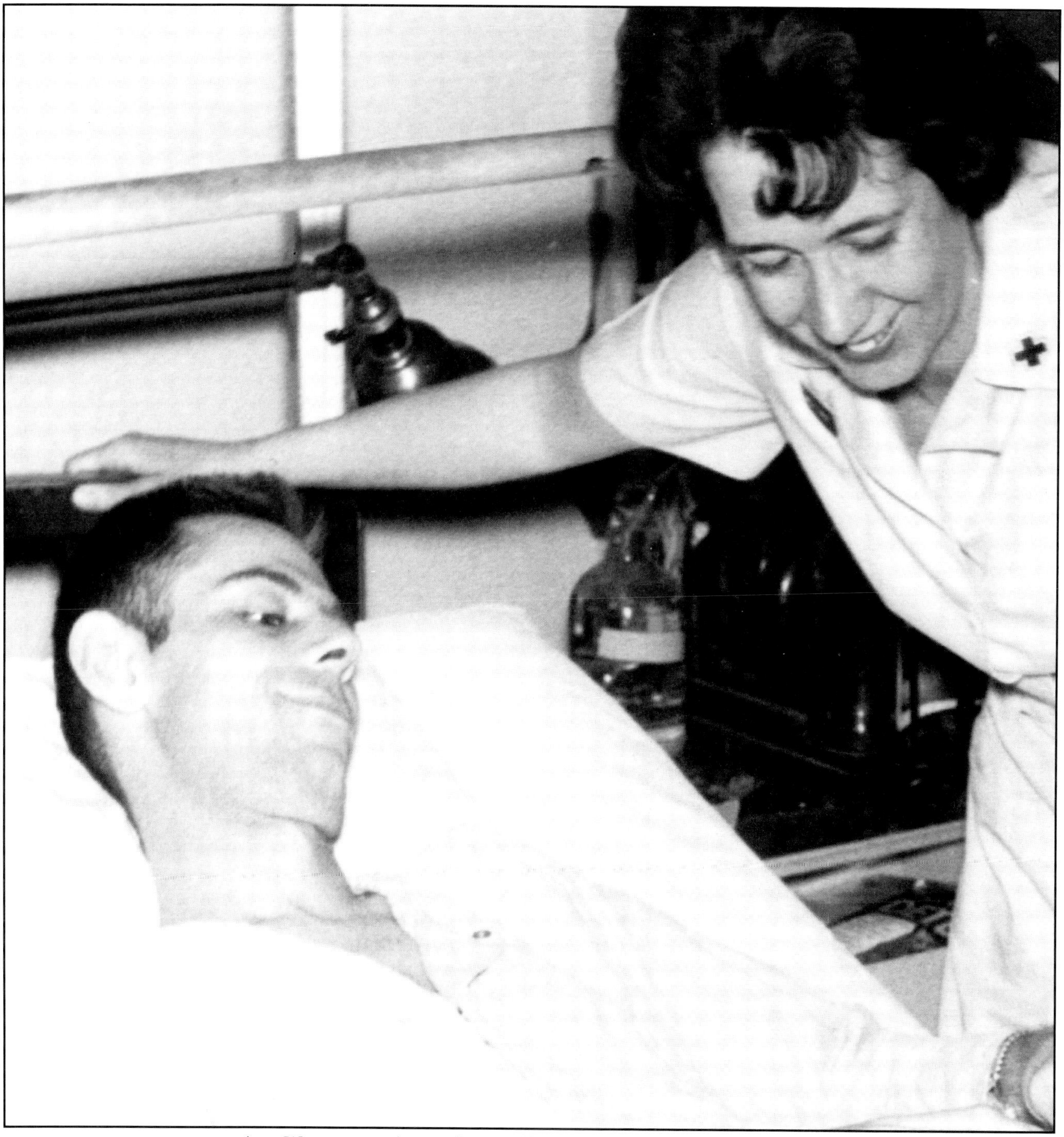

Ann Woessner assists patient at 121st Evac. Hospital, Korea, 1963.

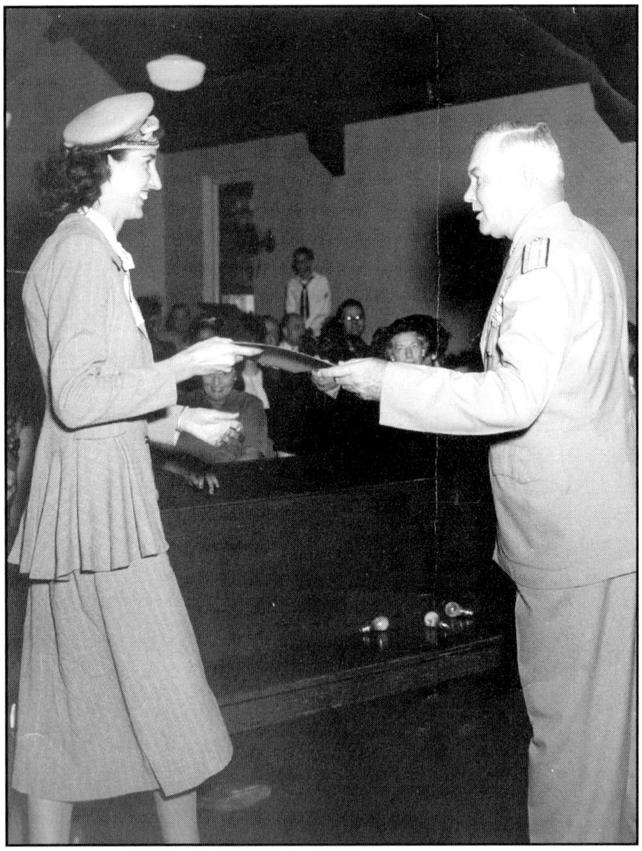

Pearl Duty receives Certificate of Achievement, Virginia Beach chapter, 1948.

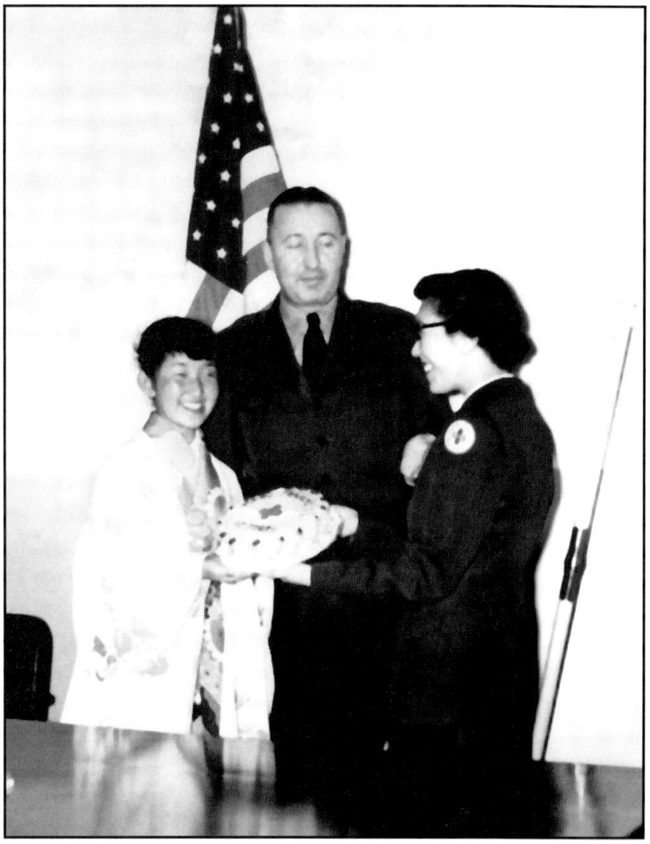

Far Eastern Headquarters, Tokyo, Japan, 1954, 10-year celebration for Mary Minamoto

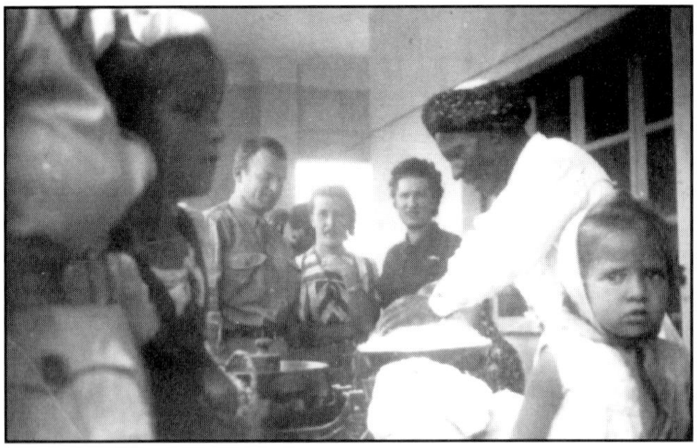

Asmara, 1942

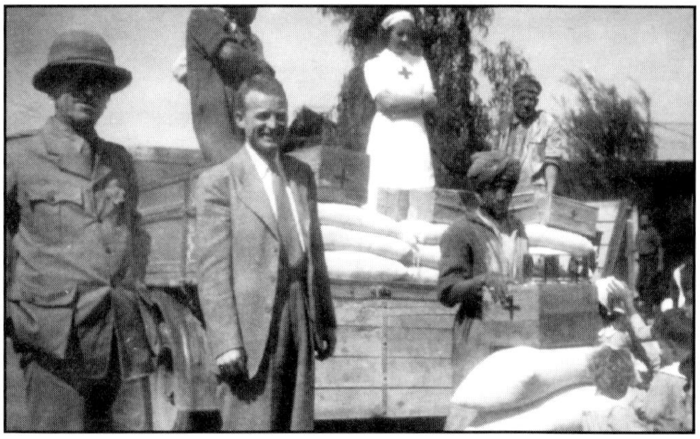

School distributions, Asmara, 1942

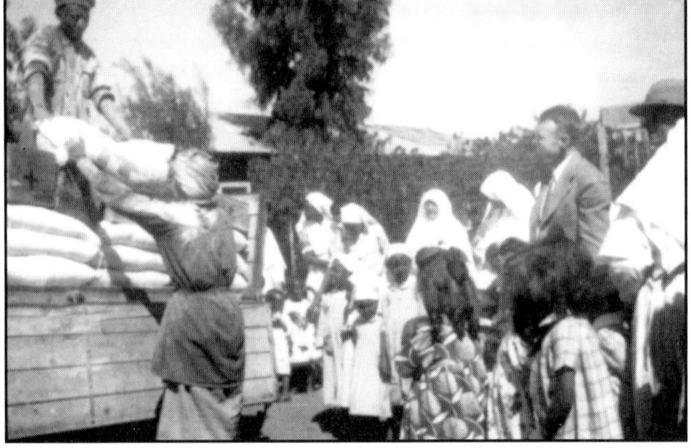

ARC supplies arrive at a school in Asmara, 1942.

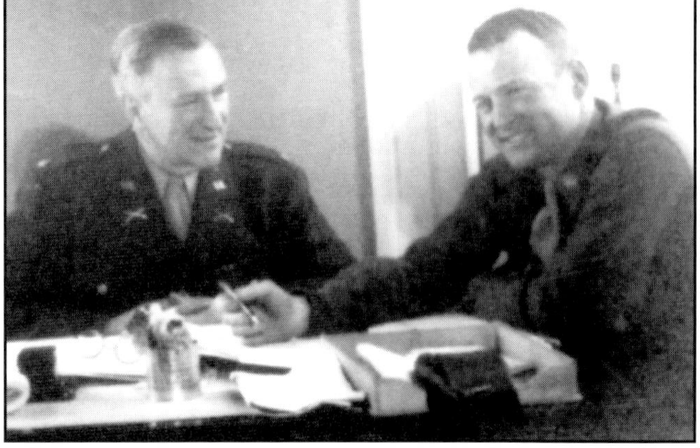

General Schuyler and James Foley, 1947

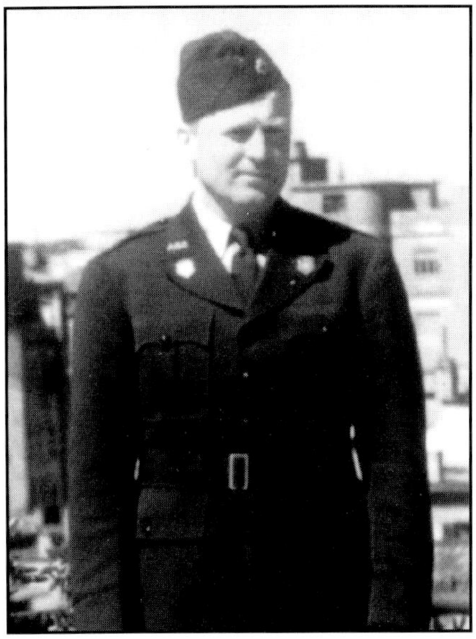

Jim Foley, Rome, 1947

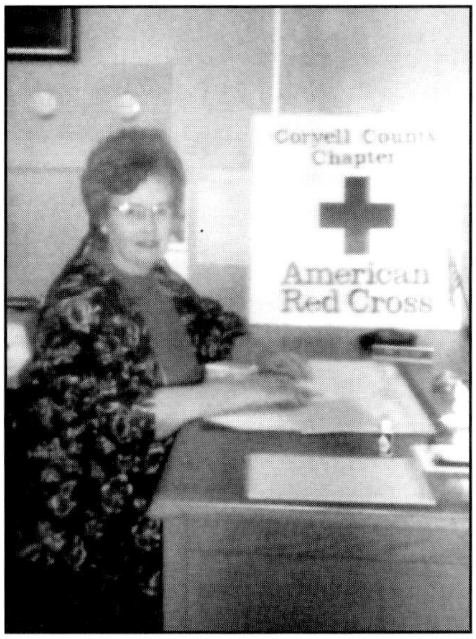

Cleo Marshall, Coryell County Chapter, TX, 1987

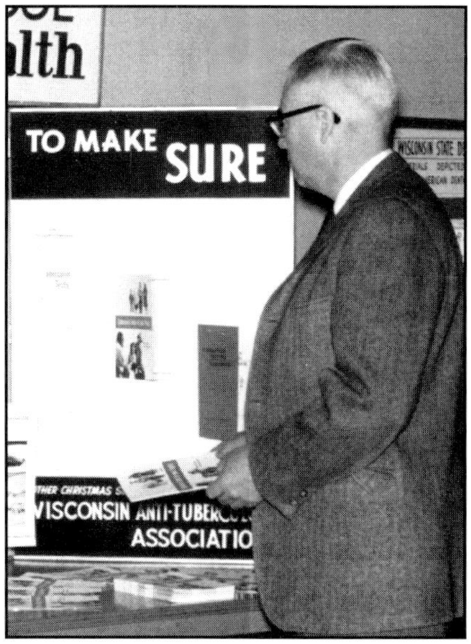

Wisconsin State School Health Council Meeting, 1961

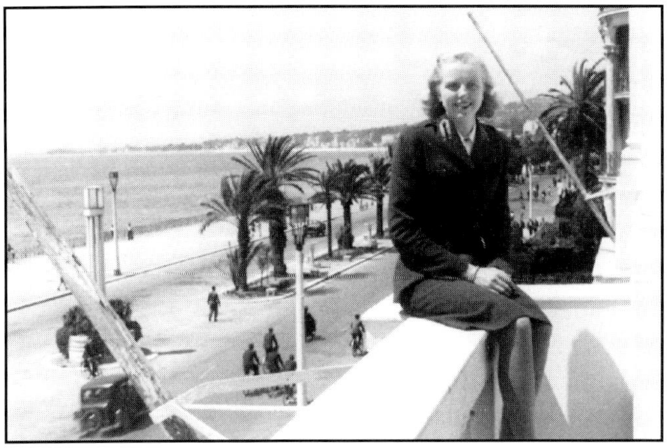

Charlotte Kilbourn Easter Kress, on duty in Nice, France, 1945

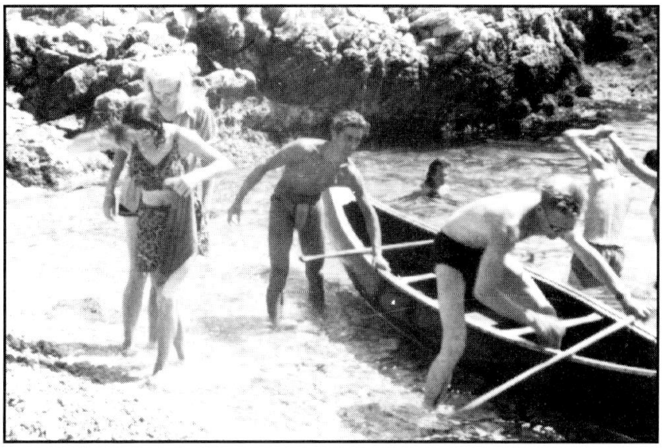

A swimming picnic, Nice, France, 1945

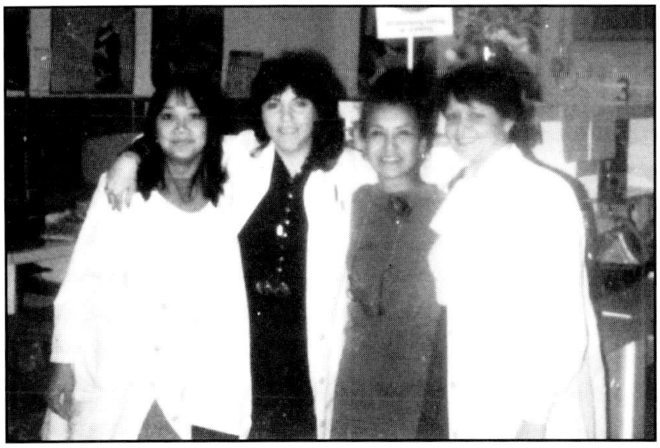

Lab techs at San Fernando Valley District Office, 1984

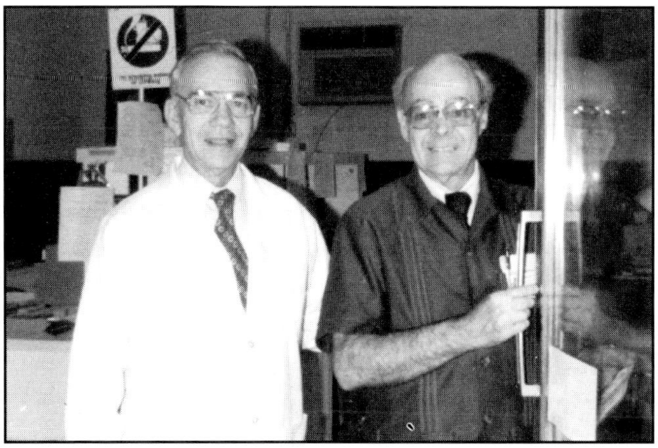

Blood Program Lab, San Fernando Valley District Office, 1982

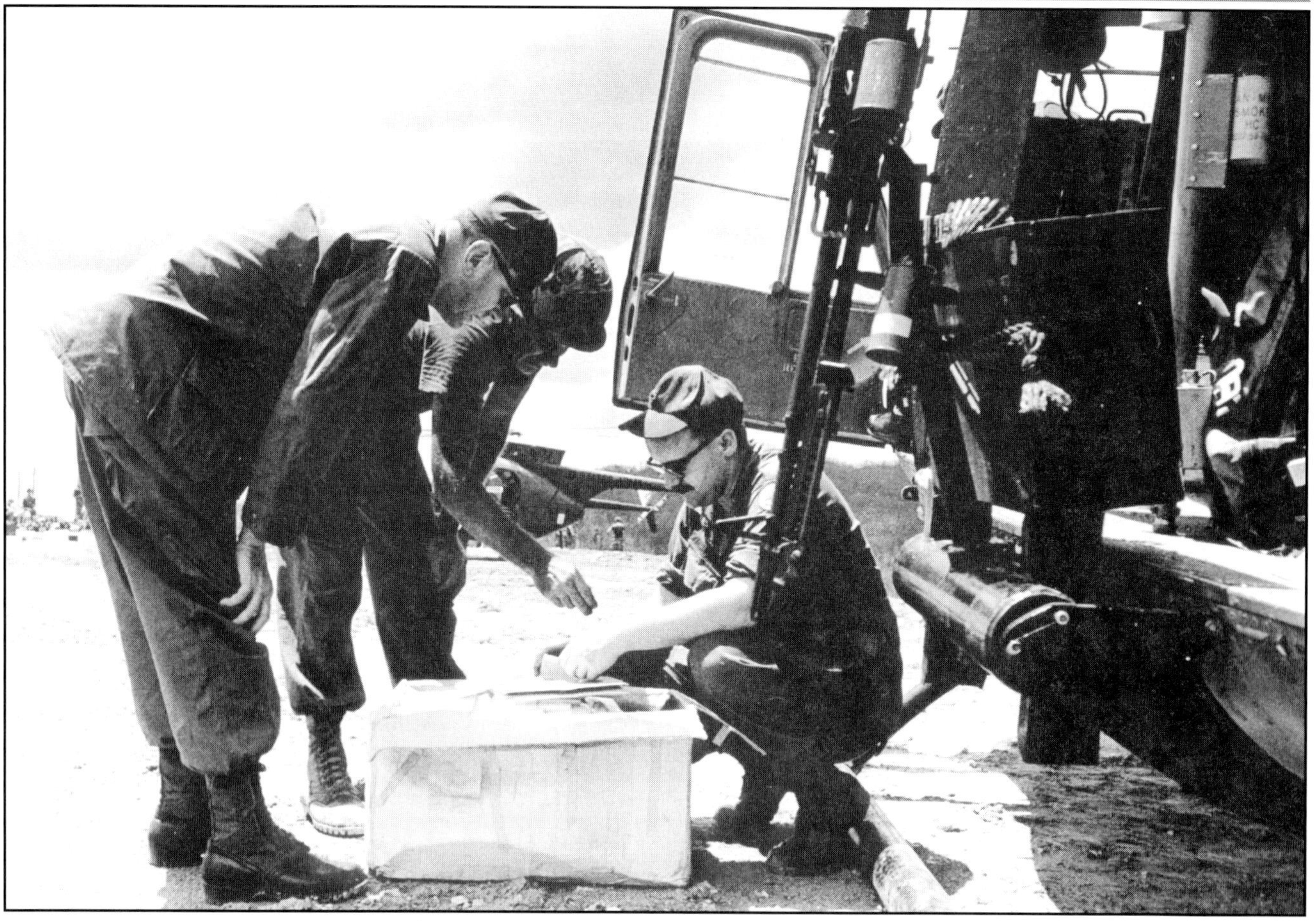

Above and below, Vietnam

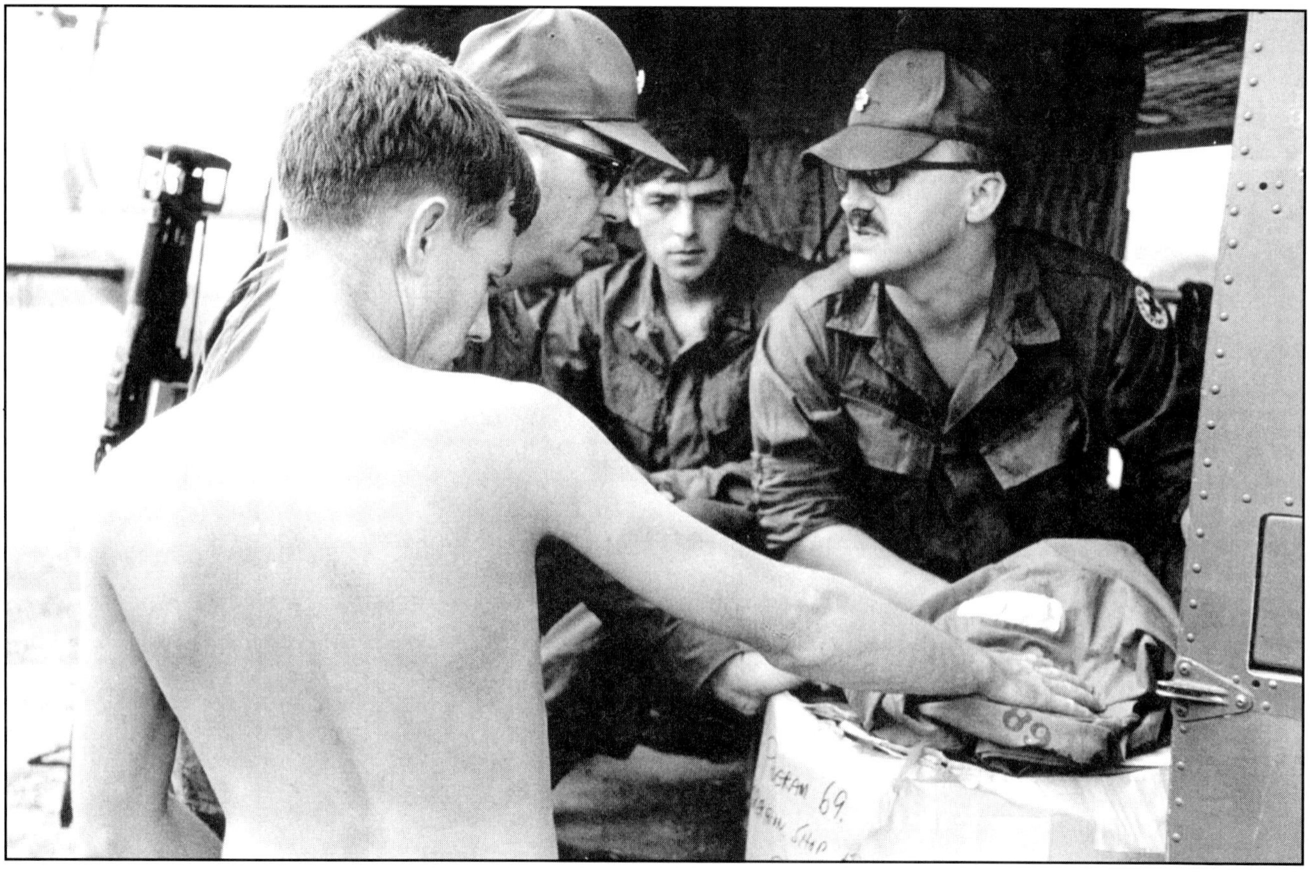

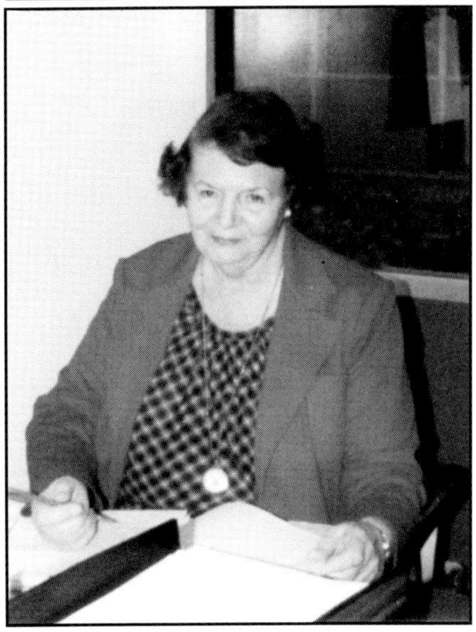

Margaret Boatright, SMF/V Valley District

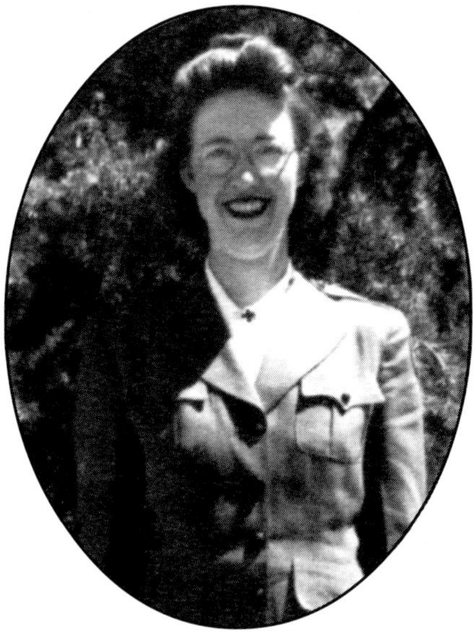

Mildred Powell, Bruno General Hospital, Santa Fe, NM, 1944

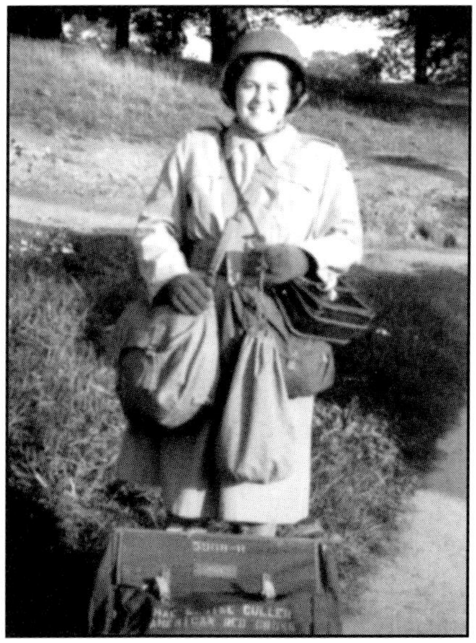

Mae Louise Culler, Camp Kilmer, NJ, ready to head overseas, 1944.

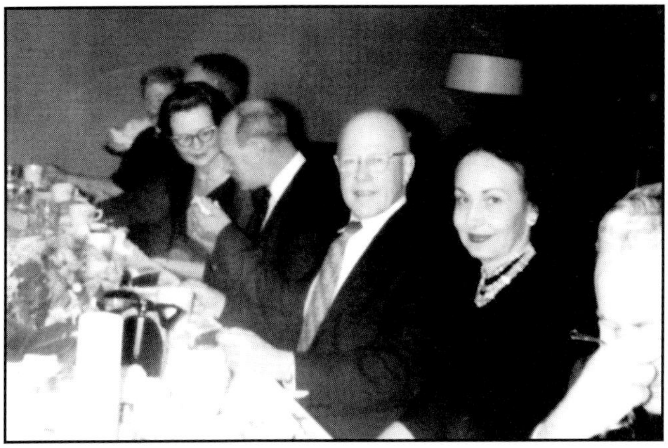

June 1959. Red Cross staff, Fort Lewis, WA, retirement luncheon. Western Area VIP, Doye Fannin, Emmit Forsythe, Walt Johnson, Mrs. Johnson, two unidentified

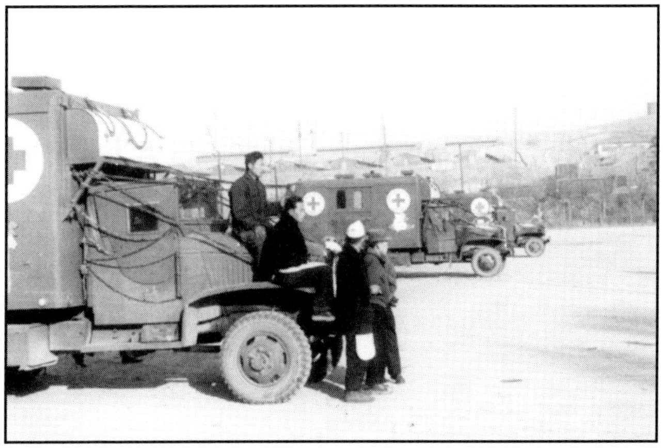

8th Army Carol Sing, Seoul, Christmas, 1954

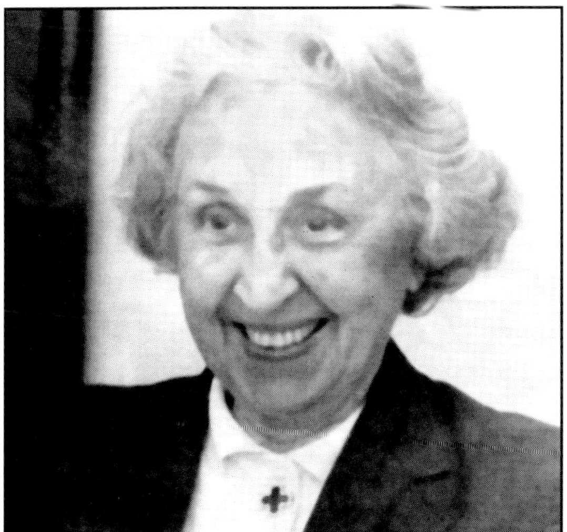

Lucile Allen, retiring after 40 years with the Red Cross

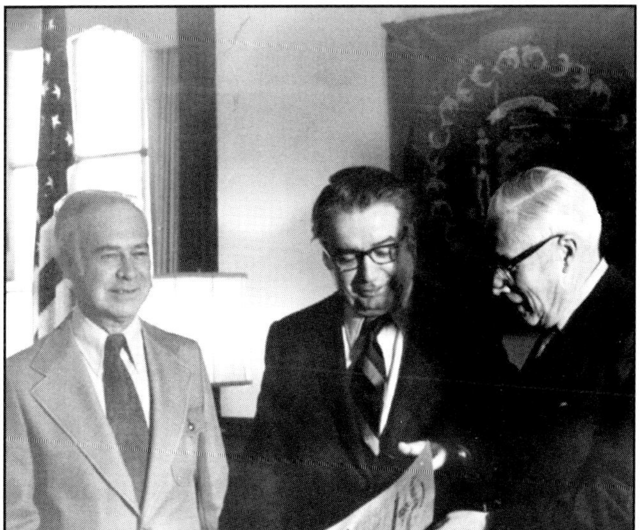

Proclamation for Human Rights Day, 1971

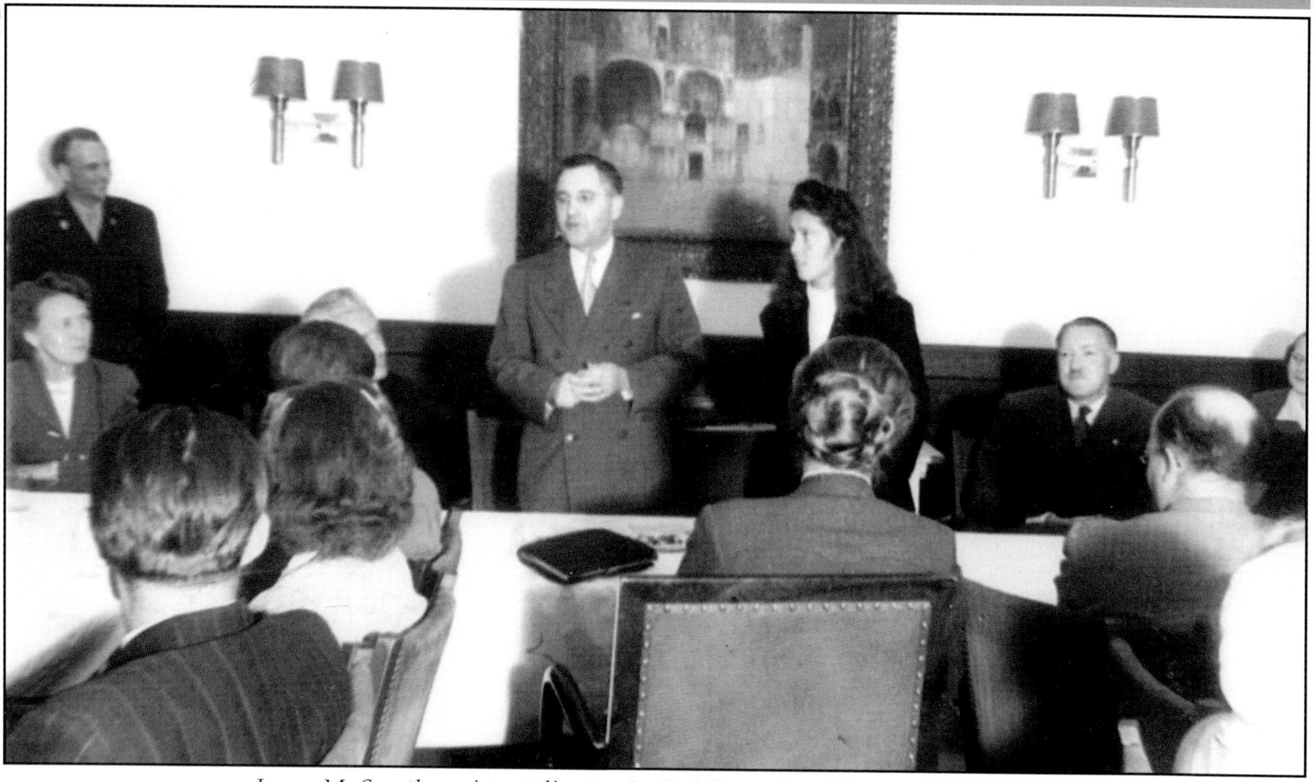

James M. Smyth, assistant director, Jr. Red Cross, Frankfurt, Germany, 1954

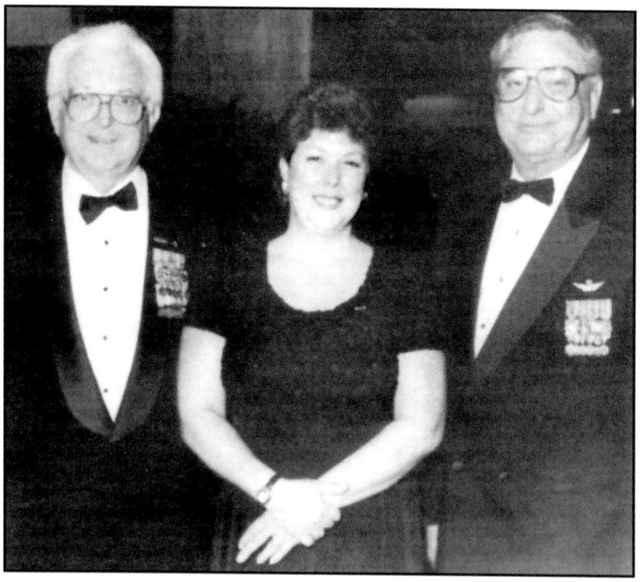

Sgt. Rebecca Pulley, Arnold, MD, wounded in Kuwait while serving as radio operator, flanked by Richard Gallant, executive director, Military Order of the Purple Heart Service Foundation, and MOPH National Commander Carroll Fylee

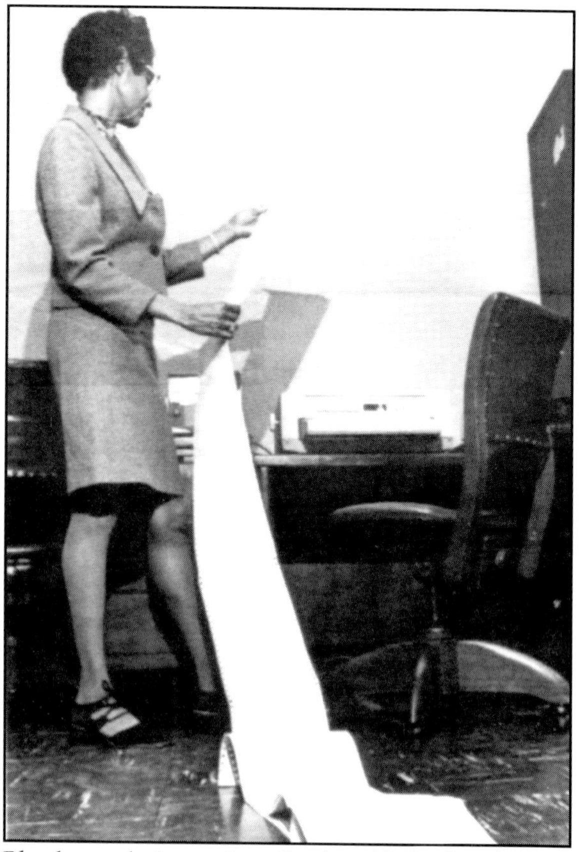

Blood records Supervisor Carolyne N. Banks, checks a day's 22-foot print-out for accuracy as it rolls off the machine.

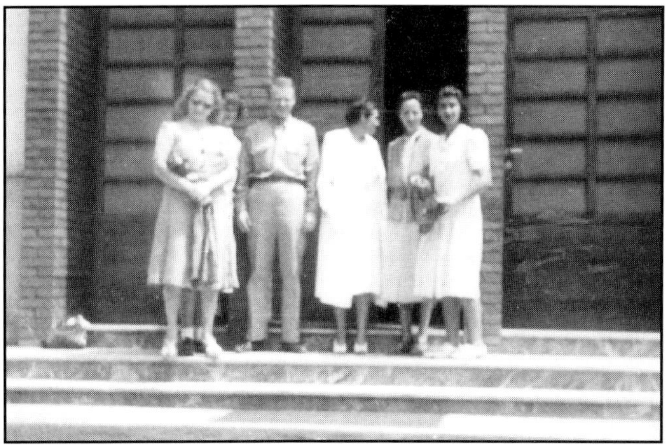

Home visitors of Eritrea, 1942

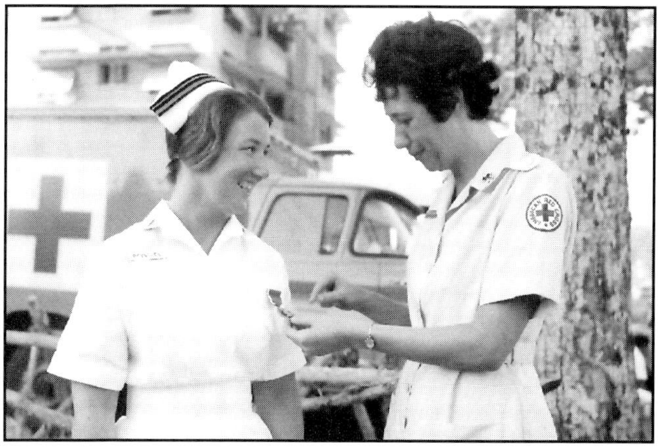

Navy nurses in Saigon

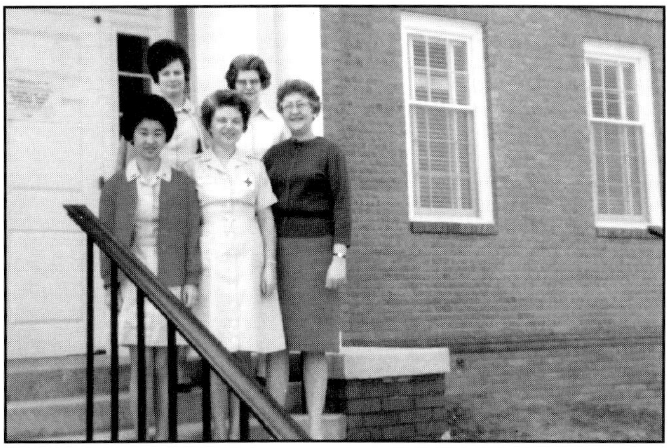

Staff at Hyattsville, MD, 1970

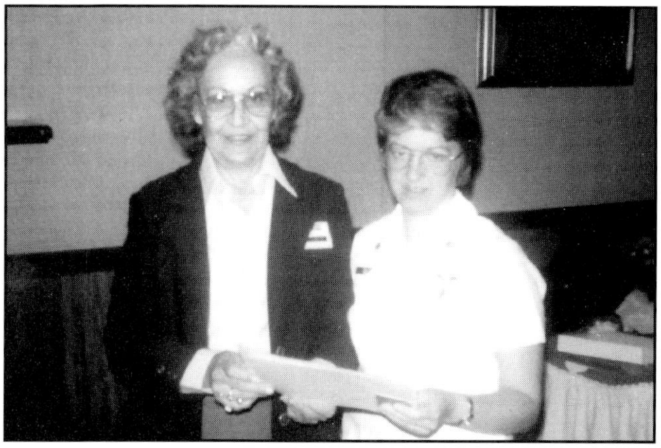

Fall 1981. Doye Fannin, presenting certificate of appreciation to USAF chief nurse, March AFB.

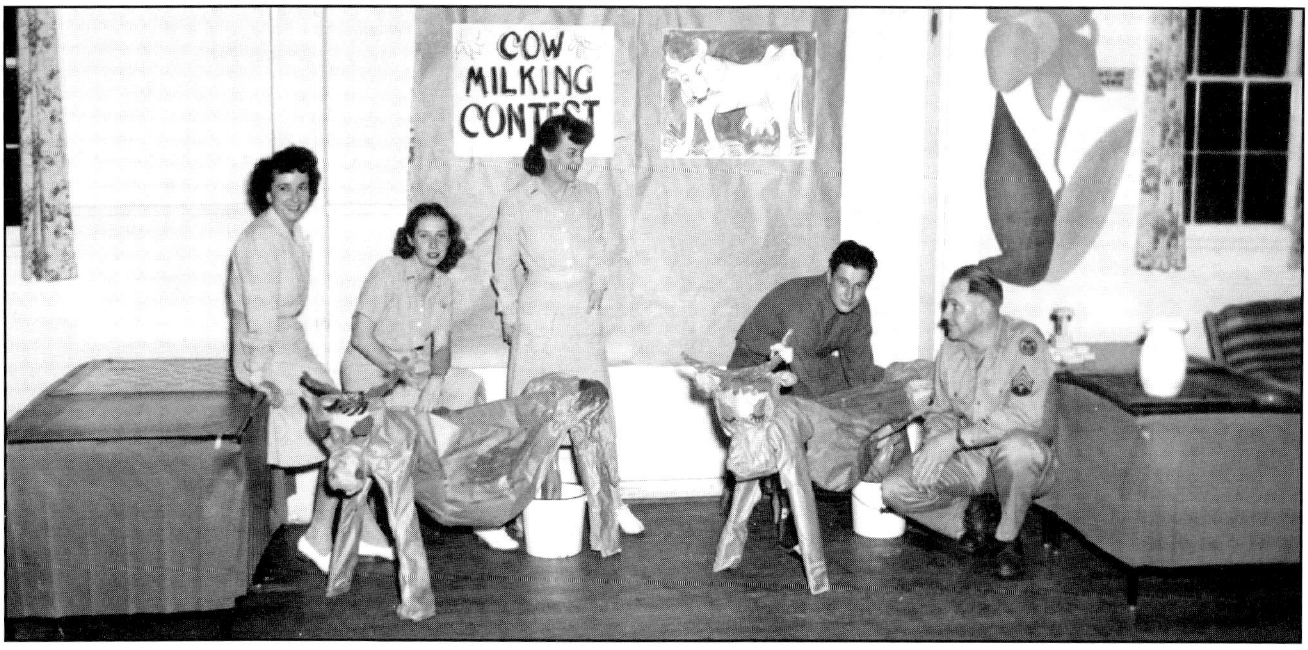

Madigan General Hospital, Carnival Night, 1945

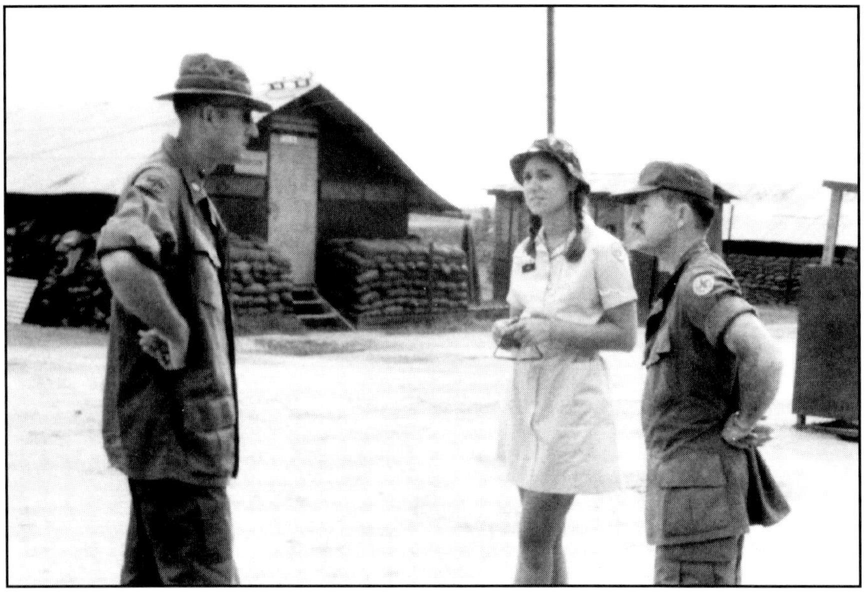

Frank Shouse with Donut Dolly, Christmas Day, 1970. Quang Tri, Vietnam

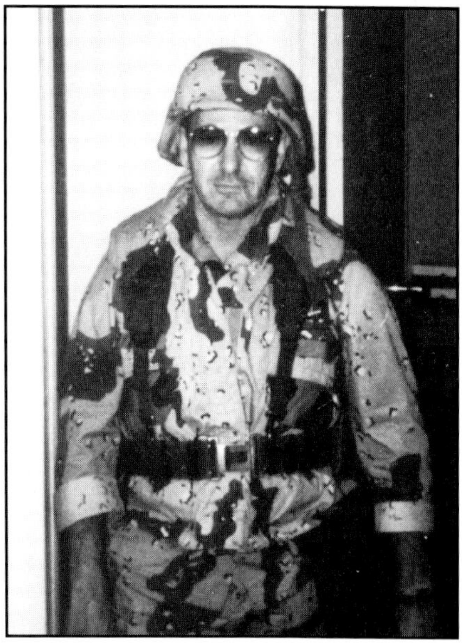

Frank Shouse, Desert Storm, 1st. IMEF, Al Jubial, Saudi Arabia, 1991

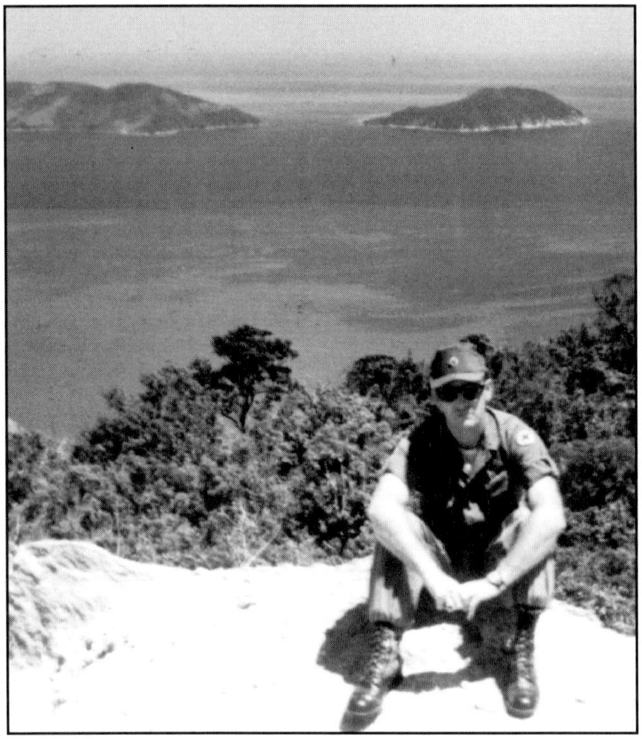

Frank Shouse, Monkey Mountain, near Danang, Vietnam, 1971

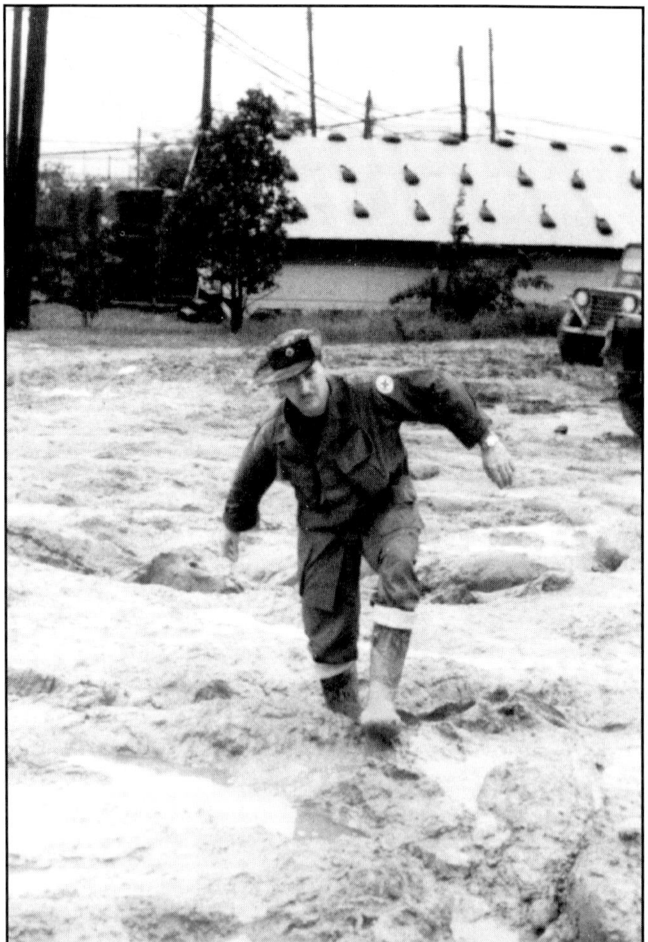

Frank Shouse in the mud in front of Red Cross office, Quang Tru, Vietnam, 1970

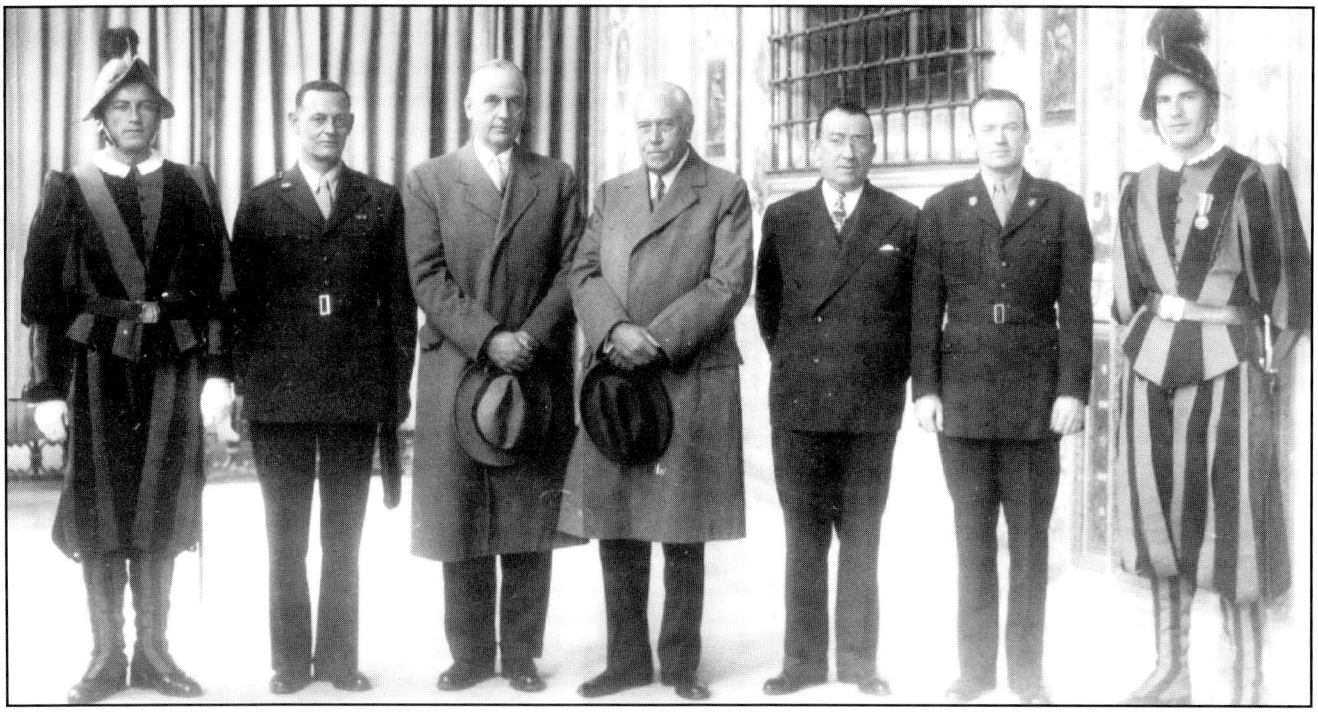

At the Vatican after a private audience with the Pope, 1944

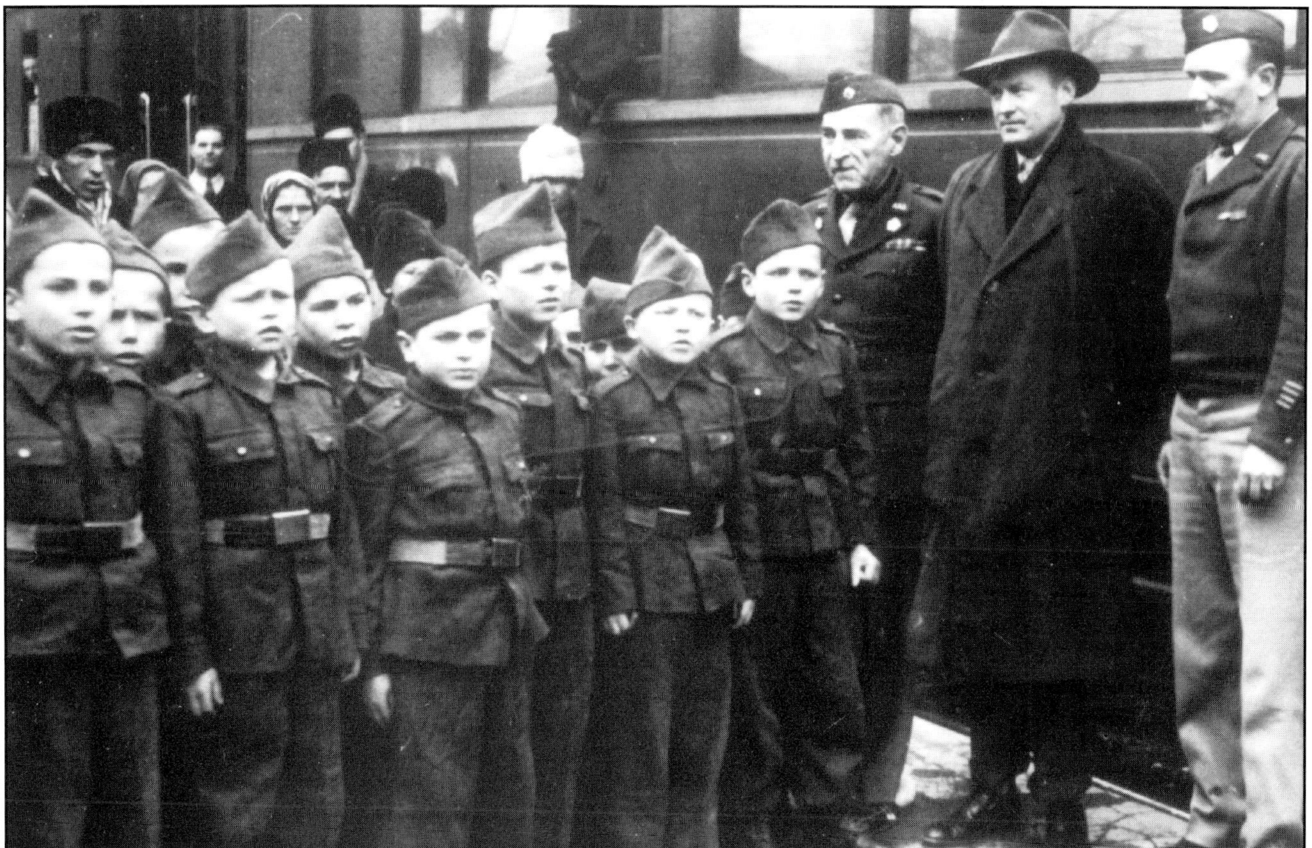

ARC reps with a group of war orphans, the Balkans

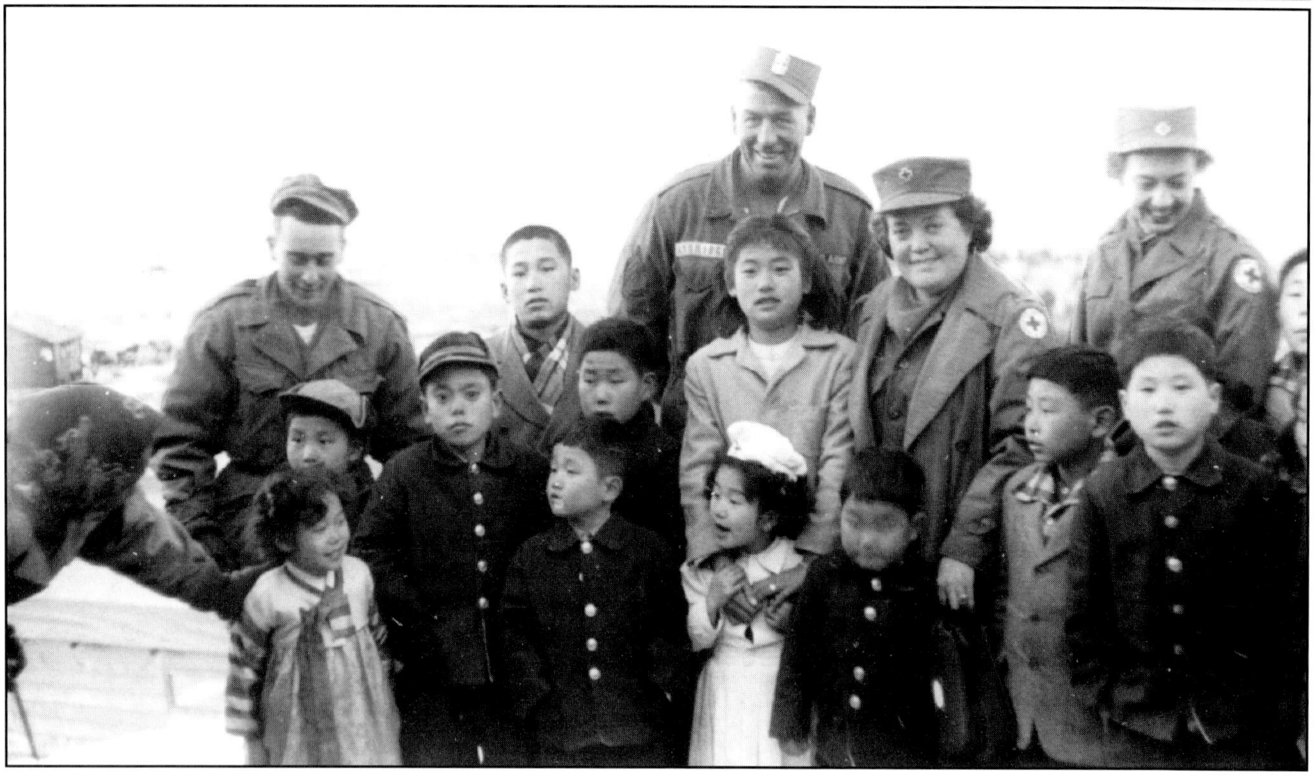

Orphans, Christmas in Korea, 1954

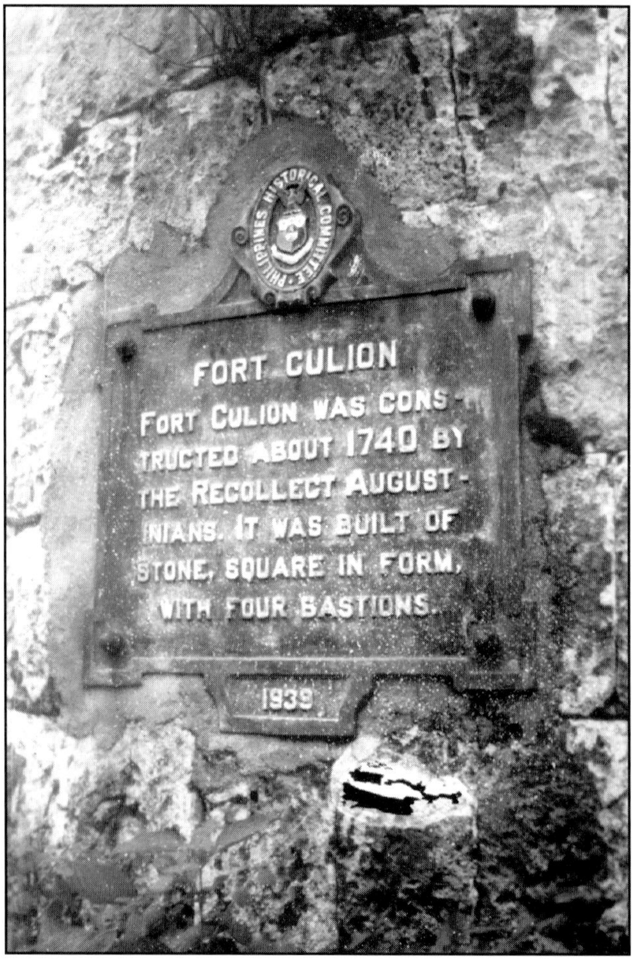
PHILIPPINES HISTORICAL COMMITTEE
FORT CULION
FORT CULION WAS CONS-
TRUCTED ABOUT 1740 BY
THE RECOLLECT AUGUST-
INIANS. IT WAS BUILT OF
STONE, SQUARE IN FORM,
WITH FOUR BASTIONS.
1939

Fort Culion sign

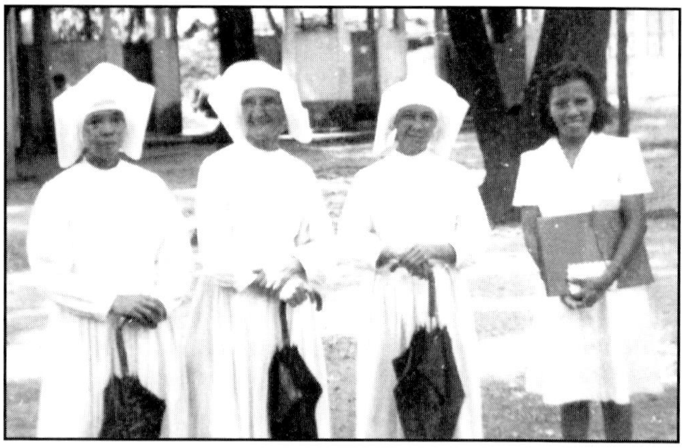

Culion

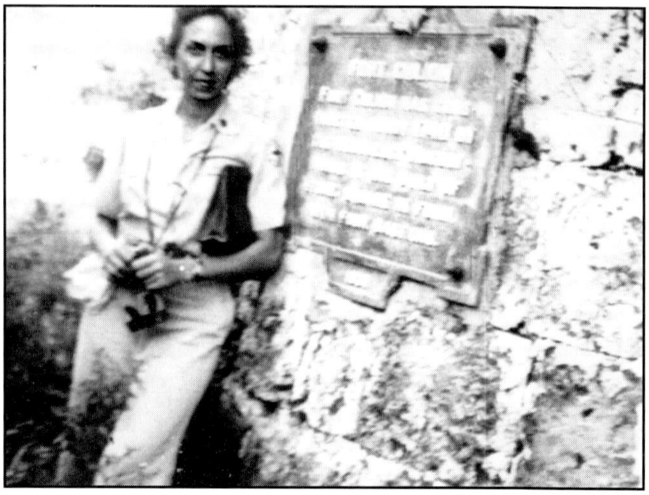

Lucile Allen at Ft. Culion, November, 1945

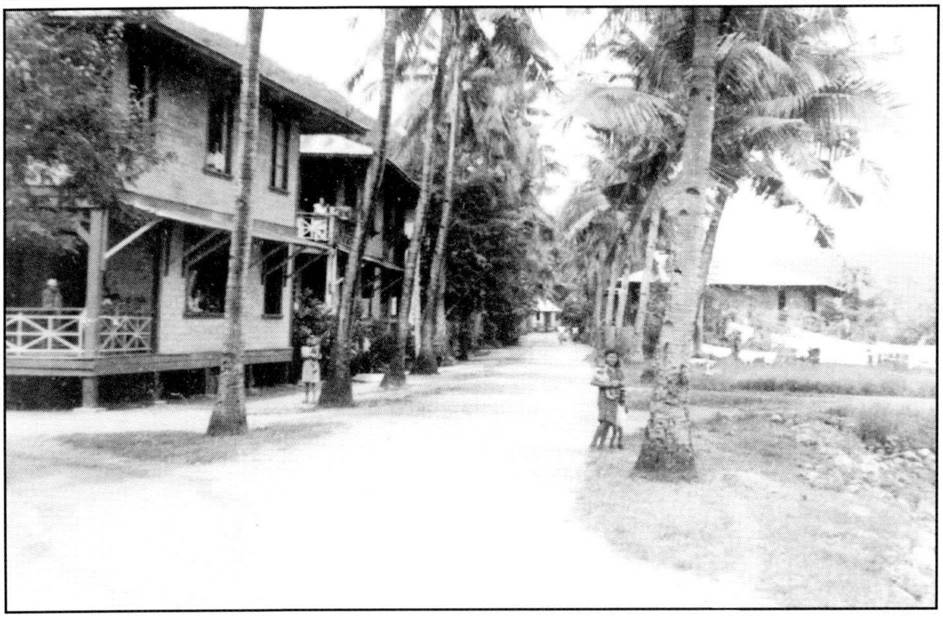

Doctor's office

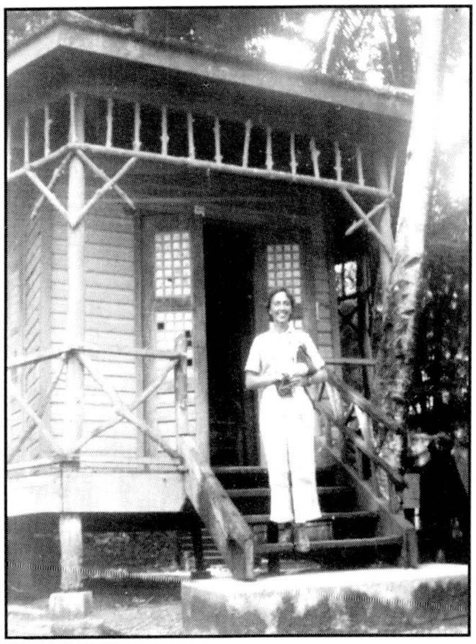

Lucile Allen at doctor's office (Windowpanes are filled with oyster shells.)

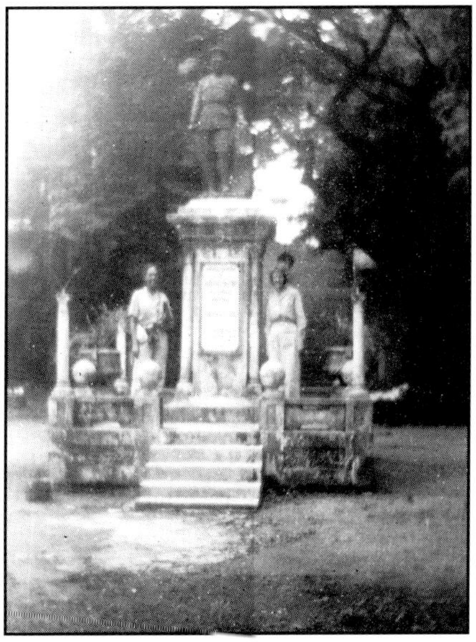

Leonard Wood Monument. Two Red Cross girls at Culion

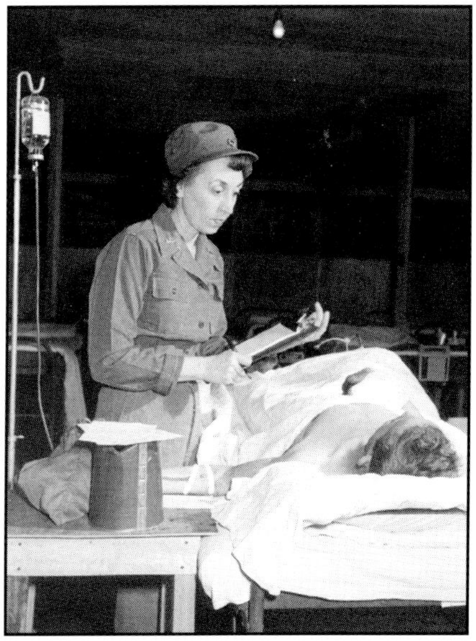

Dec. 1951. 4th Field Hospital, Taegu. PFC Dwight Darky, frostbite victim, dictating letter to fiance.

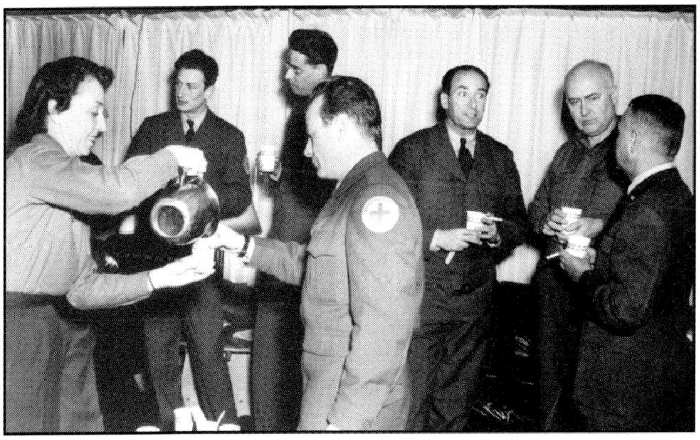

Six doctors from International Red Cross in Geneva, Switzerland

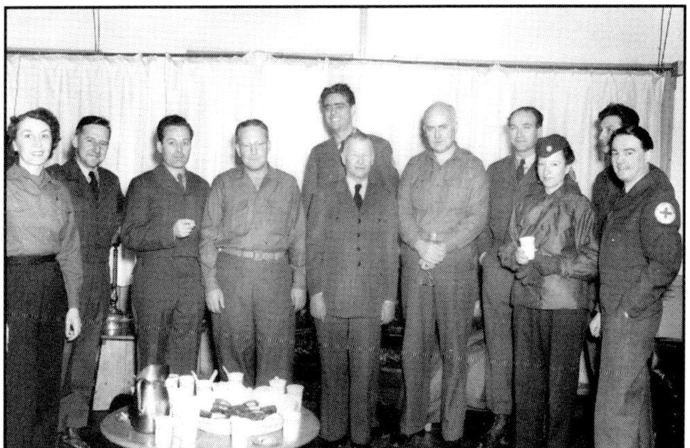

January 9, 1952

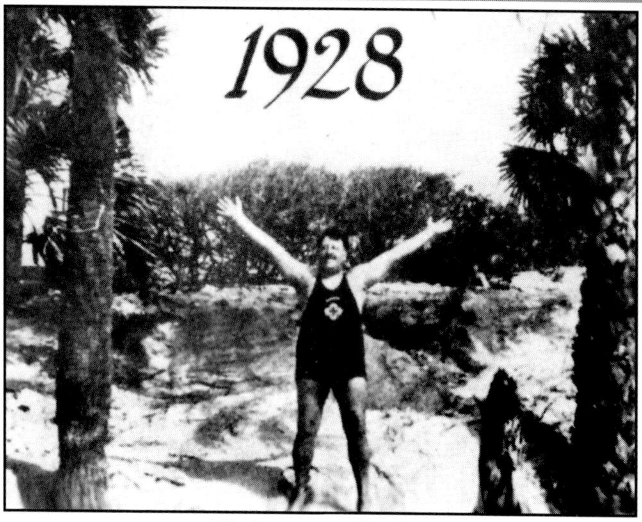
1928

Christmas card, 1928

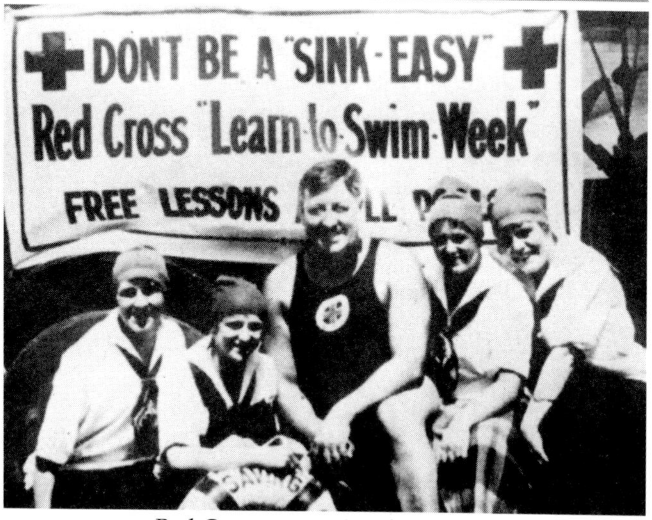
DONT BE A "SINK-EASY"
Red Cross "Learn-to-Swim-Week"
FREE LESSONS

Red Cross promotional post card

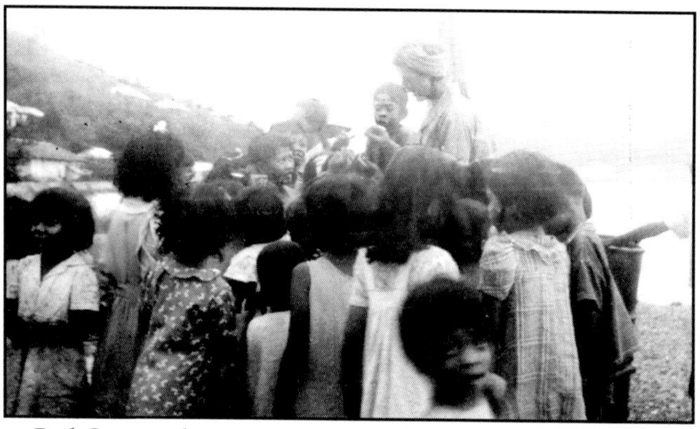

Red Cross volunteers giving candy to children at Culion

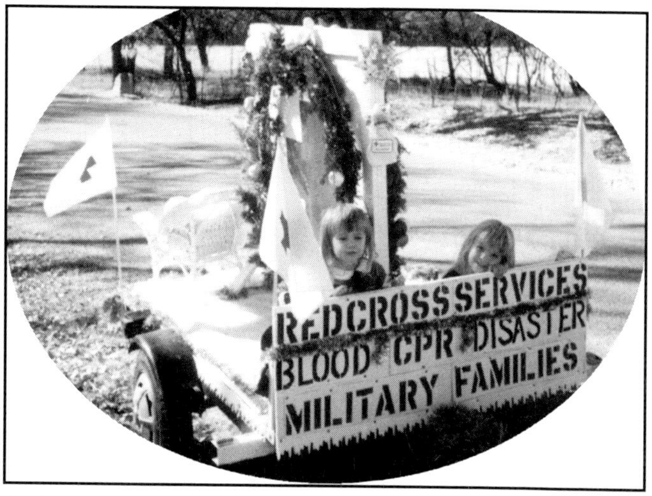
REDCROSS SERVICES
BLOOD CPR DISASTER
MILITARY FAMILIES

Red Cross youth, Christmas Parade float, 1988, Mindy Marshall and Amy Schilman

ARC President Elizabeth Dole and 99-year-old Robert H. Watson

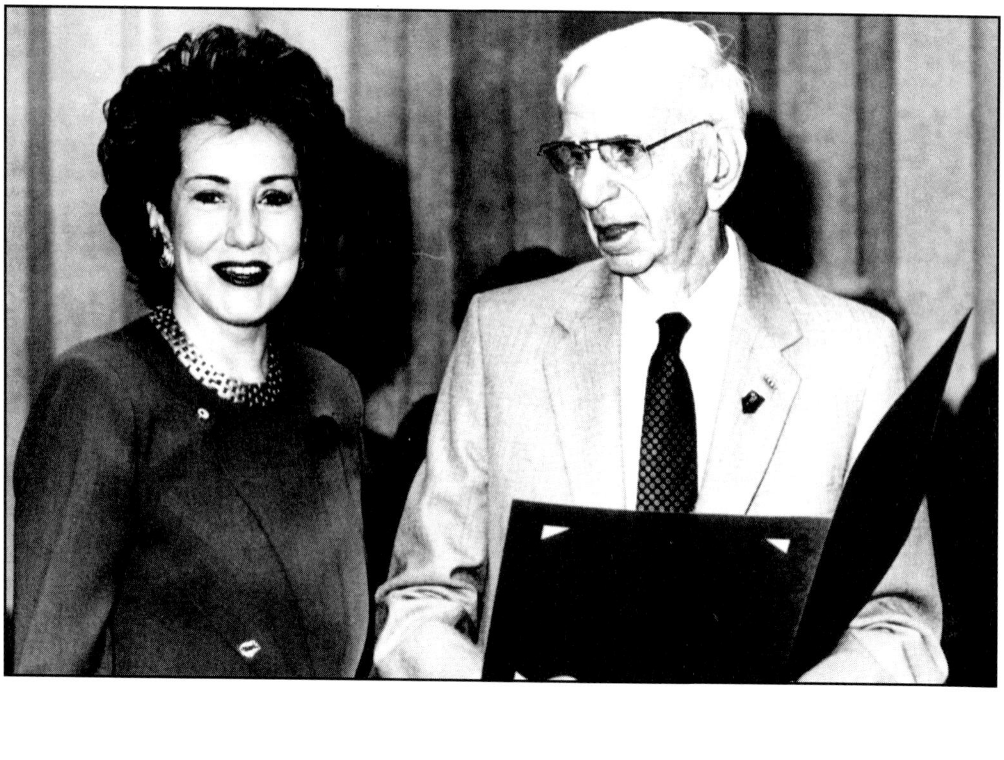

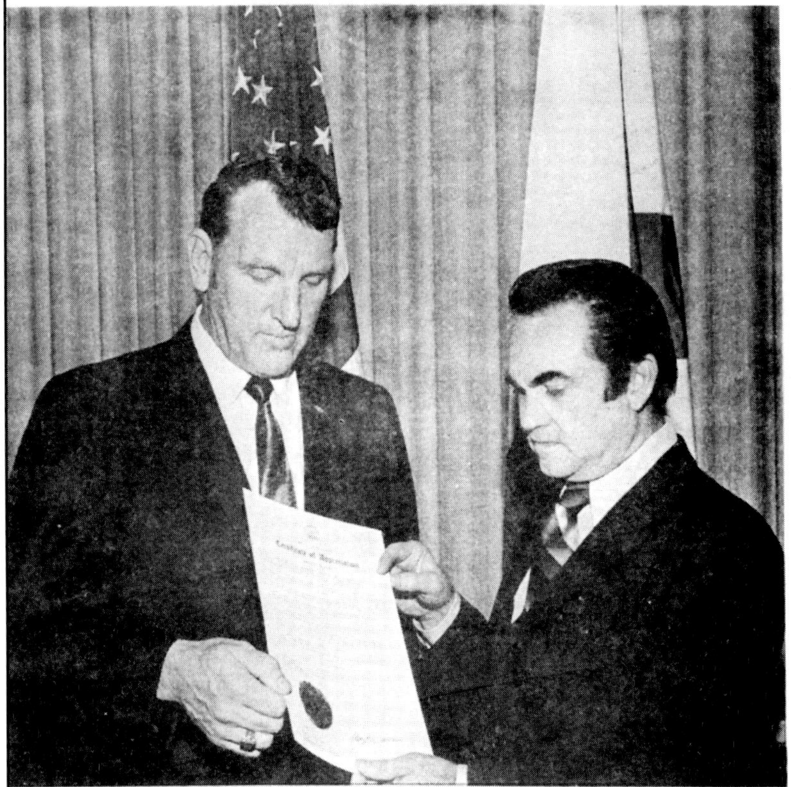

Clyde Earnhardt Honored

Clyde H. Earnhardt, Red Cross Safety Services Director, has been awarded a Certificate of Appreciation by Governor Geo. C. Wallace for saving the life of a 14-year-old boy. The youth was participating in the OEO 'Learn to Swim' program being taught by Red Cross instructors at Maxwell Air Force Base when he slipped, hit his head on the side of the pool, and sank to the bottom. Earnhardt rescued the boy from the pool and applied mouth-to-mouth resuscitation for ten minutes before the youth took his first breath. The boy suffered a cerebral concussion but due to the instructor's immediate action, had no brain damage. The human brain can generally service only 4 to 6 minutes without oxygen before brain damage occurs.

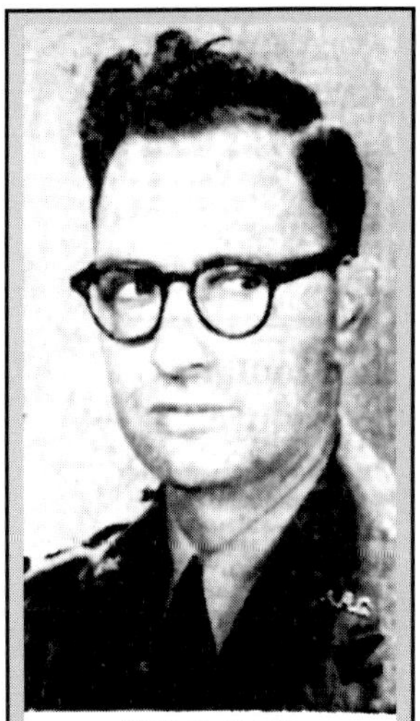

NEIL M. CLARK
. . . Joins Red Cross

• • •

Boisean Accepts Overseas Post With Red Cross

Neil M. Clark, son of Mr. and Mrs. Clifford H. Clark, Boise, route 9, has reported to the Canal Zone for overseas assignment with the American Red Cross in the Caribbean theater, according to word received in Boise.

He worked for export-import firms in San Francisco for three years before accepting the position with the Red Cross.

Clark served six years as an Army infantry officer in World war II, with three years service in the Pacific theater.

He attended Boise Junior college and the American Institute of Foreign Trade in Phoenix, Ariz.

Cadets Given Awards Of C.M.T.C.

Parade at Fort as Visitors and Regulars Look on

Youth of the intermountain sector—some 130 husky, bronzed specimens of health—were rewarded with varied awards Thursday morning at a visitors' day honor assembly and parade by the C. M. T. C. at Fort Douglas. The camp demobilizes Friday afternoon.

More than 300 persons—parents, sweethearts and friends—and a handful of regular enlisted men withstood a sweltering sun as 202 khaki clad cadets staged their final parade.

Brigadier General Walter C. Sweeney, commandant of Fort Douglas, presented the outstanding prizes.

Two Salt Lake City youths, Joseph H. Anderson, battalion commander, and Paul H. Brown Jr., battalion adjutant, were presented with regulation officers' sabers "for distinguished service."

Nineteen-year-old Bud Clarke of Boise, Idaho, won a $500 scholarship to the Hill military academy, Portland, Ore., as the outstanding trainee in camp. He will leave for the school September 1. He is a son of Mr. and Mrs. C. H. Clarke. The post commandant decorated him with the scholarship and "Order of the Rose" medal.

Wins Decoration at Camp

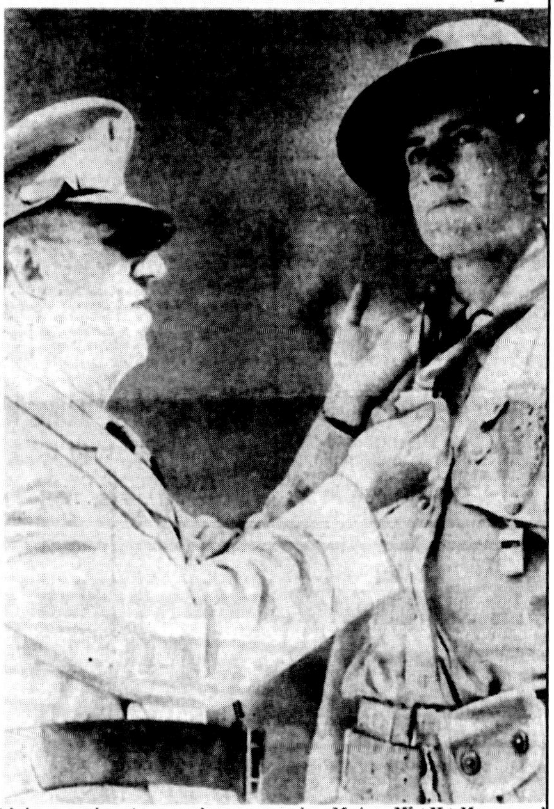

Idaho youth wins academy award. Major W. H. Hammond decorates Bud Clarke, Boise, Idaho.

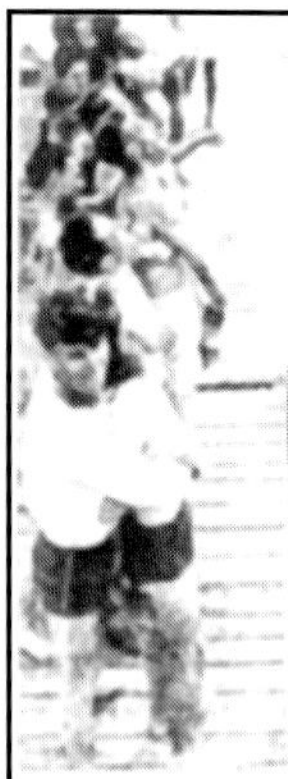

Fort Bragg boys get training

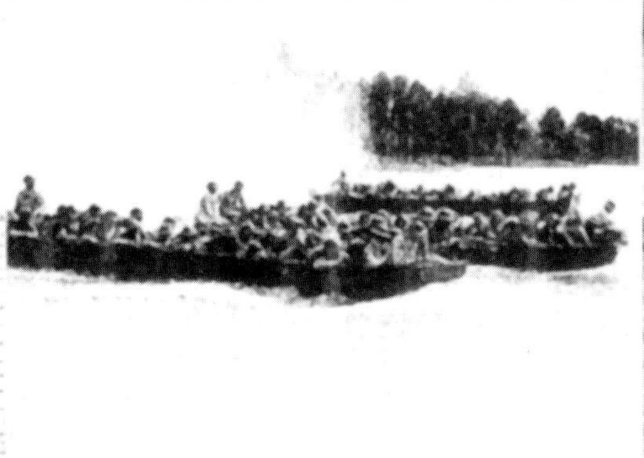

To point up value of Red Cross life saving training, soldiers simulate landing under combat conditions

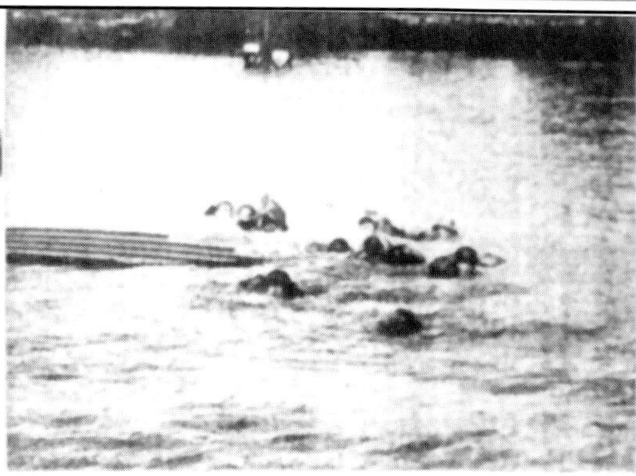

Keeping afloat in full equipment after capsizing to test Red Cross training

Men le

THE RED CROSS IS TEACHIN

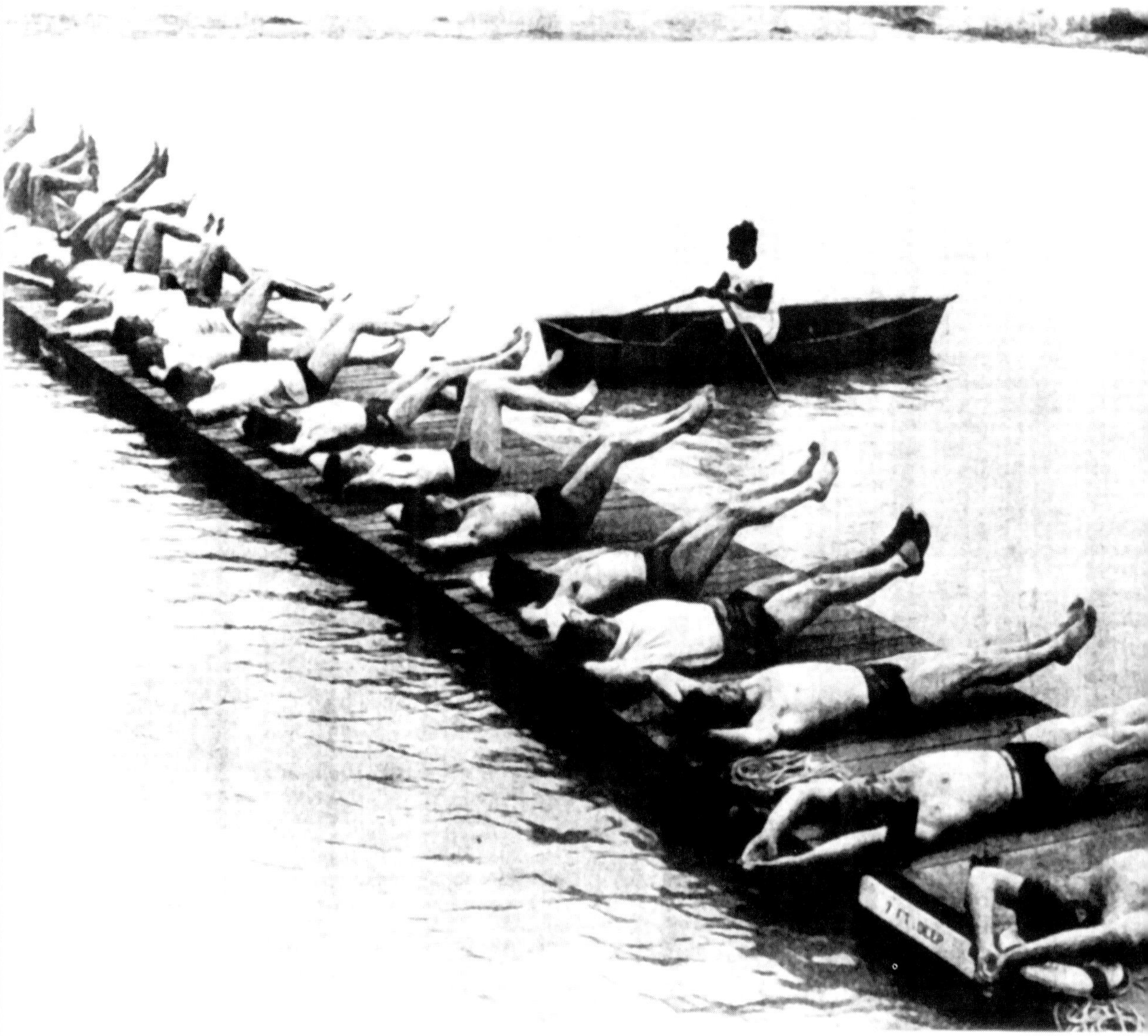

Soldiers learn to swim on their backs. This is extensively used in life saving because it is a most effective means of towing a "v and because it also affords the swimmer an opportunity to rest, thus preventing exhaustion. Furthermore, the soldier, if p incapacitated by an arm wound, can propel himself on his back, using only his legs for locomotion

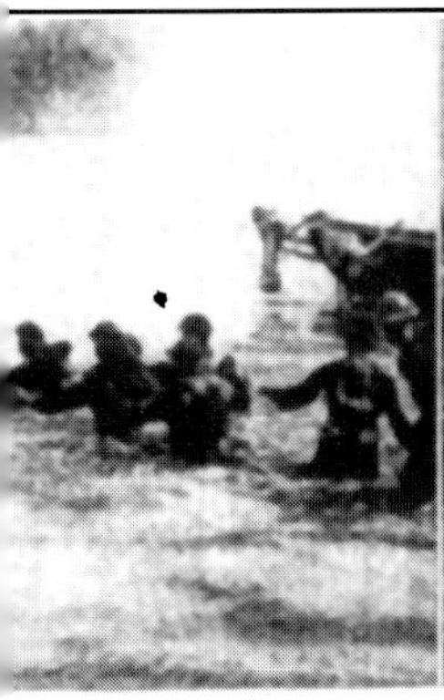

" method of rescue—aids
el who get in trouble

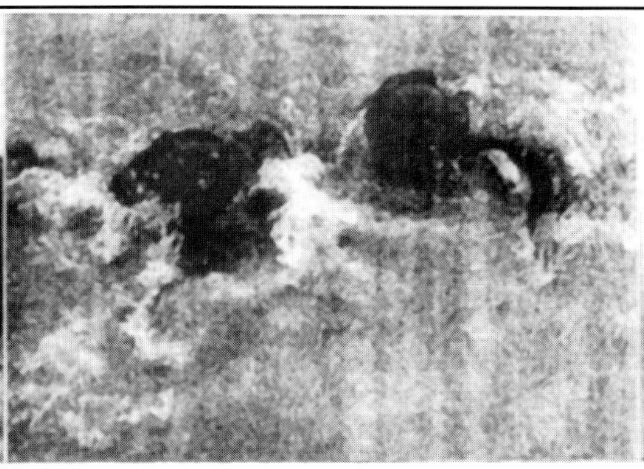

Two Red Cross trained embryo instructors prove that men, properly taught, can swim in full field equipment

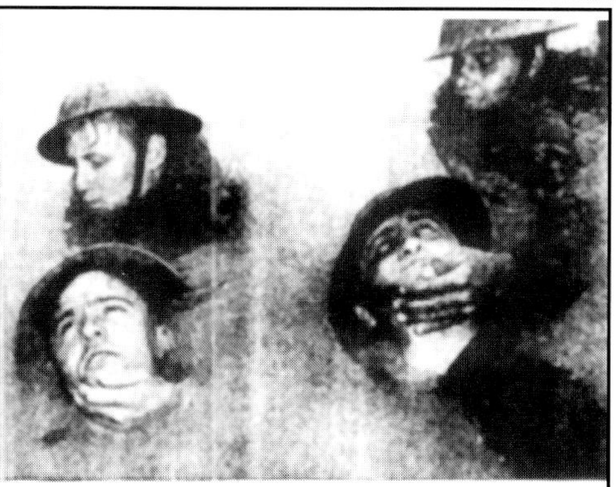

Not only that, but after mastering Red Cross skills they can tow injured comrades to safety

ARMY TO SWIM

Photos and Story by

HARRY POAGUE

THERE is little doubt in the minds f those who have seen the maneu- ers of amphibious Army units in raining at Fort Bragg and other amps that the Commando influence as really taken hold in this man's Army. The life saving and water afety program of the American Red Cross plays a major role in the future maneuverability of these amphibians. Figures have been quoted that only 0 per cent of Army personnel are xpert swimmers; the balance are ovices or non-swimmers.

Red Cross instructors are training lasses of soldiers to be swimming in- tructors in Army camps. These po- ential teachers will in turn teach wimming and life saving under ac- ual service conditions.

The Red Cross program of both wimming and life saving begins on dry land, with study from textbooks and instructors' manuals. The men are then taught to master all swim- ming strokes and life saving technique efore venturing into the water. The rogram then gets its feet wet, but n shallow water where the potential nstructor has the opportunity of ap- plying his knowledge with the great- st degree of safety. After the shal- ow water period, training moves into deep water, and then the men are given an opportunity to demonstrate their ability under actual combat conditions, and really go to town.

The program has disproved the widely believed theory that it was not possible for soldiers to swim with safety under service conditions. Actually, the uniform and pack lend buoyancy to the soldier in the water. Don Northey, Red Cross Life Saving and Water Safety Service field representative, has been enlisting service men of better than average swimming ability and has been turning out a class a week of certified instructors. These men are qualified to instruct Army personnel to handle themselves safely in the water under actual combat conditions.

In the one-week training program the soldier-instructor devotes the entire day to swimming instruction and textbook study. It has been found that by carrying on the training so intensively the soldier is better able to coordinate the various steps in the program. The swimming day begins at 8:30 in the morning with an hour out for lunch and ends at 4:30.

At the end of the one-week training period the men are given both written and actual swimming examinations before they are certified as Red Cross instructors in life saving and water safety. The pictures on these pages were taken at Fort Bragg, North Carolina, under actual training conditions. This is but one of the Red Cross Water Safety and Life Saving programs for the instruction of soldiers in the Army camps of the United States. It has already been shown that the hazard of loss of life through the activities of amphibious units thus will be greatly reduced.

■

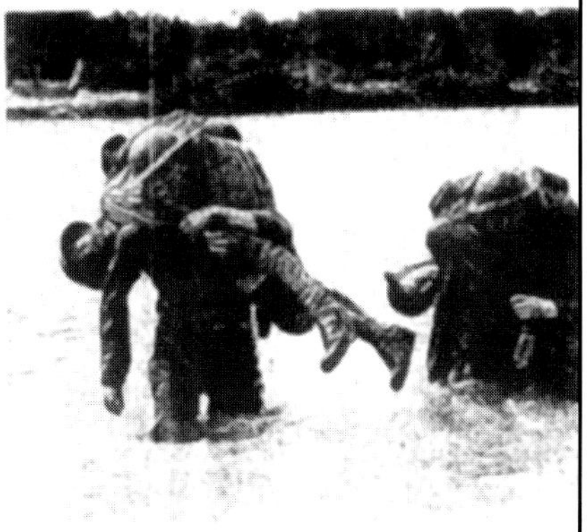

By using fireman's carry, soaking wet "victims" are brought safely through shallow water

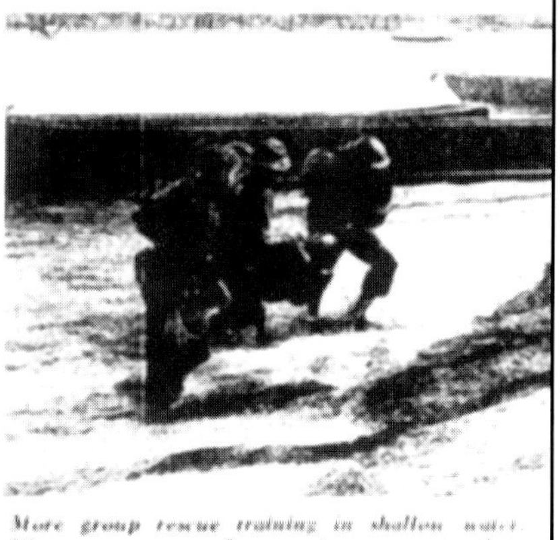

More group rescue training in shallow water. These men are to become instructors in their own right

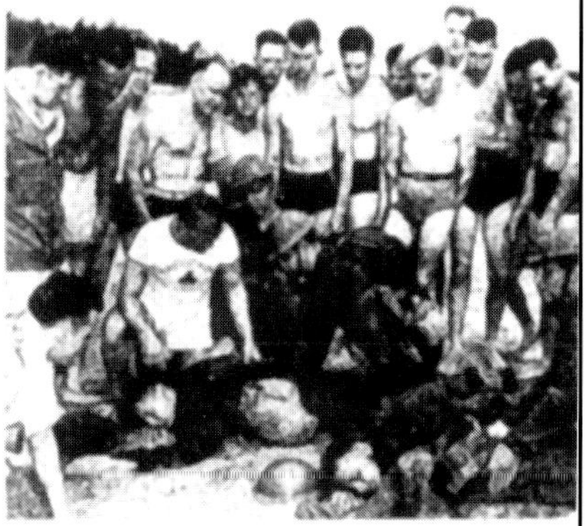

Red Cross expert stresses value of starting artificial respiration immediately when immersion has stopped victim's breathing

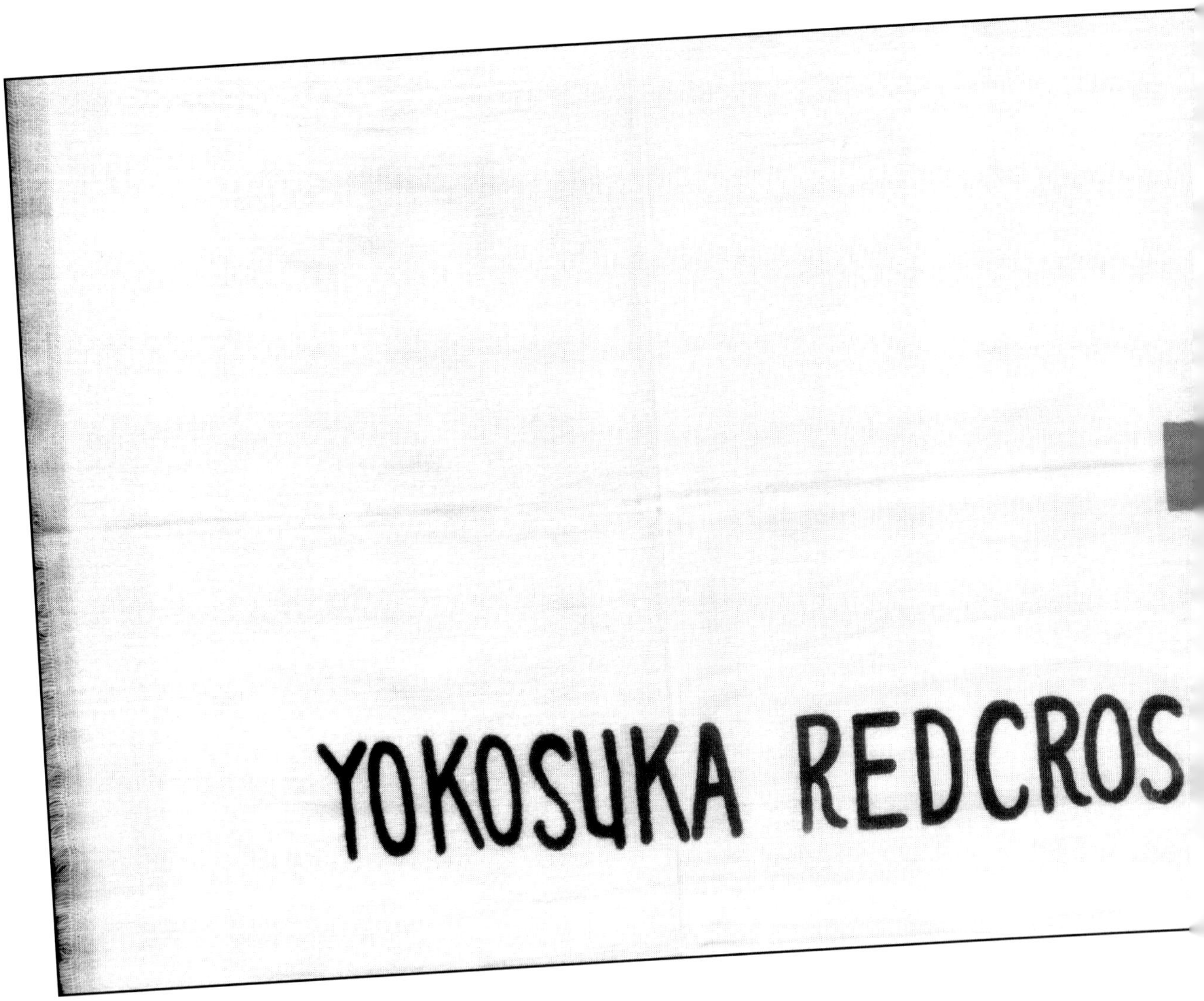
YOKOSUKA REDCROS

American Red Cross Presidents

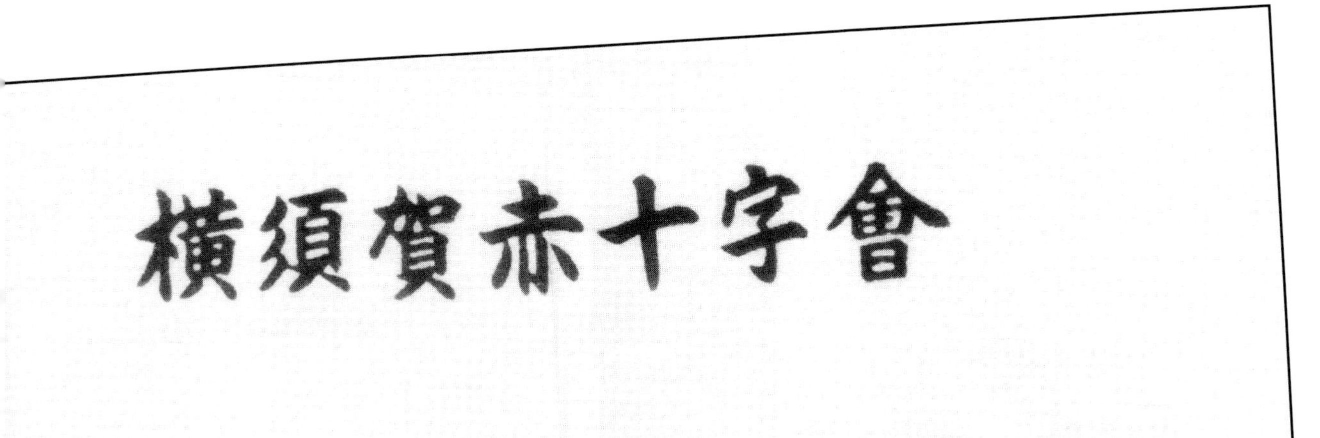
横須賀赤十字會

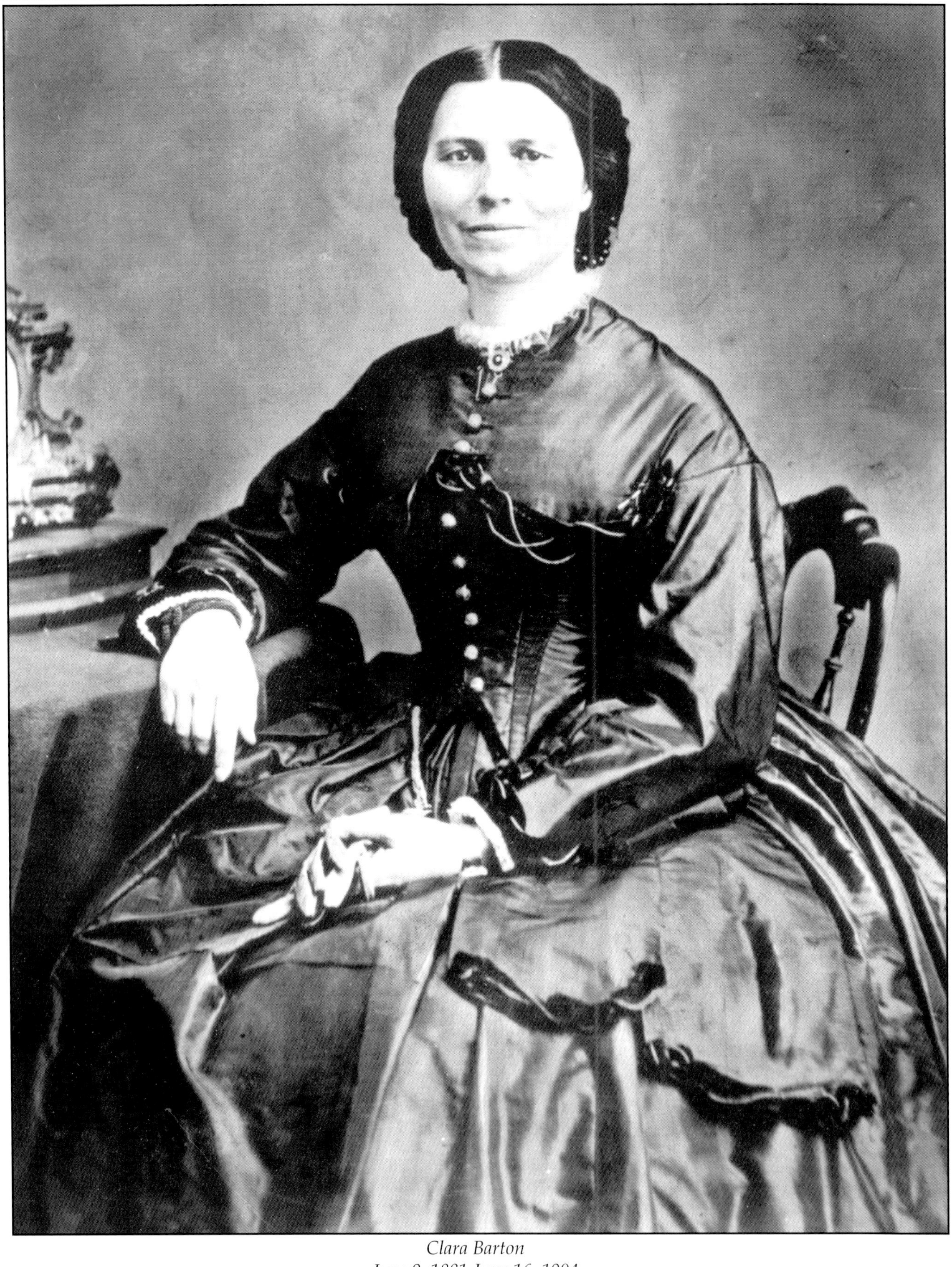

Clara Barton
June 9, 1881-June 16, 1904

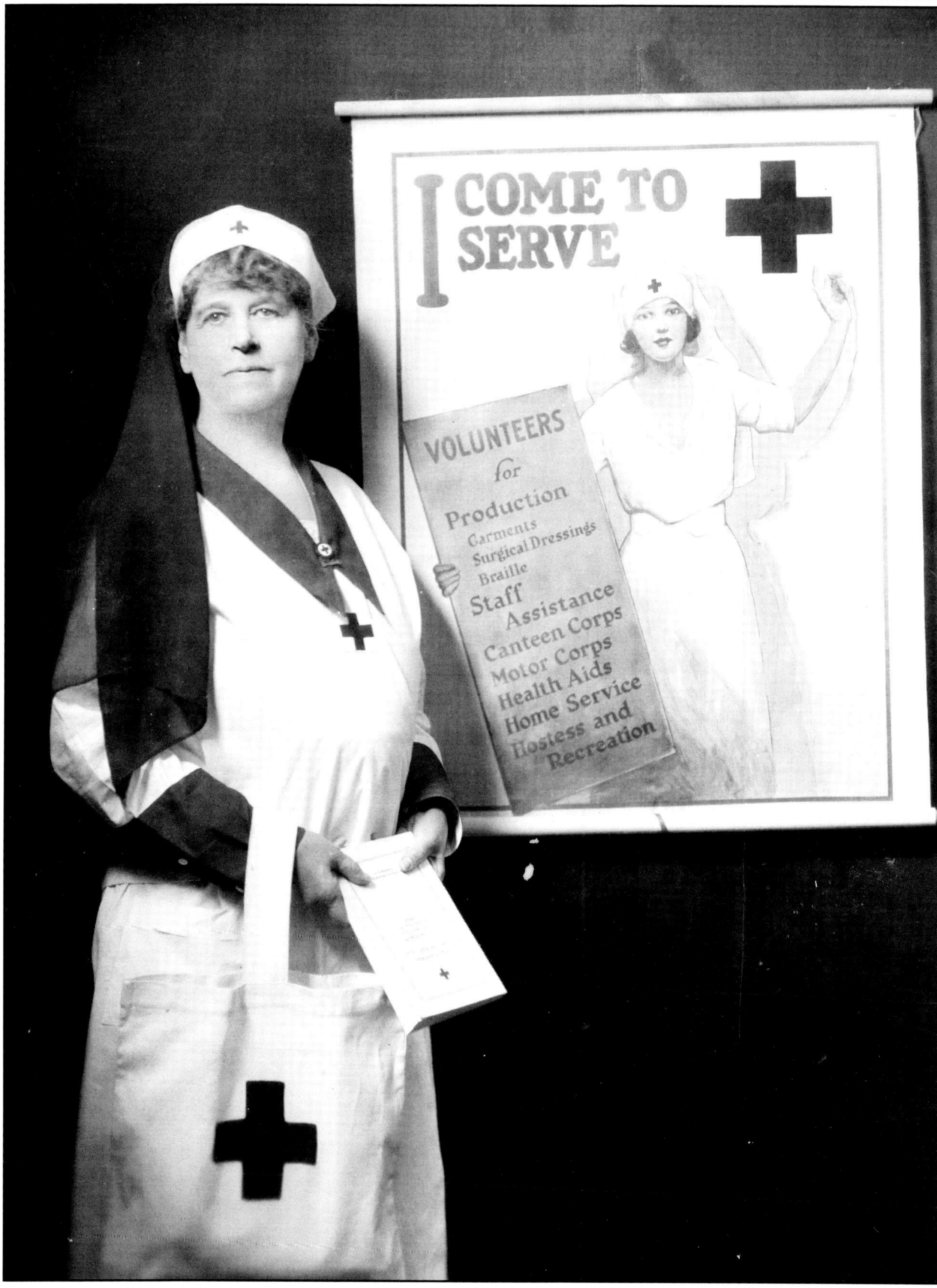
I COME TO SERVE
VOLUNTEERS
for
Production
Garments
Surgical Dressings
Braille
Staff
Assistance
Canteen Corps
Motor Corps
Health Aids
Home Service
Hostess and
Recreation

Mabel Boardman
June 1904-1919

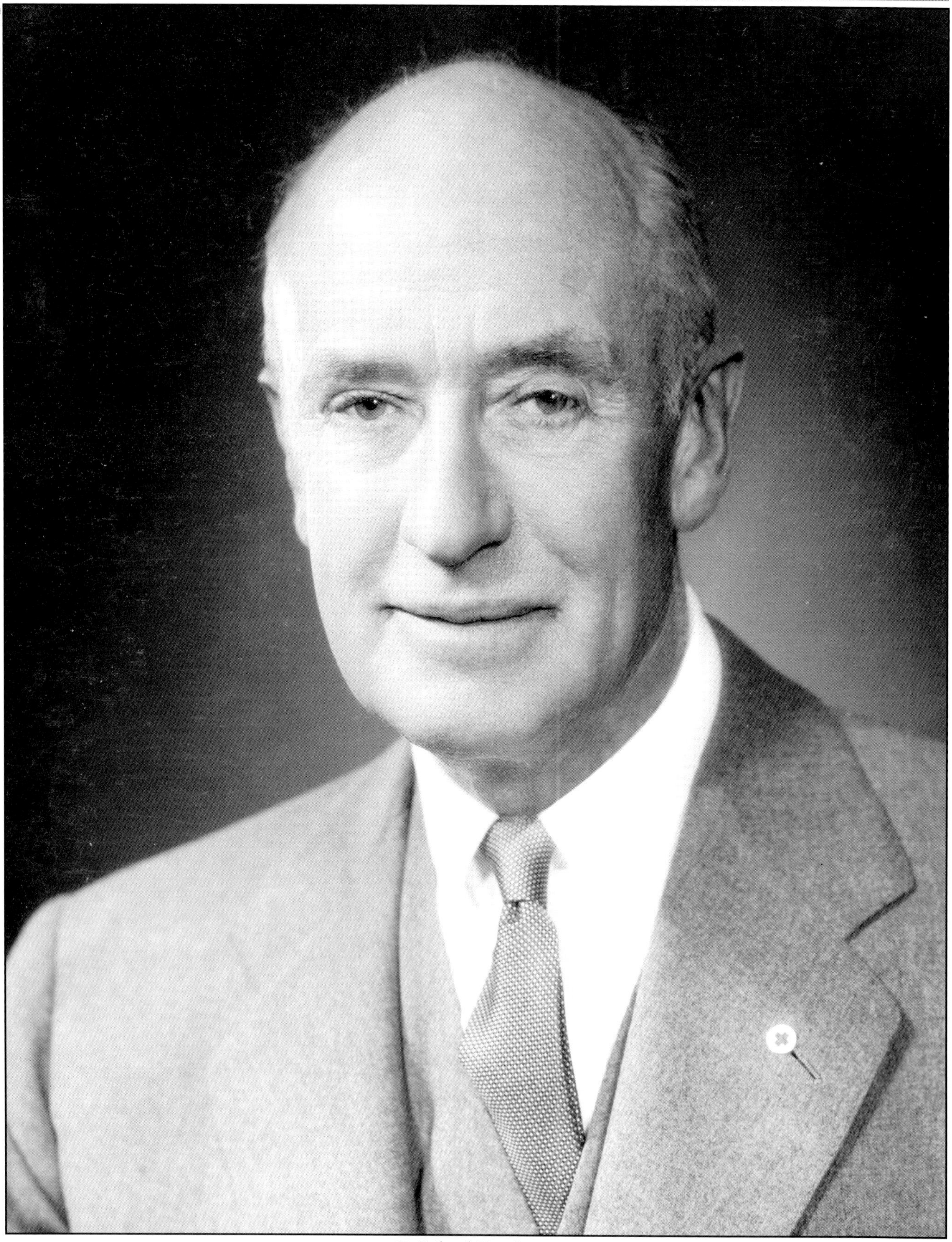

E. Roland Harriman
December 1, 1950-December 31, 1953

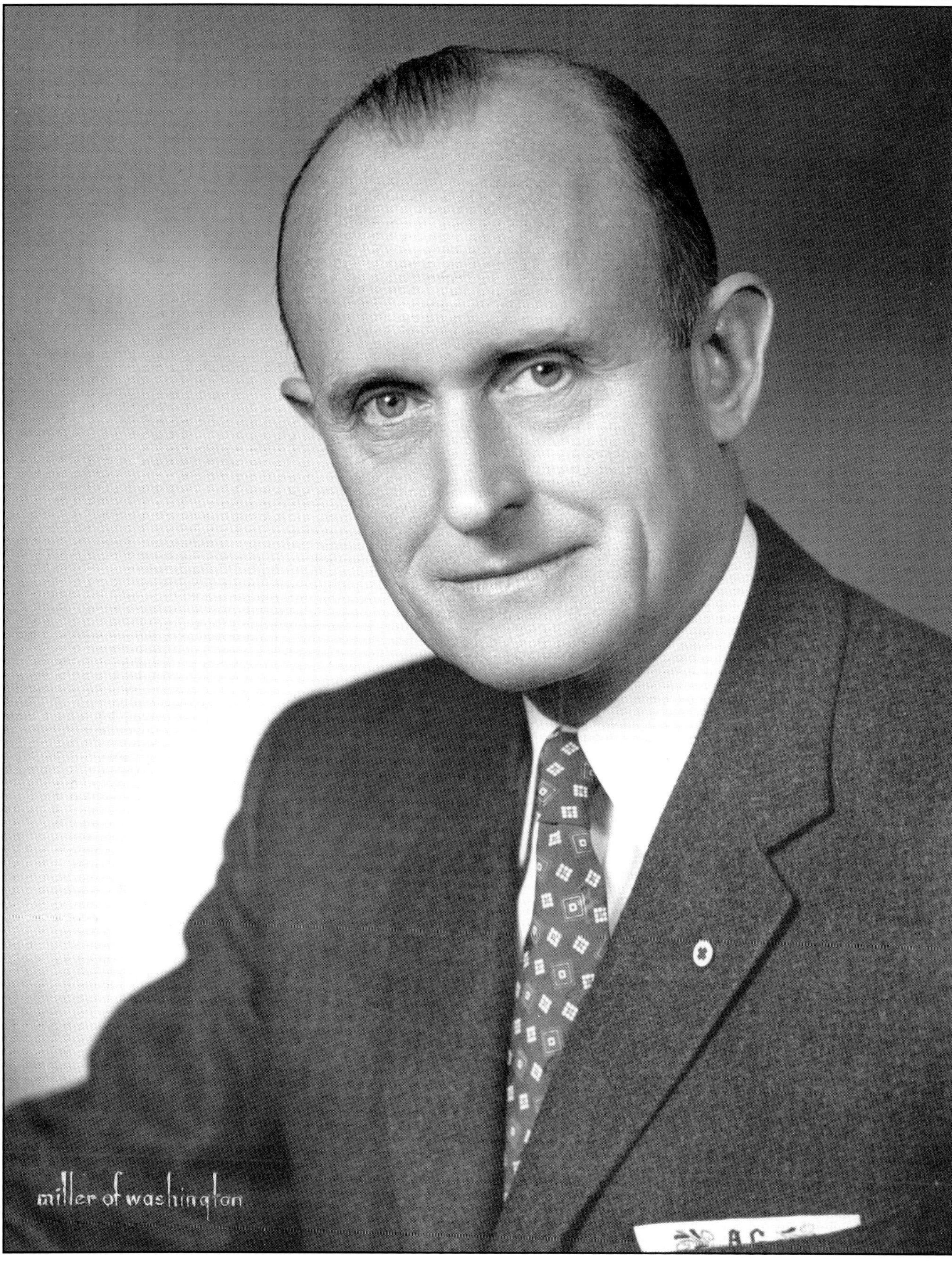

General Alfred M. Guenther
January 1, 1957-March 31, 1964

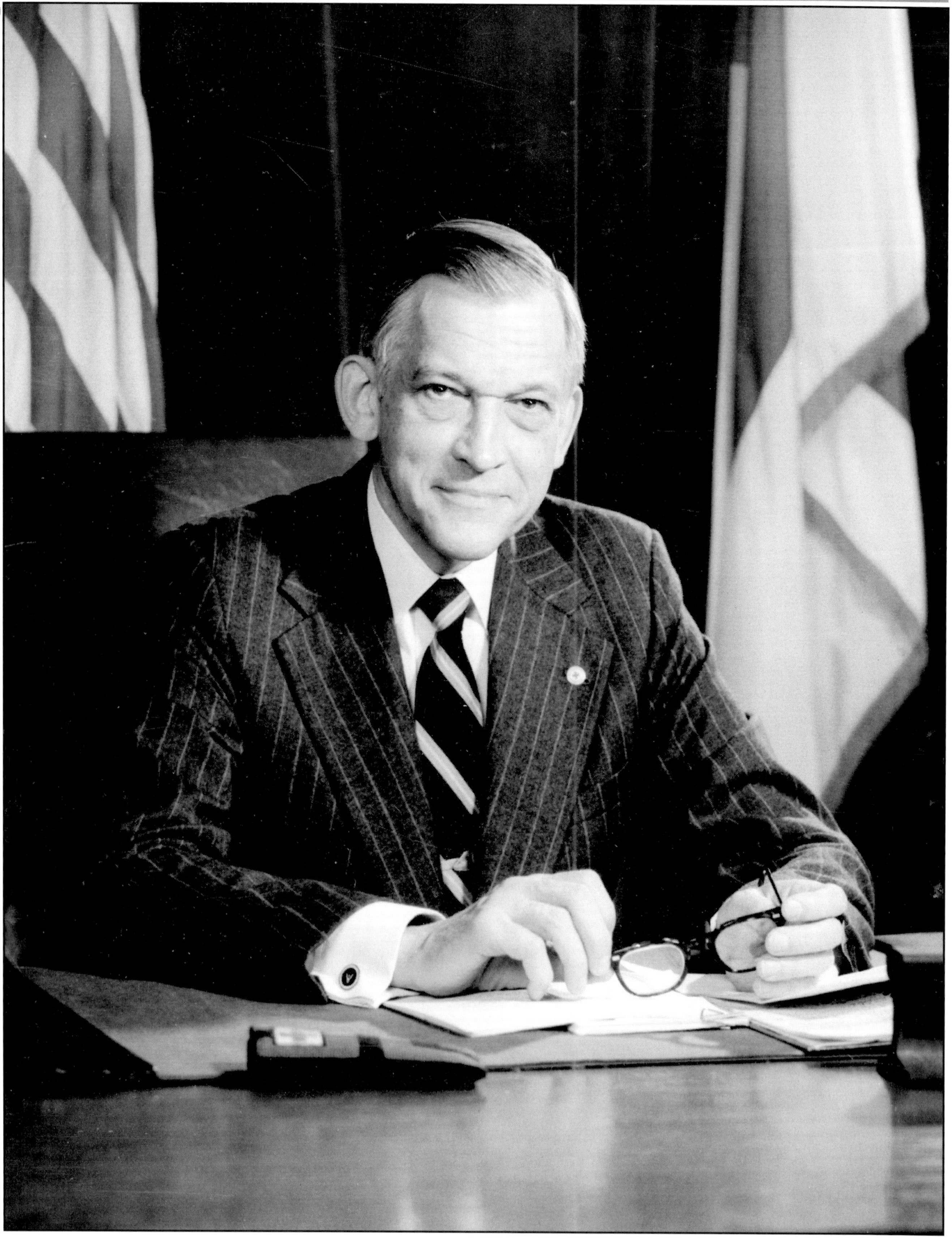

George M. Elsey
October 1, 1970-December 31, 1982

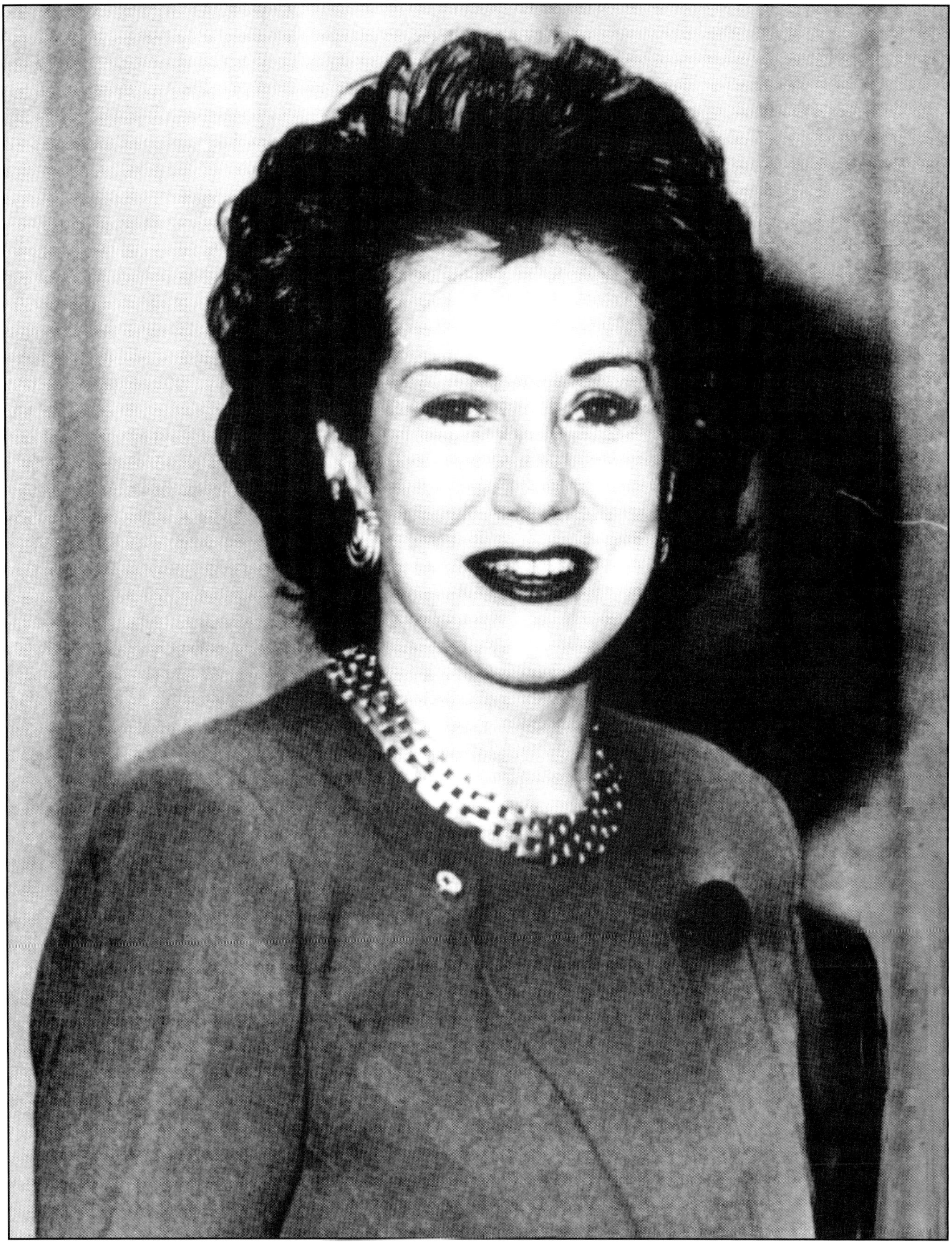

Elizabeth Dole
February 1991-November 1999

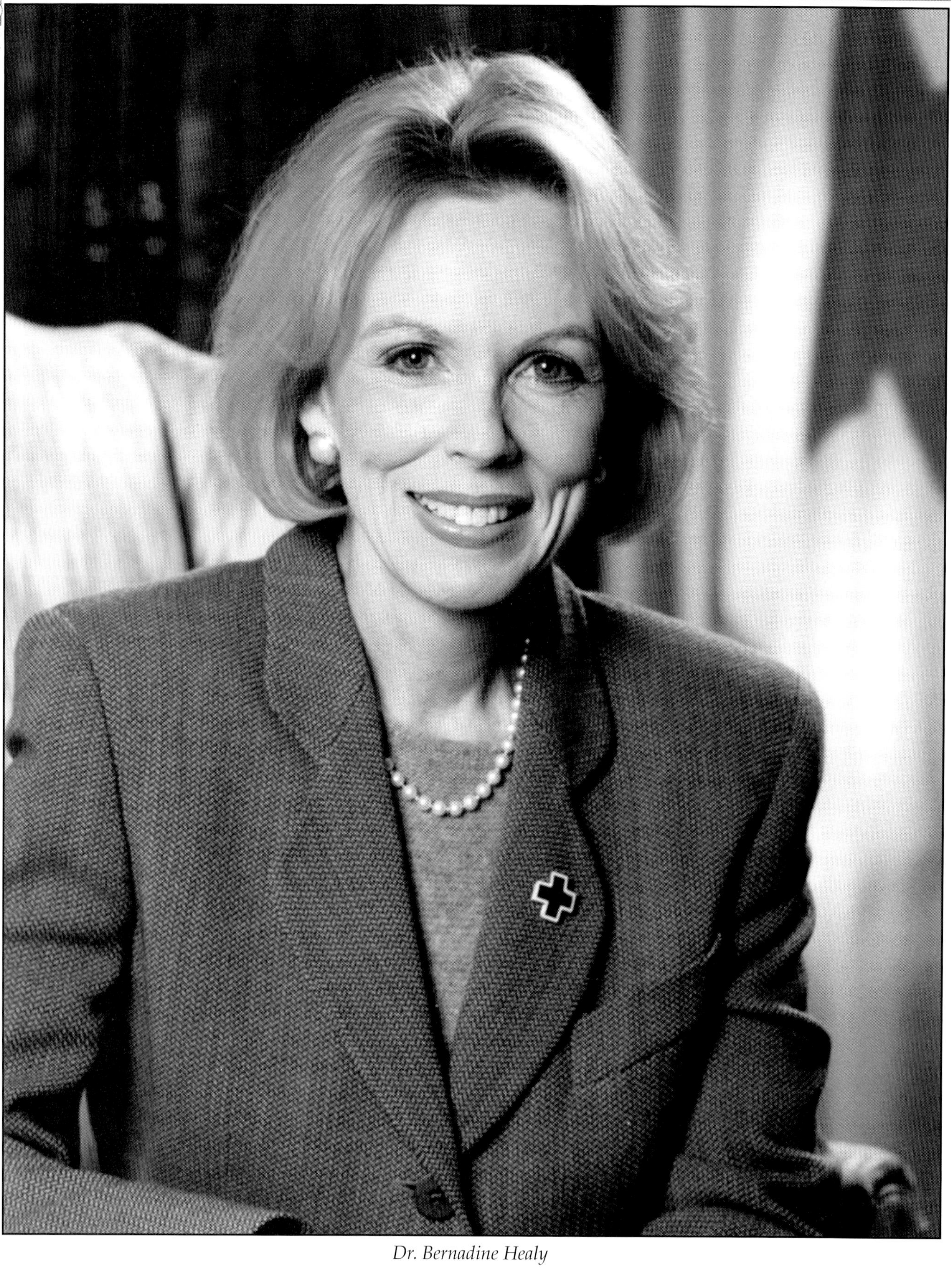

Dr. Bernadine Healy
1999-present

American Red Cross Retirees

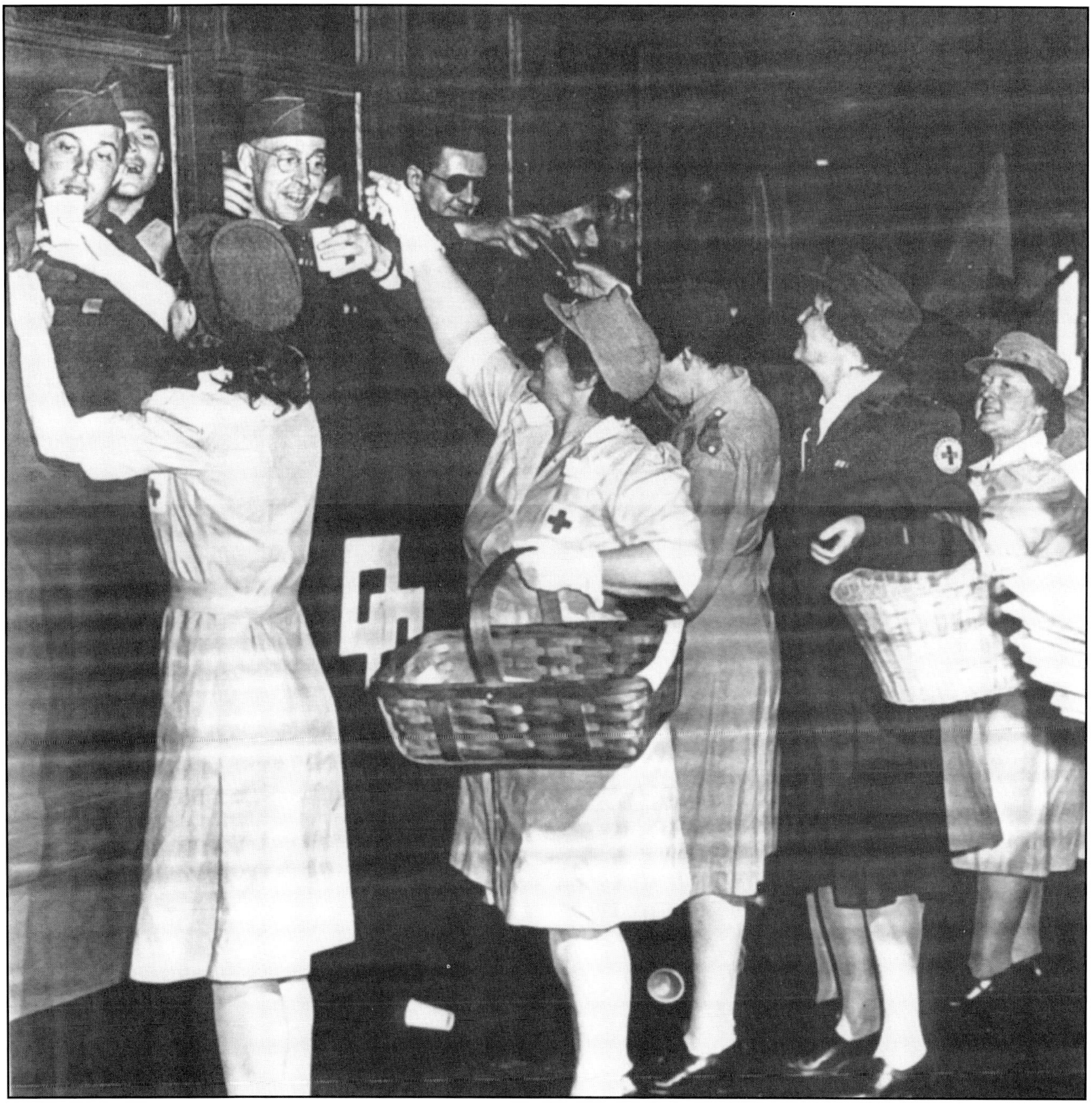

New York, May 29, 1945, American Red Cross canteen workers serving milk, coffee, ice cream, and daily newspapers to returning soldiers

ORGANIZATION AND LEADERSHIP OF THE ASSOCIATION OF RETIREES FROM THE AMERICAN RED CROSS (Jan. 2001)

8111 Gatehouse Rd., 2nd Floor
Falls Church, VA 22042
Office Telephone: (703) 206-7184
Fax: (703) 206-8545
E-Mail: mailto:wagnerb@usa.redcross.org
(For mail to officers, administrator, and Retiree editor)

NEWSLETTER EDITOR
Roy Popkin
2111 Hanover Street
Silver Spring, MD 20910-2108
(301) 587-5079
mailto:rmpopkin@att.net

RETIREE ADVISORY COUNCIL PRESIDENT
Mary Penny
449 E. Canon Green Dr.
Santa Barbara, CA 93117
(805) 685-5526
mailto:marypenny@usa.net

ADMINISTRATOR
Betty R. Wagner
7568 Cloud Ct.
Springfield, VA 22153
(703) 644-5192

EX OFFICIOR
Dexter Galusha (2001)
59 Lawrence Road
Salem, NH 03079
(603) 898-1702

OFFICERS
(Year terms expire, December)

President
Marjorie L. Miller (2001)
12 Grant Lane
Wayne, PA 19087
(610) 687-2849
mailto:ammiller12@aol.com

Vice President
James J. Hladecek (2001)
26 Pinewood Ct.
Port Townsend, WA 98368
(360) 379-0306
mailto:jamesh@Olypen.com
jim@hladecek.com

Secretary
Mary Penny (2001)
449 E. Canon Green Dr.
Santa Barbara, CA 93117
(805) 685-5526
mailto:marypenny@usa.net

Treasurer
John T. Goetz (2001)
1758 Little Conestoga Rd.
Glenmoore, PA 19343
(610) 286-6273
mailto:jamesh@Olypen.com
JohnThomasGoetz@aol.com

Assistant Treasurer
Myra Halpin (2001)
4921 Seminary Rd. #1605
Alexandria, VA 22311
(703) 845-1691
mailto:myra4921@juno.com

Mid-Atlantic Region Representative
Anthony J. Dombroski(2002)
RR#1; Box 29 Harding
Pittston, PA 18643
(570) 388-6104

STATES: Washington, D.C. (DC), Delaware (DE), Maryland (MD), New Jersey (NJ), Pennsylvania (PA), Virginia (VA), West Virginia (WV)

Eastern PA Unit
Lorraine Spencer
359 Rural Avenue
Chester, PA 19013
(610) 874-3594

Gr. Wash.-Baltimore Unit
Sally Ann Stewart
3608 Isbell St.
Silver Spring, MD 20906
(301) 946-7399

Northeastern PA Unit
Jean Bartley
324 South Hancock Street
Wilkes Barre, PA 18702
(570) 825-5321

Western PA Unit
E. Dale Jones
201 Waterdam Rd.
McMurray, PA 15317
(724) 941-6771
mailto:Zeke@nb.net Zeke@nb.net

Midwest Region Representative
Lou Gillespie (2003)
1142 Belmont Ave.
South Bend, IN 46615
(219) 234-1571
mailto:louisbg@michiana.org

STATES: Illinois (IL), Indiana (IN), Kentucky (KY), Michigan (MI), Ohio (OH), Wisconsin (WI)

Greater Cleveland Unit
Evelyn Faulkner
17213 Fernshaw Ave.
Cleveland, OH 44111
(216) 941-6898

Illiana Unit (IL & IN)
James L. Call
97 N. 656 W.
Valparaiso, IN 46385
(219) 759-6931

Indiana Unit
George Drew
1705 Forest Valley
Ft. Wayne, IN 46815
(219) 749-9743

Trumbull Co. OH Unit
Patricia C. Treisch
366 Willard Ave., S.E.
Warren, OH 44483
(330) 393-0376

Mountain West Region Representative
Ira B. Huggins (2002)
715 S. Clinton St., 7A
Denver, CO 80231
(303) 341-0779

STATES: Arizona (AZ), Colorado (CO), Idaho (ID), Montana (MT), Nevada (NV), New Mexico (NM), Utah (UT),Wyoming (WY)

Colorado Unit
Harry W. Shade
8517 West 8th Ave.
Lakewood, CO 80215
(303) 234-9389

North Central Region Representative
Madeline R. Merriman (2002)
4075 West 51st St. #310
Edina, MN 55424
(952) 927-4413

STATES: Iowa (IA), Kansas (KS), Minnesota (MN), Missouri (MO), North Dakota (ND), Nebraska (NE), South Dakota (SD)

Upper Midwest Unit
Gordon Heininger
796 E. Bellwood Ave.
St. Paul, MN 55117
(651) 772-2300

Gr. St. Louis Unit
James E. Bowling
12447 Leigh Lane
Maryland Heights, MO 63043
(314) 878-2078
mailto:jbowling@freewwweb.com
bowlingjebb@juno.com

Northeast Region Representative
Philip Chapman (2003)
408 George Washington Tnpk.
Burlington, CT 06013
(860) 673-8813
mailto:chapmanp@cre8v.com

STATES: Connecticut (CT), Maine (ME), Massechusetts (MA), New Hampshire (NH), New York (NY), Puerto Rico (PR), Rhode Island (RI), Vermont (VT), Virgin Islands (VI)

Buffalo New York Unit
Helen Schweitzer
6 East Spring Street
Williamsville, NY 14221
(716) 632-3018

Connecticut Unit
Officers being selected April 2001

Gr. New York Unit
Angelo R. Cinti
27 Ashley Drive
Delran, NJ 08075
(856) 824-0248
mailto:nancycinti@aol.com

New England Unit
John H. (Jack) Carroll, Jr.
5 Sherry Dr.
Andover, MA 01810
(508) 475-2737

Pacific Region Representative
Lee Pritchard (2003)
8424 N. Nevada St. Apt.345
Spokane, WA 99208
(509) 465-3094
mailto:Jstroud6@aol.com
LPritc466@aol.com

STATES: Alaska (AK), California (CA), Hawaii (HI), Oregon (OR), Washington (WA), Guam (GU)

Evergreen State (WA) Unit
Corinne Barnes
1200 Lincoln St. #115
Bellingham, WA 98226
(360) 734-5548

Northern CA Unit
Pete Ashen
67 Cityview Way
San Francisco, CA 94131
(415) 550-8196
mailto:ashen@crossnet.org

Oregon Unit
Helen Penk
22530 NW Gillihan Rd.
Portland, OR 97231
(503) 621-3542

Southern CA Unit
Kay Lorance
21852 W. Alamogordo Rd.
Saugus, CA 91350
(661) 296-4771
mailto:kayjim@greenheart.com

Southwest Region Representative
Harold D. Denny (2001)
6153 Masters Dr.
Shreveport, LA 71129
(318) 686-5525
mailto:breid19191@aol.com

STATES: Arkansas (AR), Louisiana (LA), Oklahoma (OK), Texas (TX)

Greater Houston TX Unit
Sherman B. Fant
12514 Hazelwood Lane
Houston, TX 77077
(281) 493-2802

Louisiana Unit
Harold D. Denny
6153 Masters Dr.
Shreveport, LA 71129
(318) 686-5525

South Central Texas Unit
Kent Hoffman
8010 Hickory Forest
San Antonio, TX 78239
(201) 946-1205
mailto:khoffman1@freewwweb.com
kenth1@netzero.net

Southeast Region Representative
Donald Northey (2001)
57 Oakview Circle
Ormond Beach, FL 32176
(904) 441-1564
mailto:nicon@gateway.net

STATES: Alabama (AL), Florida (FL), Georgia (GA), Mississippi (MS), North Carolina (NC), South Carolina (SC), Tennessee (TN)

Carolinas Unit
Doug Ambrose
6025 Crabtree Rd.
Columbia,SC 29206
(803)787-6955
mailto:ambrosed@bellsouth.net

Central Florida Unit
Margaret Tinkham
4032 Yacht Court
Winter Park, FL 32792
(407)671-4764

Florida Suncoast Unit
Barbara Hamilton
4145 Moss Oak Place
Sarasota, FL 34231
(941) 921-9250
mailto:BAH2762@aol.com

Georgia Unit
Chet Somerville
3605 Henley Park Court
Atlanta, GA 30340
(770) 723-9511

Gulf Coast Unit
Lee Kemp
3062 Aspen Drive
Mobile, AL 36693
(334) 666-7337

Representatives at Large

Edgar C. (Bud) Good (2002)
187 Sawlog Rd.
Gore, VA 22637
(540) 858-3307
mailto:gooderth@mnsinc.com

Ervin R. Oberschmidt (2003)
29 Fairway Dr.
Southgate, KY 41071
(606) 781-7433
mailto:janervo@gateway.net
JVOberschmidt@Juno.com

Gil Tills (2003)
15 Gagama Court
Brevard, NC 28712
(828) 884-5250
mailto:gtills@juno.com

Committees and Chairmen
Membership

Finance
James Hladecek
26 Pinewood Ct.
Port Townsend, WA 98368
(360) 379-4172
mailto:jim@hladecek.com

Nominations
Philip Chapman
408 George Washington Tnpk.
Burlington, CT 06013
(860) 673-8813
mailto:chapmanp@cre8v.com

Financial Development
Angelo Cinti
27 Ashley Drive
Delran, NJ 08075
(856) 824-0248
mailto:nancycinti@aol.com

Services and Programs
Barbara Hamilton
4145 Moss Oak Place
Sarasota, FL 34231
(941) 921-9250
mailto:BAH2762@aol.com

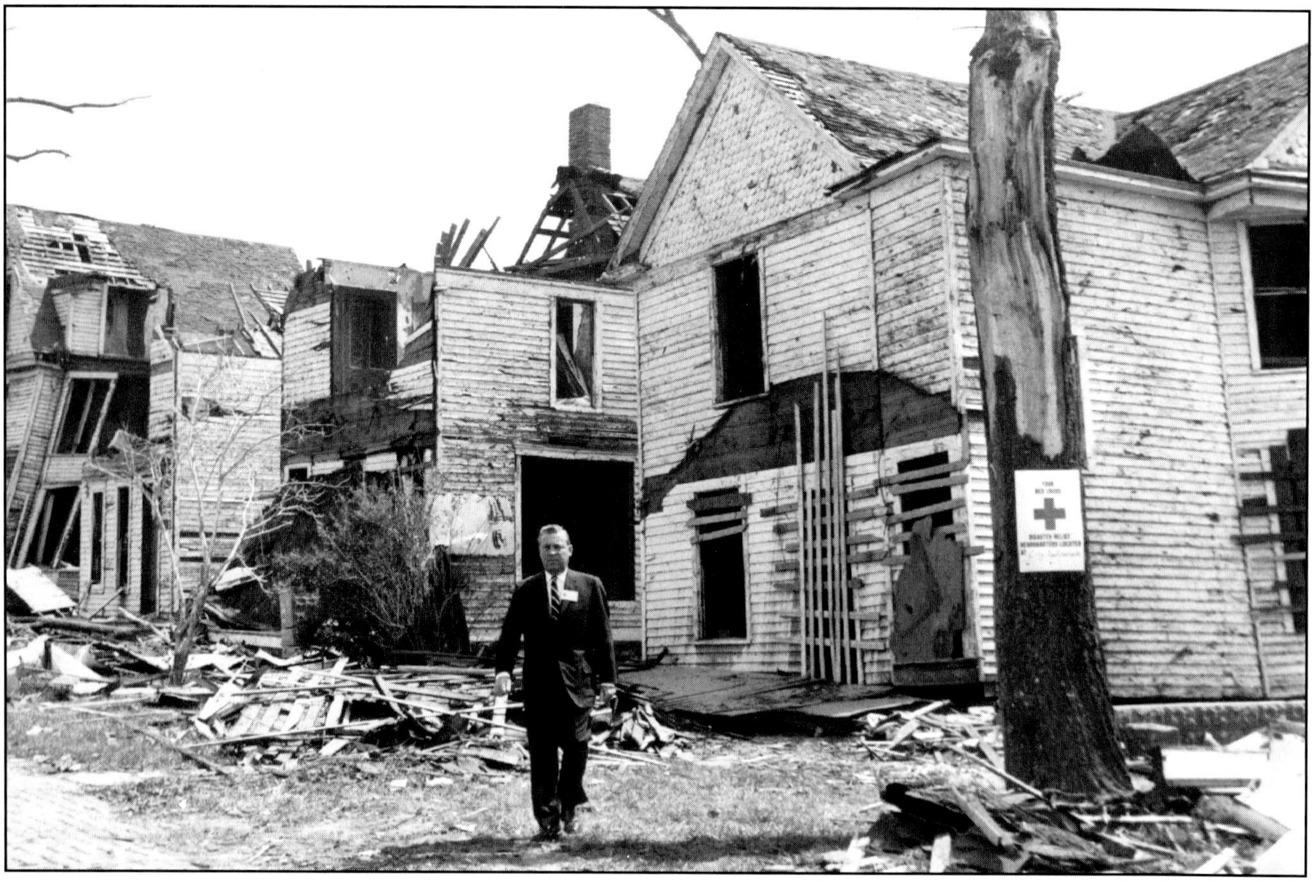

Kansas tornadoes, 1966

Red Cross Retirees...

**Editor's note - This is the official roster of the ARARC as provided to the publisher. It was the most current version available at time of publication.*

Rebecca D. Abernathy
Irene Abplanalp
Evelyn M. Abrams
Blossom B. Ackerman
Myrna H. Adam
Alice R. Adams
Carol Adams
Faith M. Adams
Jo Ann Adams
Lillian M. Adams
Mamie F. Adams
Caroline T. Addison
Cecelia (Mickey) Adelhardt
Mary E. Ahern
Amy Akagi
James T. Akiyama
Edith M. Albano
Verna G. Aldous
Margaret Allee
Aileen T. Allen
Carolyn B. Allen
Lucile M. Allen
Mary L. Allen
Priscilla Allen
Willie B. Allen
Nancy Allis
Sylvia Allred
William J. Ambrogio
Douglas W. Ambrose
Richard W. Ambruster
Raymond J. Amiro
Nancy J. Amsden
Iva F. Amundson
Audrey A. Anderson
Beverly J. Gerkin Anderson
Frank R. Anderson
Gayle M. Anderson
Harlan Anderson
Hildur H. F. Anderson
Linden N. Anderson
Lisette M. Anderson
Marjorie G. Anderson
Mary Lee B Anderson
Paul M. and Gene Anderson
Roy Anderson
Virginia Ann Anderson
Frances K. Andrews
Gloria M. Applegate
Margaret B. Arazi
Vincent Arlotta
Jean W Armstrong
Ruth E. Armstrong
Nancy M. Arnebold
Marilyn Arras
Margaret B. Arthur
Marilyn F. Asby
Pete Ashen
James C. Ashley
Don R. Atkinson
Jimmy R. Atkinson
Connie M. Augustine
Mr. Norman R. Augustine
Isobel C. Auld
Bertha I. Axtell
Lucille L. Babroski
Ferne E. Bachman
Margaret E. Badaracco
Amon L. Baer
Lorean E. Bahls
June E. Bailey
William A. Bailey
Bobby Baines
Rachel Keene Bair
Dora Elizabeth Baker
Dorothy M. Baker
Mary B. Baker
Katarina Bakic
Melva B. Bakkie
Carolyn N. Banks
Susan C. Bauman
Lorene M. Barber
Nell D. Barker
Patricia S. Barker
Miriam A. Barnard
Corrinne L. Barnes
Elena M. Barnes
Dorothy Reiss Barros
Lois V. Barth
June L. Barthol
Ann E. Bartholomew
Jean G. Bartley
Mary C. Basile
Ina Bass
Ruth M. Bateman
Joyce M. Battell
Mildred W. Battin
Maxine Bauer
Margie B. Beare
Fannye Beaty
Robert P. Beaver
Gary A. Becker, M.D.
Helen L Beckman
Ruth J. Beckman
Gloria Beckwith
Sidney M. Beeson
James P. Begansky
Mary R Behr
Eileen M. Beier
Ellen D. Belcher
Bertha E. Bell
Ida Bell
Mary V. Bell
Mildred A. Benaski
William G Benavitz
Janet L. Bender
Laura B. Bennett
Shirley A. Benskin
Eleanor C. Bent
Nancy H. Bentley
Robert L. Berg
Ruth H. Bergeson
Sheldon I. Bergeson
Marie G Bernier
Selma M. Bernstein
Evelyn P. Berrigan
Jean D Berry
Frances Beuttel
Helen J. Bewick
Betty L. Bianco
Vinnie M. Biberdorf
Lawrence L. Bickford
Everett Bidwell
Enso V. Bighinatti
Beatrice E. Binner
Ruth E. Binns
Helen Birr
Donald B. Bishoff
Richard Bjurberg
Robert and Dorothy Blackburn
Chandler J. Blackington
Wilma Blakeman
John W. Blaker
Joseph M. Blassie
Julia M. Blaszcak
William G. Blau
Herbert L. Blom
Judy A. Blume
Rosanna Blunt
Theresa C Boehm
Norman T. Boggs
Ruth P. Bogorad
Richard M. Bolyard
Rachael L. Bond
Lewis G. Bondurant
Ida Borgstedt
Zora P. Borich
Adella A Bosler
Helen V. Bosserman
Carol D. Bostrom
Norman G. Bottenberg
Robert E. Bouffard
Mary C. Bowers
Kathryn M. Bowler
Rich Bowles
James E. Bowling
Virgina F. Bowser
Dorothy Boyce
Charles Scaife Boyd
Maria K. Boyd
Donald H. Boyette
Marjorie J. Boylan
Neal J. Boyle
Margaret L. Bradfield
Nannie Bradley
John R. Brady
Regina F. Brady
Marie C. Brandl
Barbara McCloud Brandt
Alice M. Brassard
William E. Braye
Joel K. Breitenhirt
Myra Bremer
Abby Brent
Frances Lee Brent
Marcia L. Breskin
Wayne J. Brewer
Elaine H. Brice
Virginia E. Bridges

Pauline A. Briesemeister
Dorothy S. Briggs
Elizabeth B. Brizendine
Laverne Brodie
Frederick A. Brodt
Ann Brokloff
Karriet F. Bronwe
Wanda S. Brooks
Eleanor M. Broomhall
Ann P. Brower
Barbara J. Brown
Gloria Brown
Jean E. Brown
Margaret A. Brown
Roy H. Brown
Sophie E. Brown
Willard L. Brown
Arlyne W. Brown-Shirk
Harriet F. Browne
Harvey G. Brugge
Cora Pauline Brumfield
Harriet Brunner
Vivien A. Bucher
Lorine B. Buckalew
Lucile A. Bugbee
Khanh Bui
J. Gary Bunch
Ellen H. Burgess
Eugene D. Burke
James J. Burke
Mary P. and Florence M. Burke
Mary R. Burke
Thomas F. Burke
Jim S. Burleson
Charles R. Burnett
A. Joyce (Joy) Burnham
Barbara N. Burns
Robert F. Burnside
Betty C. Burton
Betty J. Butler
Emily Nord Butler
Hyatha B. Butler
Pearl E. Butler
Peggy Butler
Louis Buttgen, Jr.
Harold S Buttman
Marguerite Buttolph
Clifton B. Byrd Jr.
Helen G. Cahill
Patrick R. Cahill

Charles W. Cairns
Bernice P. Caldwell
Lynette F. Caldwell
Narce Caliva
James L. Call
Jane E. Call
Gloria A. Callahan
Esther W. Cameron
Janice Camp
Edvia Campbell
Joan M. Campbell
Yoshiko M. Campbell
Ella M. Campilongo
Enrique J. Canas
Anne E. Cappello
Irene Caprari
Rhea Lee Carey
Jean Carlson
Ralph E. Carlson
Elsa Gunvor Carlsson
Mildred Carney
Joseph P. Carniglia
Eliette G. Carroll
John H. Carroll Jr.
Betty A. Carron
Benito Cartagena
Agnes N. Carter
Dorothy M. Carter
Mary E. Caruthers
James Casey
Billie J. Cass
John B. Cataldo
Vincent J. Celeste
Floyd S. Chadwick Jr.
Donald A Chapman
Mary Louise Chapman
Philip H. Chapman
San Gabriel Valley Chapter
Edna J. Charles
Charles W. Chase
Ruth T. Chase
Mr. Pete Chavez
Desun Chen
Patricia L. Chen
David J. Chesney
Rosemary E. Childers
Doreen K.M. Ching
Frances M Chiossi
Alice A.. Chittick
George M. Chitty

Ann Rhoda Chopick
John M. Christensen
Shirley Christensen
Daniel G. Christenson
Ella Jane Christenson
Mary W. Christian
Marion N. Church
Richard L. Church
Angelo R Cinti
Anthony Ciotola
Claranell W. Clark
Dolores C Clark
Ellen L. Clark
Mary H. Clark
Neil M. Clark
Shirley J. Clark
Marian L. Clarke
Moussja Clason
Robert F. Clayton
C. Frances Cleary /Duffy
Maxine Clements
Eugene A. Clervi
Margaret B. Clifford
Maureen Y. Clinton
Elizabeth Clowes
William T. Coakley
Francis H. Cobb
Edith Cocek
Patricia D. Cochell
William F. Cochran
Mrs. Dale E. Cockrell
Thaddeus R. Cocot
Marlene B. Cohen
Jule Cohets
Sue C. Coker
Martha H Colbourn
Edward F Colburn
Ann Cole
Lucille H. Cole
Mabel W. Cole
Idalene S. Coleman
Isabel S. Colky
Gaylord W. Colle
Eva F. Collier
Donald R. and Louise Collins
Geraldine E. Combis
John J. and Phyllis Conaboy
Dorothy M. Conde
Mary E. Conlin
Raymond J Conly

Wilber D. Conn
Eleeda G. Connors
Jean P. Cook
Leola E. Cook
Marion D. Cook
Lillian Cooper
Marylou G. Cooper
Ruth Cooper-Alston
Edgar P. Copelan
Lucille E. Copenhaver
Roanne C. Coplin
Helen Copper
Alice Marie Cornet
Dr. F. Jane Cotton
Wynne H. Cotton
Katherine A. Coupar
Elizabeth D. Covey
Dale Cox
Dorothy Jean Cox
Rosemary A.Crane
Janis E. Cranford
James R. Craven
Charlotte Crawford
Martha L. Crawford
Diana H. Creecy
Loren C. Crews
Dorothy Crocker
Huron L. (Kitty) Crosby
Jean K. Crosley
Nancy Crosson
Russell D. Crouch
Jeanne S. Crumb
Laurie L. Crump
Helene Cselle
Ann M. Cumor
Elvis L. Curb
Margaret B Curlee
Odell S. Curran
Kathleen R. Curry
Gloria Curtis
June W. Dahl
Miriam B. Dahlke
Dorothy G. Dammarell
Margaret R. Danielson
Mildred B. Dantzig
Fleeda Darby
Robert L. Darling
Martha A. Darrow
Yvonne K. Daubenspeck
Helen G. Long Davidson

Hattie Sue Davies
Anjalette K. Davis
Doris M Davis
Edna L. Davis
Ralph E. and Sara Davis
Joyce R. Dawson
Mary Jane Day
Georgina De Los Rios
Virginia De Simone
Barbara M. Dean
Margaret P. Dean
Darlyne P. Deckant
Edith Decker
Reno W. Del Grande
Santos L. Dela Pena
Mary J. Dell
Barbara Delong
Elizabeth Denman
Harold D. and Lois Denny
Richard O. Denston
David A. and Kathleen Denton
Rose Depoian
June M. Dermody
Marjorie J. Deroy
G. Deruiter
Jordan Derwin
Jo Ann E. Deslandes
Grace W. Despot
Katharine H. Destler
Marjorie M. Detsch
Edward L. Deutch
Monica H. Dewulf
Sharon L. Dibble
Wendell D. Dibrell
Janet L. Dick
Olive M. Dickinson
Roger W. Dickson
John A. Didsbury
Ethel E. Diefendorf
Susan M. Dikeman
Richard V Dillenbeck
Dorothy A. Dilley
Dorothy D. Dimmick
Regina M. Dinser
Agnes J. Ditsky
Robert E. Doan
Robert E. Doan
Jackson E. Doar
Aloysius J. Dobosh
Ellamae (Kip) Dodds

Catherine B. Doehler
Grace M. Dolan
Anthony J. Dombroski, Jr.
Frank Donahue
Michael J. Donlan
Gloria W. Donnan
Margaret A. Donnell
Mary Donovan
Helen B. Dopsovic
Beverly Doran
John L. Doran
Patt Dorrell
Adine E. Douglas
Frances P. Douglass
Norma M. Dowdle
Mary Louise Dowling
Mary Louise Dowling
Grace Downie
Ruth N Doyle
Ruth Draper
George D. Drew
Roger I. Drew
Dorothea Driscoll
Margaret G. Duffy
Jean M Dugan
Marcella L. Dugan
Mary Pritchard Dugan
Clarke R. Duncan
Priscilla C Dunn
Rose N. Dunn
Rowlyn W. Duprey
Dorothy L. Duval
May F. Dykes
Elinor Eakin
Robert O. Earl
Sadie Earl
Frances M. Easley
Ted Easley
Charlotte K. Easter
Jane C. Ebert
Marian A. Ebner
Susan C. Edgerton
Eleanor F. Edgington
Bob L. Edwards
Jean M. Edwards
Violet Whitaker Edwards
Hazel A. Eggleston
John J. (Jack) Ekin III
Mary M. Eldridge
Norma S. Eldridge

Glenn M Ellis
Dr. Inez W. Elrod
George M. Elsey
Charles M. Elsom
Pauline C. Endress
Emma S. Enoch
Frank J. Erbacher
Virginia C. Erwin
Catherine R. Estep
Willie B. Estes
Patricia A. Ettensohn
Helen L. Ettlin
Myrtle A. Evans
Nicholas Fachilla
Geneva H. Fadeley
Gordon M. Fader
Betty J Falzgraf
Doye L. Fannin
Sherman B. Fant
Donna Farley
Henry B. Farley
Johnnie L. Farrier
Evelyn Croft Faulkner
Evelyn L. Fay
Anne M Fears
John J. Featherstone
Edna Jo Fecht
M. Joan Fedewa
Gertrude R. Feinstein
Theresa Feldman
Suzanne F. Felix
Janice C. Fellman
Glenn Ferges
George N. Ferguson
Palmore A. Ferrell
Lucille B. Ferrier
Helen Finch
Myrtle D. Fine
Julius Harry Finkle
Patricia Ann Fiske
Maurice Flagg
Virginia A. Flaherty
Marian E. Flanagan
Frances C. Flannery
Gwendolyn M. Floro
Ruth T. Flynn
Charles S. Fodor
Helen M.P. Foehner
Robert E. Foiles
Genevieve C. Foley

Paul J. Foley
Alexander G. Fontas
Cheryl L. Ford
Joan Foreman
Frances M. Forrester
Doris G. Forson
Patricia J. Forst
Vivian L. Forsyth
Patricia A. Fosdick
Raymond L. Fosselman
Kathleen M. Foster
Marion R. Foster
Greta W. Fountain
Marcella M. Fountain
Freda Fox
Ruth M. Franklin
Joann H. Frazier
Donald Fredell
Virginia M. Freeman
William J. Freeman
Ruth A. Freitag
Betty Freshwater
Rayma L. Fretwell
Deborah L. Frey
Ronald I. Frick
Leonard I. Friedman
Jeannette M. Fritsche
Ethel M. Fritz
Virginia H. Frizzell
Marie M. Fuess
Mary E. Fugate
Berenice B. Fugge
Elizabeth Furman
Alorson W. Fussell
Alorson W. Fussell
William Robert Gabehart
Robert E. Gaddis
Virginia W. Gaddis
Walter Gagola
Marie L. Gailus
Lavonne E. Galbraith
Tecla E. Galdo
Pamela S. Gall
Daniel Gallagher
Bert E. Galloway
Dexter D. Galusha
Joan A. Gane
Barbara J. Gardiner
Virginia Lee Gareri
Mabel H. Garner

C. B. Garrett
William Andrew Garrison
Jack P. Garver
Bernice W Gaskins
Marjorie E. Gaunt
Ernest W. Gayman
Gertrude A. Gee
C. Paulette Geer
Natalie C. Gerace
Julia H.M. Germ
Betty A. Gesek
Salvadore Giammona
James S. Gibb
Marion L Gibson
Robert R. Gibson
Dorothy F. Gilbert
Jane H. Gilbert
Kathleen V. Gilbride
Kathleen V. Gilbride
Ann C Gilfillan
Bonnie J. Gill
Margaret Bowers Gill
Otis M. Gillaspie
Louis B. Gillespie
Margaret H. Gillespie
Mary E. Ginnan
Arline Glatzer
Barbara J. Gleason
Gladys M. Gleason
Gladys Gleich
Kathleen M. Glossner
Ralph E. Gode
Marie J. Godleske
John T. Goetz
Eva Gold
Nelle Gold
Henrietta Goldfeder
Alice B. Gollnick
Amelia Gomez
Freda W. Gomez
Susie A. Gonzalez
Patricia J. Good
Edgar C. Good Jr.
Howard Goodman
Margaret W. Goodman
Rob G. and Vera Gordon
Ruth Straub Gordon
Stanley A. Gordon
Annabella Gorham
Kathleen Gorin
Jacqueline S. Gorman
Margaret Gormley-Chapman
Marilyn A. Gosser
Henriette C. Gould
Loretta Goydos-Hrdlicka
Orice F. Gracey
Nancy J. Graham
Karen E. Gramke
Marguerite J. Grams
June Granahan
Helen M. Grandcolas
Bernard M. Grandjany
John O. Grant, III
Myrtle F. Grauer
John W. Gray
Diana H. Greecy
Barbara R. Green
Daniel Green
Elizabeth L. Green
B. Gwendolyn Greene
Martha M. Greene
Mr. Ainsworth Greene
Opharitta Greene
Lennora B. Greenwell
Mildred G. Gregorie
Wanda K. Gregory
Robert A. Gregson
Ethel V. Greiman
Geneva P. Griffin
Georgia Griffin
Marie G. Griffin
Helen V. Grim
Margaret B Grimes
Shirley C. Grimes
Evelyn R. Grinyer
Louise M. Groome
Fred S. Groseclose
Joan M. Gross
Paul C. Grubb
Mary F. Gulliver
Mary Lynn Gully-Guettler
Virginia O. Gunter
Eugene D. Guy
Edward W. Guyette
George H. Guyette
Carolyn W. Guyn
Gerda A. Haas
Marjorie P. Hacking
Robert P. Hager
Constance Hagger
Brendan Haggerty
Barbara L. Hahn
Dorothy A Haines
Barbara J. Hall
Ella K. Hall
Jean F. Hall
Lynn H. Hall
Ruth H. Haller
Margaret P. Halligan
Myra Halpin
Barbara A. Hamilton
Joyce S. Hamilton
Rose Marie Hamilton
Linda D. Hammack
Laura I. Hammann
Dolores Hammer
Julia C. Hammersley
John K. Hamrick
Ladene Hancey-Gordyn
Eleanore P. Hand
John A. Hand
Dorothy M. Handley
Stephen V. Hanich
Betty A. Hannan
Dorothy E. Hansen
Mildred P. Hansen
Mary P. Hanson
Phillip E. Harbarger
Alice N. Hardie
Edward J. Hardy,Jr.
Thelma E. Harmon
Marian L. Harrell
Suzanne M. Harrington
Dorothy G. Harris
Price F. Harris
Ruth M. Harris
Theodore A. Harris
Iluminada Y. Hartman
Simon S. Hartman
Florence M. Harton
Virginia Lee Harvey
Lorraine E. Haulund
Frances C. Hayden
Frances E. Haynie
Lina S. Hazle
Frances Head
Rae C. Heath
Mrs. Nellie Hedberg
Patricia Crane Heider
Mary Ann Heilweck
Jean L. Heinberger
Gordon A. Heininger
John A. Held
Mrs. Charles W. Helmick
James R. Helmly
Harold D. Helms
Robert R. Helms
Johnnie N Henagan
Mollie M. Hench
Davis Henderson
Gertrude E. Hendra
Dorothy M. Heneberry
Raphael A. Henry
Winston E. Henry
Bertha Hensley
Fabiola Hensley
Hildegarde J. Herfurth
Mardella Hermann
Virgil Herring
Frances C. (Kitty) Hess
Mary E. Hess
Lorna B. Hetherington
Mildred Hethington
Clarice B. Hewitt
Joan M. Heybruck
Betty Ann Hickey
James R. and Barbara Hickey
Evelyn M. Higgins
John F. Higgins
Frances H. High
Glenn R. Hikes
Elizabeth F. Hilgert
Claire Helene Hill
Lisa R. Hill
Pearl A. Hill
Rolland Hill
Sophia M. Hill
Eleanor P. Hiller
Constance F. Hines
Lila E Hink
Frances D. Hiteshew
Alice D. Hixson
James J. Hladecek
William E. Hockman
Mary Lou Hodge
Jan H. Hodgin
Sarah M. Hodgkins
Ethel P. Hoffman
Kent Hoffman
Margaret E. Hoffman

John E. Hogan
Mary C. Hogan
Anna Cook Hohl
Florence A. Hojnacki
Charlotte V. Holcomb
Louise C Holdeman
Frank B. Holland
Mary S. Holloway
Mr. Ronald W. Holt
Bernice D. Holtz
Alice Hons
Jennings M. Hooks
Howard D. Hoops
Dorothy Hoover
Marcella L. Hopps
Virginia L. Hordinski
Thelma J. Horgan
Julian A. Horgen
Betty O. Horn
Darlene E. Horne
Ruth S. Horne
Albert C. Horrocks
S. Capps Hoshour
Arthur E. Hosker
Jeannette Hosler
Doris L. Hostetler
Mary G. House
Pauline Hovey
Bernice C. Howard
John F. Howard
William C. Howard Jr.
Martha L. Howe
Mary S. Howell
G. Mike Howes
Clarence T. Huffman
Imogene M. Huffman
Stephen T. Huffstutler
Ira B. and Charlyn Huggins
Sarah E. (Betty) Hugh
Arthur E. Hughes
Margaret A. Hughes
William F. Hughey, Jr.
June G. Hulse
Marcella J. Humphrey
Agnes E. Hunt
Shirley Ann Hunt
Martin Hunter
Mary J. (Judy) Hunter
George Hutchens
Richard F. Hutchinson

Dorothy Hutchison
George A. Hyde
Pauline Iammarino
Juanita B. Ibrahim
Helen T. Ignes
Marianne Imm
Mary O. Ingles
Sue T. Inouye
Janeen Irrgang
Thomas W. Irving
Richard C. Irwin
Mary R Ives
Fannie May Izard
Eloise D. Jackson
J. C. Jackson
Nadine R. Jackson
Paul D. Jackson
June M. Jacobs
Paul R. Jacobsen
Bette A. James
Gertrude M. James
Marie C James
Marion Woll James
Grace Jamisongordon
Cora Jenkins
Lewis Jenkins
Joan S. P. Jensen
Patricia M Jermon
Alice L. Jernigan
Joan Joesten
Alice A. Johnson
Anna L. Johnson
Harold L. Johnson
Joan Johnson
Johnnie M. Johnson
Lloyd Johnson
Rose R. Johnson
Terry C. Johnson
Vera D Johnson
Florence M. Johnston
Susan M. Johnston
John W. Johnstone
E. Dale Jones
Jo Anne Jones
Lawrence L. Jones
Linda J. Jones
Myrtle Blanche Jones
Rev. Daniel G. Jones
Judith G. Josephson
Helen Jovanovic

Richard M. Joyce
Robert M. Joyer
Janette R. Julien
Bette A. Juneau
Albert S Justus
J.A. and M.Jane Kaczmarek
George J. Kaffenberg
Roxie M. Kalashian
Teru Kanba
John T. Kane
Alice T. Kaneko
Jane V Kappel
Mary L. Karabaich
Harold M. Kase
Rosemary A Kaskie
John Kassab
Lola E. Kathcart
Carole K. Kauffman
Fonda Kaylor
Louise J Keating
Joan M. Keenan
Sarah E. Keene
Shirlee C. Kegerreis
Thomas J. Kelleher
Richard Kellman
Betty G. Kelly
Brian V. Kelly
Dorothy J. Kelly
Esther C. Kelly
Irene Kelly
Mary E. Kelly
C. Eugene and Ethel Keltner
Lee and Opal B. Kemp
Jerome M. Kennedy
Sheila A. Kennedy
Sandra Kennedy-Owes
Alberta C. Kenny
Hyla E. Kensler
Shirley A Kenworthy
Joan E. Kessler
Elbert E. Kiefer
Ruth J. Kiely
Kathleen Kienstra
Robert E. Kilbride
Martha Killebrew
Rachel T. Kimel
Carol A. King
Loretta King
Patricia King
Juanita V. Kingdon

George and Marian Kingston
Katherine V. Kingston
Ernest J Kinney
John W. Kirby
Bertha Kirkendall
Louise A. Kirkpatrick
Gladys Kitchen
Margaret J. Klass
Patricia A. Kline
Dorothy Kloepper
Joan K. Klopf
Rosemary Kmiecik
E. Gail Knight
Elizabeth B. Knox
Horst Koeppen
Fred H. Koeth
M. Helen Koleff
Selma Kolend
John J. Komp
Emelie L. Konold
George S. Koontz
Betty Koplin
Kathryn C. Kopp
Eileen M. Kraft
Mary G. Kramer
Florence H. Krauska
Margaret M. Krell
Marjorie Kroupa
Gloria F Kuczminski
Michael J. Kudelka
Christine A. Kuhn
Joanne A. Kulp
E. Patricia Kunst
Felix Kurtsman
Arthur F. Kussman
Pearl M. Kusunoki
Madeline E. Laake
Dr. R. Howard Lackay
Eleanor Lacquement
Norbert B. Lacy
Dale Laforest
Ann Marie Lally
J. Sam Lamb
Eleanor B. Lammers
Anne C. Lancaster
Michael R. Lander
Edith M. Lane
Georgia Lanier
Marie R. Lantz
Romeo A. Laramee

Ida L. Larkin
Irene E. Larson
Kalen M. Larson
Margaret W. Larson
Willamae Larson
Helen Latimer
Leslie L. Lauderdale
Idalyne G. Lawhon
John Lawless
Hilda I. Lawrence
Joanne Lawrence
Olga M. Lawson
Paul Lawson
Lyle J. Layer
Wilda M. (Jody) Layton
Joan K. Lazarus
Pauline Lazarus
Patricia Leary
Arnetta L. Leas
Barbara J. Leatherwood
Rosamond B. Lebeau
Edythe Lebosky
Katherine P. Lechthaler
Grace A Leckliter
Bess M. Lee
Carlos E. Lee
Emily R. Lee
Eunice M. Lee
Robert A. Lee
Virgilena Lee
F. Elizabeth Lefeber
Ruth E. Lehman
Elsie F. Lehr
Penny K. Leistiko
Claire A. Lemere
Anne T. Lemieux
Leona Lenicheck
Dorothy L Lepine
Mary D. Lesho
Elma M. Leslie-Petroff
Cecil D. Lettis
Johanna M. Levan
Dr. Jack J. Levin
Annette Levine
Edith Gold Levitt
Phyllis J. Levy
Suzanne D. Lewandowski
Doris E Lewis
Emil F. Lewis
Sue M. Lewis

Mary Virginia Lewitz
Cora Lillian
Walter J. Lincoln
Daniel C. Lindstrom
Ruth B. Linvill
Betty J Lisle
Eleanora A. Little
Janet Livingston
Pat Francis J. Lloyd
Ruth S. Lloyd
Lucille M. Loftis
Shirley W. Loggans
Nina Lombardo
Anne M. Longo
Gladys L. Longoria
Warren Looker
John W. Loomis
Margaret C. Loos
Louise M. Lopez
Kathryn L. Lorance
Marie B. Lottinger
Georgann Lowe
William C. Lowe
Dolores M. Lowery
Robert H. Lucey
Catharine Luhman
Jean L. Lundquist
Nellie F. Luther
Jack Luttrell
Dorothy I. Lyles
Elaine M. Lynch
Margrethe Lyngholm
Mildred Lynn
Pauline R. Lyon
Mary E. Lyons
Margaret M. Lytton
Roberta W. Macaulay
R.E. MacConnell
James M. Macdonald
Sally C. Macdonald
Rose Mack
Eileen C. Madigan
Louise Madigan
Luigiana Maganuco
Robert L. Magee
Yvette C. Main
Marilyn A. Majewski
Linda E. Majul-Zayek
Florence G. Malicki
Pearl D. Mallory

Gwena L. Malody
Kathy K. Malt
Barbara Mancuso
Joan M. Mangan
June S. Manning
Edna Marcus
Helen Marine
Dr. William M. Markel
Ruth Marler
Carlton E. Martin
Elizabeth J. Martin
Ellen Martin
John H. Martin
Margaret G. Martin
Joseph C. Martinelli
Ursula J. Martinez
Helen W. Martinson
Amelia G. Martsfield
Meyer Mathis
Dorothy K. Mattern
Edna M. Matthews
Mary L. Matthews
Robinette M. Mattox
Philomena R. Matts
Jane P. Mattson
Barbara Jane Maxwell
Kathryn J. May
Sarah E. May
Barbara O. Mayne
Margaret Jeanene Mayson
Stella M. Mazur
Vickie M McCabe
Gertrude McCafferty
Irene E. McCall
Virginia G. McCall
Rita M. McClean
Myrtle R. McComas
Dorothy McCourt
Sara L. McCullough
Mary Ann McCurdy
Genive McDaniel
James P. McDaniel
Mrs. Jane V. McDonald
Mr. D. Richard McFerson
Richard L McFeters
Doris McGaffin
Howard F. McGee
Bernice C. McGhee
Olga P. McGhee
Joseph B. McGinnis

Lee Michael McGowan
John M. McGraw
Maryrose A. McGroarty
Frank A. McGurk
Shirley McLallen
Dorothy H. McLaughlin
Mary K. McLellen
Barbara W. McLeod
William H. McNeely
Elizabeth M. McNeill
Jane McNeill
Mary C. McQuillen
Malcolm L. McRae
Lois A. Meadows
Nancy A. Means
Betty J. Mechler
Genevieve A. Meehan
Vallorie C Meehan
William E. Mehling
Judith A. Melicks
Colleen C. Meller
Angelo F Menna
Clarella H Menner
Rita Merrigan
Madeline Merriman
Anna Messina
Dorothy O. Metoxen
Audrey S. Metzler
Dorothy A. Meyer
Matthew D. Meyer
Shirley Meyer
Zelma L. Meyer
Ray Meyers
Virginia A. Mezzera
Shirley E. Michael
Rodney A. Mickelsen
June R. Middleton
Beulah I. Miles
Marvin R. Miles
Mary Ellen Miles
Donald M. Millar
Barbara A. Miller
Charlotte H. Miller
Everett W. Miller
George C. Miller
Marie C. Miller
Marjorie L. Miller
Raymond R. Miller
Robert M. Miller
Thomas D. Miller

Karoline W. Mills
Mary Minamoto
Sharon L. Minick
William J. Miracle
Beulah E. Mitchell
David E. Mitchell
Elizabeth K. Mitchell
Marvin Mitchell
Leo Mize
Vera Grace Mobley
Mary O. Mock
James R. Mockbee
Freda Mockenhaupt
Frederick W. Moeller
Sally M. Mohler
Ray W. Mohney
Gertrude Mohr
Lucia E. Mojica-Daly
James D. Monahan
Yolanda C. Monarchy
Esperanza Montero
Barbara A. Montgomery
Elizabeth A. Montgomery
Alice I Mooney
Flora Alice Moore
Horace W. Moore
Janet A. Moore
Louise B. Moore
Mary Helen Moorling
Blanche L. Morgan
Emma R. Morgan
Ella Virginia Morman
Margaret W. Morris
Mary Joan Morris
N. Patricia Morris
Ruth Morse
Hazel I. Morton
William E. Mottice
Anne K. Moye
Lila M. Muck
Bertha Mudd
Ramona Muerdter
Martha J. Mull
Mary Mullen
Brian R. Muller
Marianne F. Muller
Helen E. Mulry
Mary Lela Munday
Ruth Mundorff
Elizabeth F. Munkres

Mercedes P. Munson
Violeta Murgado-Lombardia
Anne E Murphy
Robert J. Murphy
Garland B. Murray
Janice M. Murray
John S. Murray
Annabelle Myers
Orin H. Myers
Helen Myrmel
Lydia G. Nanney
Mary D. Needham
Gladys L. Neff
Herbert C. Nelson
Marcella S. Nelson
Carlotta D. Nemeth
Joan T. Nesgoda
Maxine Newlander
Billy G. Newsome
Gail S. Newton
Jere A. Nichols
John Irvin Nichols
Kathy A. Nicolini
Marie L. Niedzielski
Miguel A Nieves
Thomas E. Noell
Tiia Nolte
Ralph and Catherine Norris
Ralph F. Norris
Donald G. Northey
Robert D. Norton
Wanda L. Norton
Stanley Gene Nudley
Waldena O'Barto
Nicole O'Connor
James F. O'Donnell
Mary D. O'Geary
Marion K. O'Hara
Margaret H. O'Keefe
Ann C O'Leary
Ruth Oberg
James F. Oberholz
Ervin R. Oberschmidt
Emily C. Ogburn
Jamie L. Oglesby
Ellen Okahara
Edith Olson
Elizabeth A. Olson
Evelyn H. Olson
James R. Olson

Roberta B. Omlor
Janet I. Oosterbaan
Rose S. Ornstein
Nola E. Osborn
Isabelle M. Osgood
Gladden Ostander
Vernon E. Ostenby
Robert M. Oswald
Lillie E. Ott
Ester Ruth Ottewell
Peter W. Overton
Margaret N. Owen
Nancy S Owen
Ralph W. Owen
Elizabeth P. Owens
Martina G. Owens
Genevieve M. Owings
Marvin W. Oxford
Doris P. Renno
Ellen V. Page
Henrietta M. Page
Tula Pagonis
Arthur B. Papineau III
Lawrence L. Parker
Robert L. Parker
Robert O. Parrish
Randi Passamaneck
Else Pasternak
Barbara Pathe
Louise T. Patrick
Heidi A. Patten
Lois J. Patterson
Ruby E Patton
Barbara R. Paul
Robert Paul
Stephen R. Pavlick
Helen K. Pawlowski
Donald T. Peak
Ethel Petersen Pearce
Lincoln E. Pearson
James W. Pecaro
Doris E. Peets
Marie Gloria Pelletier
Joseph H. Pendleton
Helen F. Penhale
Mary M. Penny
Robert K. Pentz Sr.
Anna Pepe
Lola Peressin
Betty Perez

Ophelia M. Perkins
William H. Perkins
Dorothy H. Perry
Muriel E. Perry
Vernon J. Person
Dr. Martha L. Peters
Virginia R. Peters-Martin
Virginia K. Peters-Verdi
Glenn R. Petersen
Mary L. Peterson
Noreen E. Peterson
Dale Petranech
Edith B. Pfeiffer
Bobby G. Phillips
Dula Phillips
Eileene C. Phillips
Helen A. Phillips
Hosea A. Phillips
Lucianne Phillips
Sylvia Phillips
William H. Phillips
William J. Phillips
James C. Pichon
Luz E.C. Pitterson
Joe A. Pittman
Theresa R. Pixler
Donna W. Placzankis
Mary N. Plaga
Helen R Poff
Michaela J. Pointek
John J. Pokorny
Jack and Janice Pokras
Rosalie J. Poland
Evelyn W. Pomeroy
Britt V. Pope
Roy S. and Mary Popkin
Alice H. Porter
Mary A. Porter
Mary Kay Porter
Marian E. Potters
Marguerite L. Potts
Mildred B. Powell
Paul Preston
Ann W. Priem
Lee L Pritchard
Laverne P. Prizner
Martha E. Probes
Charles A. Prohaska
Marie Alice Prsha
William O. Pugh

Virginia Pullen
Dolores Mary Purvis
Katherine W. Purvis
Helen A. Putur
Lorraine C. Pyne
Rita M. Quane
Dora A Quarles
Leonor A. Quiliza
Marie V. Quillin
Mary P. Quinlivan
Eileen Racklin
Thelma Gibson Radden
Dilys Radke
Ruth F. Rafner
Susan B. Raftery
Robert D. Ragsdale
Dorothy E. Raine
Theodore H. Rainey
Alvin B. Rakow
Eustacio Ramirez-Molina
Dale Ramsey
Mrs. Patricia J. Ramsey
Esther H. Rand
Doris Ransier
Ella M. Rast
Milton R. Rathke
Edward T. Raymond,Jr
Cynthia S. Reardon
Claude M. Reeves Jr.
Eleanor P. Reif
Karl P. Reiser
Trini F. Rendon
Waldemar Ernst Renken
William H. Reno
Mary Lou Reynolds
Nora F. Rhodes
Irene L. Rhoton
Ludmilla F. Rice
Robert W. Richard
Elizabeth B. Richardson
Rita Richardson
Womeva Richardson
Harriet B. Ridgill
Lenora O. Riggan
Patricia Riggs
Dorothy S Riley
Fern E . Riley
Marie L. Riley
Evalyn M. Ringer
Gus H. Rissman

Richard F. Roach
Leroy A. Robberson
Eleanore Robbins
Jacqueline H. Robbins
Beverly B. Robein
Ken Roberson
Dorothy Nash Roberts
Jerry C. Roberts
Mildred B. Roberts
Helen Lee Robertson
Harriet M. Robinson
Melbern Joe Robinson
Shirley A. Robinson
Sara M. Robison
Georgina (Cookie) Rodante-Spoto
Marcia A. Rodgers
Marjorie E. Rodrick
Dale E. Roe
Martha V. Roehner
Nedra M. Rogers
Barbara J. Romeiser
Donna L. Ronn
Carl A. Ross
Carol D. Ross
Mernice R. Ross
Rose Roth
Edwin D. Rounds
Thomas R. Rounds
Martha L. Royse
Helen E. Rue
Elizabeth M. Rush
Dorothy M. Russell
Grace M. Russell
John R. Russell
June M. Russell
Rina Ruttinger
Rina Ruttinger
Yolande M. Ruzak
Joseph R. Sacca
Anita J. Sadowski
Constance C. Saitta
Lillian Sakowski
Barbara B Ourand Salvani
Ernest G. Sanchez
W. J. Sande
Stephen H. Sanderson
Virginia L. Sandlin
Margaret Sanfelice
Naomi E. Casa Santa

Pete Sapon Jr.
Aphrodite F. Sarelas
Doris M. Satre
Martha V. Sauve
Doris L. Saxerud
Mary Helen Schaeffer
Zira Scheer
Rosemary A. Scheutzow
Mildred R. Schildmeyer
Ray L. Schindell
Arthur E. Schlak
Virginia M. Schmedes
Arnold P. Schmidt
Charles M Schmidt
Lorraine J. Schmidt
M. Caroline Schnabel
Elsie B. Schnier
Mary Anna Schoenfeld
Paul H. Scholz
Julian B. Schor. MD
Georgette Schottland
Edmund V. Schroback
Katherine M. Schroeder
Robert H. Schuelke
Rebecca G. Schultz
Helen A. Schulz
Douglas A. Schumacher
Marjorie L. Schuster
Edna R. Schweitzer
Helen M. Schweitzer
Marjorie Ann Schweitzer
Wanda Schweitzer
Alice R. Scipio
Linda D. Scorgie
Cory G. Scott
Katherine Scott
Linda J. Scott
Richard H. Scott
Gwenellen Scupholm
Mary Lou Seamens
Agnes C. Sears
Andrew M. Sedlack
Gene and Elinor Seevers
Dolores B. Sefchik
John L. Seibel
Virginia J. Seiler
Margaret T. Sellmayer
Helen L. Senior
Margaret Serene
Josephine M. Servitto

Mary B. Settle
Mary Helen Seymour
Harry W. Shade
Doris E Shapiro
Joan H. Shassian
Mary Ann Shaw
Gloria Sheaffer
Jane H. Sheehan
Ethel Walsh Sheldon
June E Shellhamer
Helen J. Shemtob
Glorene Shenberger
Harry A. Sheridan
Joseph A. Sheridan
William C. Sherwood, M.D.
Jessie B. Shipp
Aline B. Shoemate
Caroline M. Short
J. Frank Shouse
Gerry E. Sickles
Marie Sigerist
Rosalyn S.Silver
Sylvan Silver
Wesley E. Sime
Vivian P. Simmons
Palmer and Eloise Simpson
Emily V. Sisser
Alfred J. Skarda
Blanche E. Skidmore
Caro H. Skidmore
Helen M. Skorupski
Olive S. Skroback
Andrew Slaten
Regina Jeanne Slifka
William C. Small
Alice Smith
Barbara R. Smith
Carol M. Smith
Donna D. Smith
Elizabeth H. Smith
Ella Louise Smith
Esther H. Smith
Frances T. Smith
Harriett N. Smith
Helen J. Smith
Henry C. Smith
Irene B. Smith
Jeanne E. Smith
Jesse J. Smith
Loretta A. Smith

Marlene C. Smith
Mary B. Smith
Richard N. Smith
James M. Smyth
Alice G. Snead
Margaret R. Snellgrove
Adrene M. Snider
Joyce A. Snider
David R. Snow
Stella M. Snyder
Geraldine Sohle
Chester R. Somerville
Agnes H. Sommermeyer
Betty A. Sonnenberg
James E. Sonnie
Michael Sorbello
George P. Spain
Robert K. Spangler
E. Lorraine Spencer
Bonita P. Sperry
Carol A. Spiering
Barbara Spooner
Elizabeth Spooner
Ernest G. Sprague
H. Jerry Spruell
Carroll L. Spurling M.D.
Janet R. Stahl
Ruth D. Stalker
Daniel M. Stango
Stan Charles Staniforth
Gladys A. Stanke
Ethel Stanwix-Hay
Louise F. Steeble
Maybelle Steele
Phoebe Steffey
Jane K. Stephans
Gloria H. Stevenson
Sally Ann Stewart
Mary W. Stilp
Mary Grace Stiner
Ethel W. Stinson
Clara Lee Stoermer
Stephanie A. Stogoski
Dorothy H. Stokley
Corry E Stolk
Adelyn A. Stone
Clara Mae Stone
Evelyn B. Stone
George R.and Ora Lee Stoner
Mary Dell Stout

Cecile M. Stowe
Alice T. Stowers
Greg Strader
Charles L. Strate
Kent R. Stratford
Virginia G. Street
Mary J. Streit
Betty Stringer
Jean Strojny
John D. Stroud
Gertrude Geiger Struble
Doris L. Stuart
Phyllis L. Stuart
Constance D. Sullivan
Muriel Sullivan
Lillian Summers
Charles E. Sumner
Charles A. Super
Joan B. Sutherland
Love W. Sutphen
O'Dell W. Sutton
Dianna B. Swann
Phyllis B. Swanton
Sylvia L. Swearingen
Marie J. Sweeney
Elaine M. Sweet
Lynn Swerrie
Virginia Swisher
Dorothy B. Taaffe
Charlotte M. Tagg
James F. Tait
Patricia A. Takacs
Frances S. Tanaka
Mark A. Tannenbaum
Betty L. Tanner
Thomas F. Tatarczuk
Jean N. Tate
Betty A. Taylor
Donna E. Taylor
Erma B. Taylor
Francis M. Taylor
Helen M. Taylor
Louise St. John Taylor
Marylou Taylor
Robert F Tedder
Sarah Louise Tedder
Marvin and Nancy Teeter
Amelia G. Temer
Wallace L. Tharp
Selma A. Thatcher

Raymond E. Thayer
Nancy L. Theisman
Myrtle R. Thigpen
Adaline B Thomas
Elna M. Thomas
Geraldine N. Thomas
James E. (Jim) Thomas
Lydia H Thomas
Margaret Ann Thomas
Sarah A. Thomas
Dorothy H. Thompson
Irene M. Thompson
Margaret V. Thompson
Marjorie J. Thompson
William T. Thompson
Beverly A. Thonburn
Roxanne P. Thoreson
Lois I. Thornton
Edith E. Ott Thorpe
Ruby E. Thorwaldsen
Lillian K. Throckmorton
Dorothy A. Tillman
Gil Tills
M.E.and Edwin E. Tinkham
Mary E. Tinsley
Charles R. Tolbert
Ayako S. Tom
George Y. Torrance
Lewis W. Torrison
Inez Tory
Naomi L. Towers
Thomas J. Tracy
Margaret Trail
Hanh Van Tran
Patricia C. Treisch
Raynerd J. Troedson Jr.
Joseph R. Trombley
Eva C. Trued
John H. Tucker
Marie A. Tully
Doris V. Tuman
Florence E. Tupper
Jo Ann Turner
Richard and Caroline Turner
Janet M. Tuttle
Carol A. Tyler
Margo H. Tyler
Norma J. Uhrich
J. Marshall Upton
Arlene A. Urbanski

Maj. Gen. William R. Usher
Edward J. Valenzuela
Katherine L. Van Auken
Gerald Van Genderen
Joyce E. Van Keuren
Lucille A. Vance
Samuel W. Vance
Evelyn G. Vanderveer
Ann V. Vare
David L. Vargo
Jacqueline D. Vaughan
Julia S. Vaughan
Catherine S. Veasey
Dorothy Veith
Lucy S. Veler
Edgar Leigh Venzke
Robert D. Vessey
Hi A. Vincent
Bonnie S. Virch
Jennie Vodopivec
Carolyn M. Voelkner
Dorothy M. Vorberg
Mildred Vossler
Marian C Waddell
Dick Wagener
Helen H. Wainwright
Eloise B. Waite
Angela G Waits
Charlotte E. Walhay
Harold A. Walker
Wilber H. Walker
Clifton Wall
Donna Marie Walla
Ramona Walla
Alice Jean Walrad
Beverly C. Walsh
Helen A. Walter
Harriet Walters
Anne Ward
Mamie B. Ward
Rosemary Ward
Howard G. Warner
Virgil L. Warner, Jr.
Mary B. Warren
Mary Agnes Washington
G. Frank Waters
Janet M. Weber
Suzanne B. Weber
Joann M. Webster
Robert B. Weekley

March 17, 1942, The Red Cross in the military hospital. A rugged soldier, confined to the Fort Dix, NJ station hospital with his leg in a heavy cast, is interviewed on his preference in books by a couple of volunteer Red Cross recreational workers, known as "Gray Ladies." The "Gray Ladies" are Mrs. J.C. Wilson and Mrs. C.G. Guthrie, both from Princeton, NJ Red Cross Chapter.

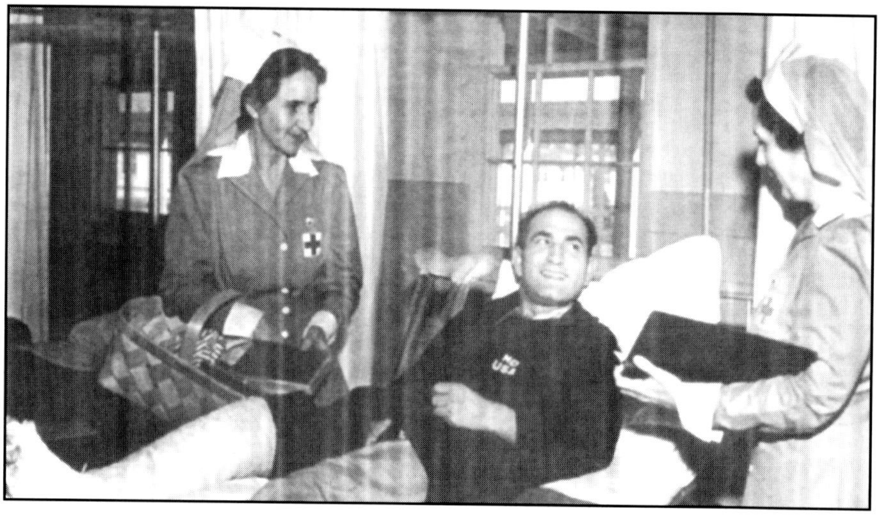

Joanne C. Weir
Norma M. Weir
Muriel Weiser
Virginia C. Weiss
Mary E. Weissbrod
Rebecca F. Welch
Dorothy Welker
Eugenia E. Wellman
William J. Wells
Margaret D. Werner
Ranghild E. Westin
Gay S. Weston
Paul D. Whalen
Erin R. Whatley
Allen W. Whear
Doris Diane Wheeler
Beulah M. White
Dortha M. White
Eileen W. Whitmire
William George Wibby
Robert G Wick
Agnes M. Widmer
Anne R. Wiesen/Brown
Guy E. Wilber, Sr.
Alice V. Williams
Angie L. Williams
Archie C. Williams
Bertha M. Williams
Catherine S. Williams
E. Janice Williams
Edna M. Williams
Elizabeth A. Williams
Eunice E. Williams
Frieda B. Williams
Herman J. Williams
James F. Williams
Marion E. Williams
Ramona Williams
Robert H. Williams
Robert J Williams
Sandra Williams
St. Elmo Williams
Johnnye Rose Williamson
Paul W. Willis
Janice L. Wilson
Margaret D. Wilson
Otis Wilson
Ruthelle Duke Wilson
Phyllis A. Wilt
Colleen S. Wincentsen
Bjarne N. Wolding
Corrine Wolfe
Mildred C. Wolfe
Nancy Wolfford
Helmer E. Wolkow
Marguerite Belz Wolter
Elizabeth H. Womer
Arlene M Wood
Eda C Wood
Frances C. Wood
Judson E Wood
Marie H Wood
Myra Jean Wood
Evelyn Jennette Woodall
Walter L. Woodward
Colleen Lee Wooley
Leanora Woolley
Mary J. Woolston
Edith M. Workman
Daniel W. Wormwood Jr.
Fern M. Worth
Ann M. Wright
Jane A. Wriston
Jean M. Wylie
Jean C. Yates
Emma Jane Yengel
Joan M. Yonki
Lucille Young
Norma G. Young
Ruth E. Young
John B. Youngs
Martha G. Yund
Mildred C. Zamiska
Dick Zamjahn
Mary Lou Zamora
Julia J Zapf
Vera Zarkoski
Ollie "Sue" Zebick
Joseph T. Zebley
Linda L. Zerbe
Paula L. Zintl
Lisa Zolar
Ann M. Zoll
Velma H. Zolzer
Robert G. Zubrod
Walter E. Zukowski

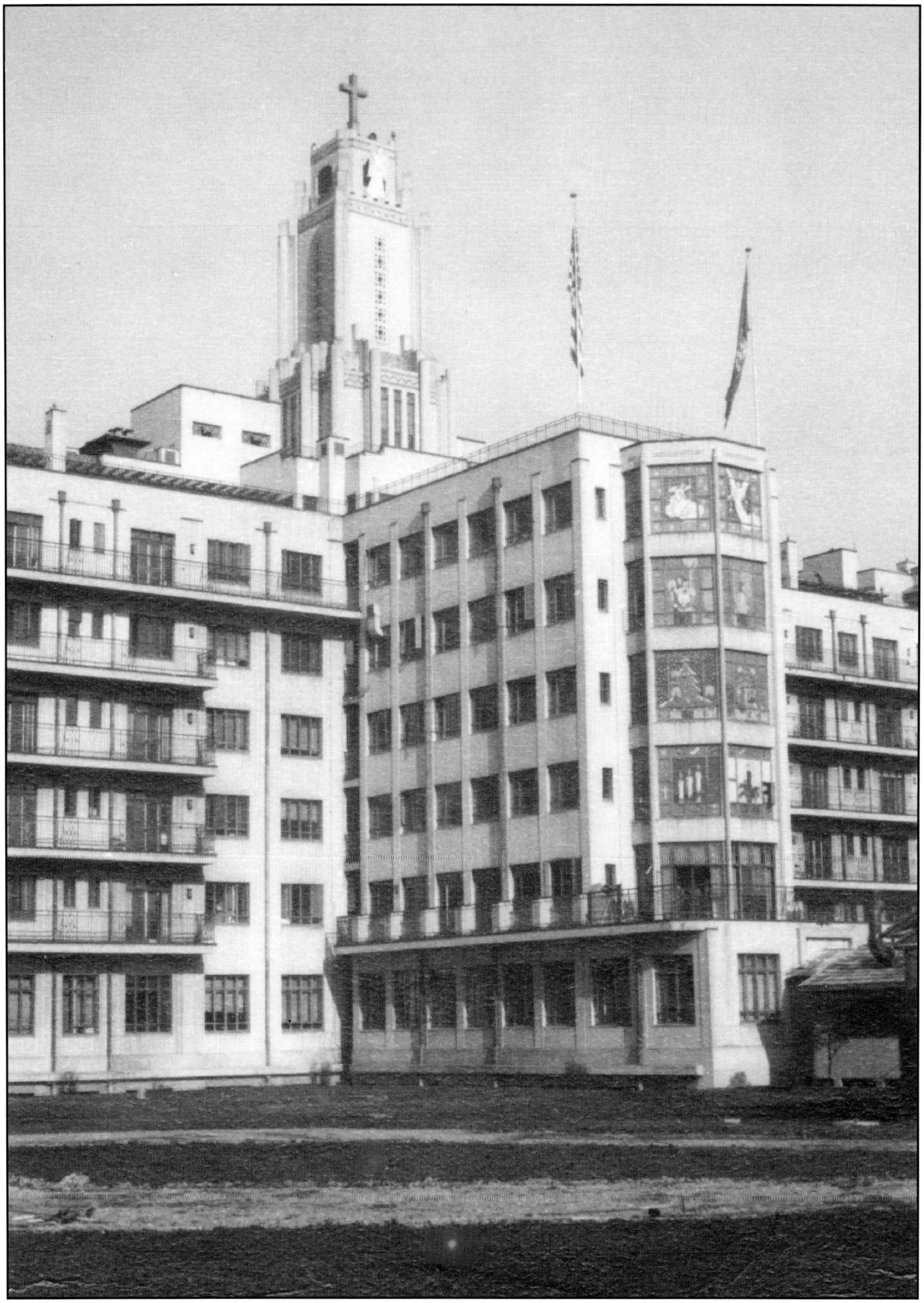

Army Hospital, Tokyo, 1950

JAMES T. AKIYAMA was born June 20, 1920, Platteville, CO. He received a Master of social work, the Graduate School of Social Work, Univ. of Denver.

Assignments with the RC included working as a caseworker, Home Service (SMF&V), Denver Chapter, Denver, CO 1954-68; field instructor, Graduate School of Social Work, Univ. of Denver; Denver Chapter, 1961-67. He also served as dir., SMF&V, Seattle-King Co. Chapter, Seattle, WA, 1968-83; division dir., SMF&V, Pacific Northwest Division, Seattle, WA, 1972-83. Akiyama has memorable experiences as a disaster relief worker in Eastern KY Floods, 1957 and AK Summer Floods, 1967.

He served in US Army Military, Intelligence Service in southern Japan with the 24th Infantry Division during WWII, retired in Jan. of 1983, and currently resides in Bellevue, WA. He is married to Dorothy, and they have two daughters and three grandchildren.

VERNA GREAVES ALDOUS joined the RC as a caseworker, then supervisor, for the Salt Lake Co. Chapter, from 1946-48. In 1964 she joined the Golden Gate Chapter, in Service to Military Families and management, retiring in 1991 as exec. dir., San Francisco.

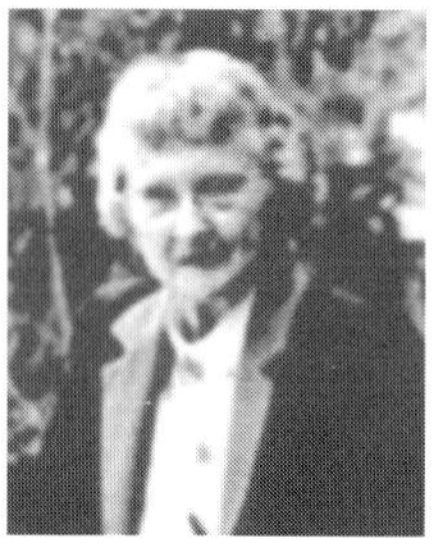

Major disaster experiences were Orphan Airlift, 1982 and 1986 floods, and 1989 Loma Prieta Earthquake.

She strongly supported community-based services for changing societal problems, believing the "troops" should be in constant readiness, and has often described her work as demanding but rewarding.

She married Newell Aldous in 1946. They have three children and four grandchildren. Since retirement she has served as president, San Mateo Co. Commission on Aging, State Council rep., and delegate to the White House Conference on Aging. She has specialized in community based long term care, strategic planning, implementation, and funding for public and private agencies.

AILEEN T. ALLEN was born Sept. 24, 1918 in DC. She was educated at the American Institute of Banking, DC. She received letters of commendation from the chairman of the Board of Veterans Appeals on Jan. 10, 1978, Dec. 23, 1981, Aug. 18, 1987. Allen served as a volunteer nurse's aide at the DC Chapter from 1942-43, and then was transferred to overseas service at the 80th General Hosp., SWPA, 1944-45. She served in the Panama Canal Zone from June 1946 to Aug. 1948 at Ft. Clayton Army Hosp., and in Germany at the 15th Evac Hosp. in Nuremberg and the 98th General Hosp. in Munich from Oct. 1948 to Oct. 1951.

In late 1951 she returned to the States, switching to Claims Counsel and Admin. Review Counsel. She became field dir., applying to VA legislation to medical data on such issues as service connection, disability compensation/pension, rehabilitation, insurance and benefits to veterans' survivors.

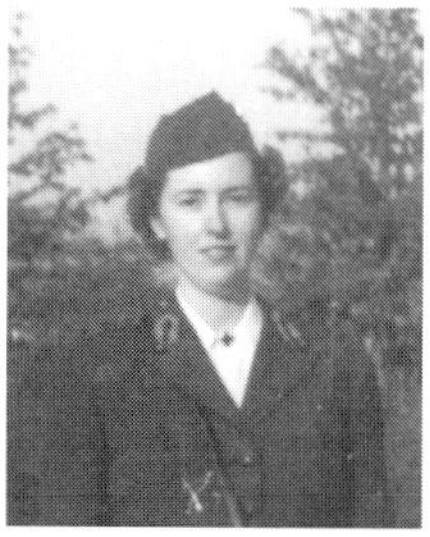

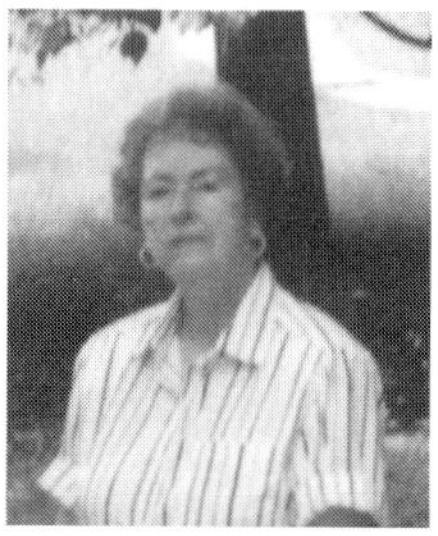

From 1975-87 she served on the Chief Appeals Counsel, as coordinator of the Board of Veterans Appeals, Veterans Advocate at the Appeals level; spending two of those years (1977-79) as asst. dir. of SVAO. She enjoyed every day of her 44-year career. She now travels extensively, and enjoys many activities.

LUCILE M. ALLEN was born in 1911 at Brocta, NY. She received her Master's degree in social work from the Univ. of Buffalo. In 1942, while a social worker, Allen heard a RC speaker and wanted to change jobs. Feb. 14, 1943 she became personal service dir. with the Foreign Service of the ARC. She trained in DC, and on May 15, 1943, sailed from NY City with other ARC personnel on the *Uruguay*, arriving in Australia June 16, 1943.

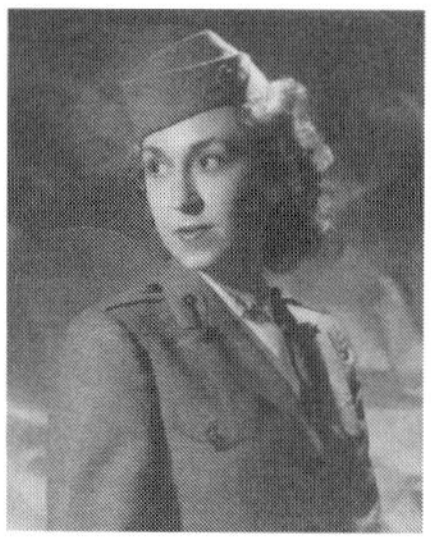

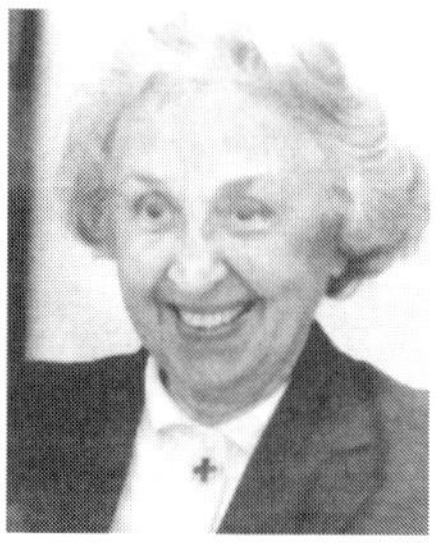

Allen served in Sydney in the club for the American and Australian Army and Navy. She served in New Guinea; Philippines; Island of Palawan; Tripler Hosp., Honolulu, HI; US Naval Hosp., Mare Island; USN Hosp., Oak Knoll; Navy Hosp., Yokosuka, Japan; USA Hosp., Taegu, Korea; Military hosp., Bainbridge, MD; USN Hosp., Yokosuka; USA Hosp., Osaka; and USAF Hosp., Clark Field, Philippines; USN Hosp., Philadelphia; USA Hosp., Neubruche, Germany; USAF Hosp., Wiesbaden, Germany; Bethesda, MD; DC Chapter; Veterans Admin. HQ; Natl. Association of Social Workers. She retired in 1976, but was rehired in 1977 to work on program to help American military and civilian men waiting for their Vietnamese wives and children to come to the US. From 1983-86 she was volunteer station mgr., Munich, Germany. At age 75 she lives in East Aurora, NY. Although legally blind, she enjoys news of ARC activities. **See Red Cross Memories story, "Leper Colony."*

WILLIAM J. AMBROGIO was born Feb. 21, 1923 in Cleveland, OH, graduated from John Hay High School in 1940 and was educated at Fenn College from 1941-43. Places of service with the RC include: 1958, Std. and First Aid instructor; 1960-pres., instructor trainer of Std.; community CPR for Pro, Blood Borne Pathogens; instructor, HIV-AIDS in work place; 1970-84, chief, First Aid Mobile Unity Corps; 1991-pres., Per Diem instructor, all health courses, Cleveland RC. Awards he has received are as follows: 1978, Hall of Fame and 1998, 40-year pin.

Ambrogio has been a staff member of RC Health and Safety, Cleveland, OH since 1991. He is married and has three sons and seven grandchildren.

BEVERLY "BEV" GERKIN ANDERSON was born Jan. 30, 1937 in Howell, MI, and graduated from Howell High School in 1954. She attended St. Lawrence School of Nursing in Detroit, 1954-57, and joined the RC in 1964. Assignments with the RC include: 1964-1971, staff nurse, Blood Mobile; 1971-97, deputy head nurse, Los Angeles ARC and supervisor, BSN, ARC, Southern CA, Los Angeles Chapter. Her most memorable experience was traveling with Blood Services Mobile Unit over the entire area of Orange and Los Angeles Counties. They covered all of the industries, ships afloat in Long Beach Harbor during Vietnam, aerospace, movie studios, radio stations and all military bases. They watched air planes being built, movies being made, newspapers being published, because they toured the places they took blood and got to know the caring people who gave blood to save lives. She saw changes in collections from bottles to plastic and even their uniforms from starch white dresses with white stockings and white shoes to colorful and casual. Anderson retired early in June 1997 after 33 years of service. She married Arthur Don Anderson in 1993 after a long loving relationship of 27 years. She has two stepsons, Wayne and Mark.

CLAUDE "PETE" ASHEN joined Golden Gate Chapter in 1961 as disaster chairman. In 1964, he helped in the 8.6 Alaskan earthquake. He assisted in relocating the Indian village of Chenega, devastated by the tsunami. He also served in the following capacities: disaster/fund dir., Golden Gate Chapter; ICRC delegate status, Nigerian/Biafran Civil War; organizer, "Orphan Airlift" —which brought children from Vietnamese orphanages to adoption families in the USA; President and Mrs. Ford flew to San Francisco to participate—; Northern CA/Western NV Division disaster dir., establishing Disaster Institute, CA State Univ., Sacramento; Disaster Institute chairman; establishing "Disaster Preparedness Information Council" (DPhilippinesC).

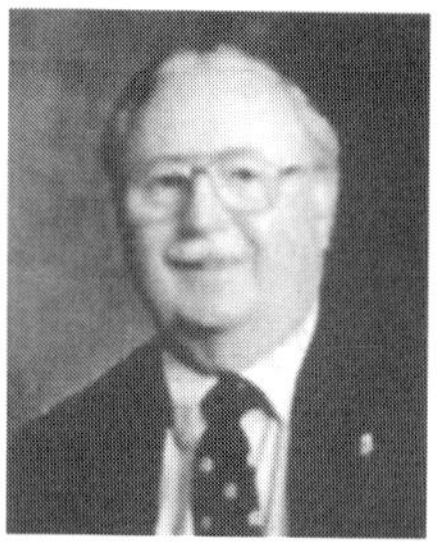

In 1994 Ashen retired from ARC Bay Area, but continues to work as a volunteer at Natl. HQ and to teach supervisory classes in Chapters and Institutes all over the USA. On Natl. Disaster Operations he serves in Admin., Mass Care, & Logistics. He lives with his wife Catherine in their home in San Francisco, CA.

AMON "LEW" LLEWELLYN BAER was born Dec. 10, 1912 in Highspire, PA. He received his BA at Bucknell Univ., 1938, and did his graduate work at PA State and Bucknell (1938-40).

Assignments with the RC include: service to military families, Ft. Eustis, VA; Langley Field, VA; Ft. Belvoir, VA; Blood Program, Johnstown, PA; field rep., Hartford, CT, Eastern NY State; administrator, Blood Program, Boston, MA; Worcester, MA; Springfield, MA and Portland, Maine.

His memorable experiences were participating in various disaster relief operations throughout the 50s in NY, NJ, PA, CA, OH, VA, WV, KY, CT, and TN; establishing and launching the RC Blood Program in ME, which is now part of Northeast Blood Program. He received the Distinguished Service Certificate, Northeast RC, Blood Program, in June 1976.

He is currently retired (since 1976), having served as president of Condo Association, and currently active on condo committee in Brookline, MA. Baer has one son, William; one daughter, Sarah; grandsons, Liam, Luke and Matthew. He married Ann in 1982. They "winter" in St. Petersburg, FL.

M. VICTORIA BAIN is KS born and a Mercer Univ. graduate, 1980. She was hired by the RC in Oct. of 1963 and sent overseas to Camp Zama, Japan. She served at Ascom, Korea; Camp Red Cloud, Korea; 7th Fleet HQ, Yokosuka, Japan; Ft. Ord, CA; Lemoore NAS, CA; George AFB, CA; Qui Nhon, South Vietnam; HQ III MAF, Da Nang, Vietnam; MCAS, Yuma, AZ; South Ruislip AB, London, England; CONUS; Redstone Arsenal, AL and Robins AFB, GA. She graduated with an associate degree in nursing in 1984, and was employed by several hospitals in the Savannah area before GA Regional Hosp., Savannah, where she was a children's and adolescent's psychiatric nurse for seven years.

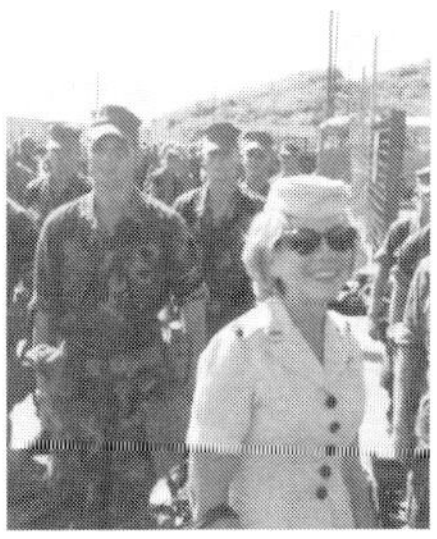

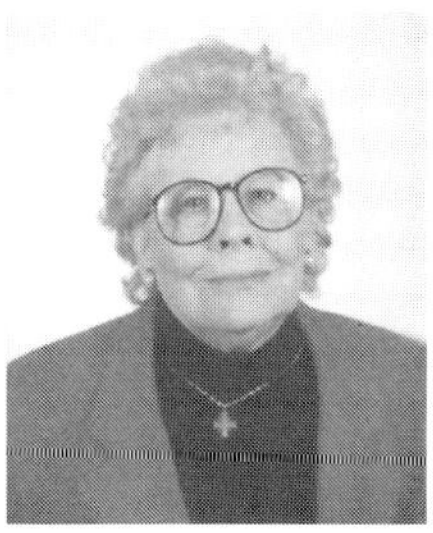

Bain has since traveled extensively and has been involved in various activities such as the Republican Women's Club and Vietnam Veterans of America, Savannah Chapter. Bain has a sister, Mary E. Levi; three nieces and nephews; six grandnieces and nephews and one great nephew. She resides in Savannah, GA. **See Red Cross Memories story, "Pianist in Vietnam."*

CAROLYNE NICKENS BANKS was born in Washington, DC, June 21, 1929. She graduated, Paul Laurence Dunbar High School, 1947, and completed one year at Miner Teachers College in 1948. She has completed numerous career studies through local universities, Career Track Training programs and ARC.

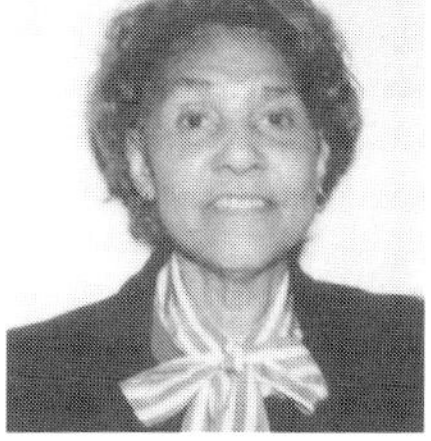

Banks was employed thirteen years with the District and Federal Governments and operated her home-based jewelry business. She began employment with ARC Oct. 7, 1968 as statistical clerk, blood records, WA Regional Blood Program. She became supervisor, May 1970. In April 1974, she was promoted to asst. controller, DC Chapter. In Jan. 1978, she left the ARC and held several financial positions through a local employment agency.

In May 1979, Banks returned to Natl. HQ as statistical asst., financial and data management. Subsequently, she received several promotions, and retired as corporate affairs analyst, Aug. 1, 1989.

Since retirement, she and her husband have traveled extensively. Their primary hobbies are photography and attending jazz concerts. Banks serves on ARARC's "Retirees Helpmate Service" committee and on her High School Class Reunion committee. Banks and her husband have one daughter, three sons, one grand-son and one great grand-daughter.

LOIS BARTH retired in 1999 after 21 years of RC service. She became known as the voice of the ARC because of her faithful, capable years at the Natl. HQ telephone switchboard. Upon retiring, she immediately began to volunteer in telecommunications and for the ARARC.

RUTH MARIE BATEMAN graduated from high school in 1942, and obtained her RN diploma in 1946. From 1951-87, she was staff nurse, supervisor, Great Lakes Regional Blood Center, Lansing, MI. Memorable experiences included seeing the growth of the blood services and working with other RC Regional Centers for special large collections at Auburn Univ.

Bateman is currently retired, volunteer coordinating nine blood drives per year, since 1992. She serves on Ogemaw Co. RC Board. She resides in Alger, MI, 150 miles north of Lansing, which she considers "God's Country," and is active in Lutheran church and other community projects. She has a son, Dr. Guy Dean Bateman, a clinical psychologist in Randolph, VT; and a daughter, Della Marie Somwaru, a dental hygienist in Minneapolis, MN. Bateman is very happy working with ARC.

ENSO V. BIGHINATTI (BIGHI) was born Dec. 18, 1921 in East Berlin, CT. Bighi attended Berlin High School 1940, and studied at Central CT State Univ. and Springfield College, MA, 1946-50. He joined the RC in 1951.

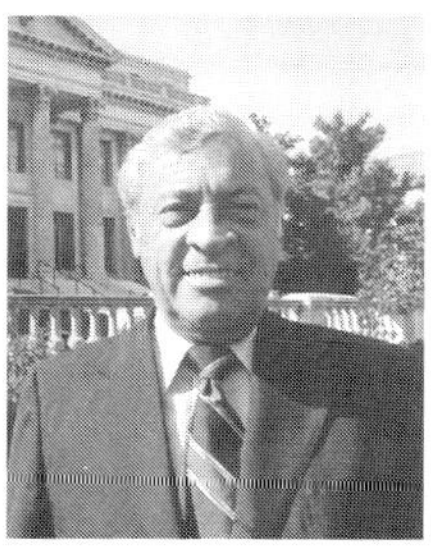

Places he served were: Alexandria, VA; San Francisco, CA; Natl. HQ; Intl. Federation of RC and Red Crescent Societies, Geneva, Switzerland. After his retirement in 1984, Bighi served as volunteer consultant; board member, DC Chapter; founder and chairman, DC Chapter Intl. Committee; member, US AID Advisory Committee on Voluntary Foreign Aid; founding member, Federal Emergency Management Agency; member, Univ. of WI Intl. Disaster Management.

During a 43-year tenure with the RC, Bighi was privileged to have served on both natural and man-made disaster operations and preparedness programs around the world. He first got to know the RC in WWII as a B24 crew member, 15th Air Force, Italy, and 8th Air Force, England, enjoying ARC coffee and donuts. He was later shot down. He would not have survived without the RC POW food parcels he received in prison camp. "My efforts with the RC are an expression of gratitude for what it did for me."

WINIFRED BLACK, born in Alabama, 1905, has a BA from the Univ. of Montevallo, AL and an MA in psychology from the Univ. of NC at Chapel Hill. She served with the RC for 33 years, interrupted only by a three-year stint as Dean of Women at the Univ. of Montevallo, her alma mater.

Her career included: 1934-39, exec. secretary, Mobile Co., AL Chapter; 1939-41, exec. secretary, Winston-Salem, NC Chapter, ARC; 1942-45, asst. dir., Office of Volunteers, Eastern Area, Alexandria, VA; 1945-48, Dean of Women, Univ. of Montevallo (AL); 1949-1956, Blood Program: responsible for developing material for chapters for recruitment of blood donors; later, asst. dir., Office of Volunteers, Southeast Area, Atlanta, GA; 1957-1959, represented Office of Volunteers and Jr. RC in Japan, Okinawa, Taiwan and South Korea, Tokyo, Japan; 1960, Office of Volunteers, designing training materials for recognition and recruitment of volunteers, Natl. HQ, Washington, DC; 1960-64, dir., Office of Volunteers, Stuttgart, Germany; 1964-70, asst. dir., Office of Volunteers, Natl. HQ, Washington, DC.

She retired in April 1970 to Magnolia Springs, AL for 20 years in her own house in a wonderful little community with new friends and a constant stream of visitors from family and ARC colleagues. "For me, Magnolia Springs was a kind of Shangri-La." In 1990, she moved to Denver, CO to be near her two daughters, five grandchildren, eight great grandchildren and lovely new friends in a centrally-located retirement club. She continues to stay in touch with many of her RC friends.

CHANDLER J. "BLACKIE" BLACKINGTON, a graduate of Boston Univ. College of Communications, holds a fifty-year RC pin for volunteer and staff service. Blackington joined the Metropolitan Boston RC as a disaster volunteer in 1948 and was later appointed Disaster Public Information chair. From 1958 to 1968 he served as public relations dir., Greater Boston Chapter. After moving to John Hancock as community relations dir.; he was appointed Disaster chair for the Greater Concord Chapter, a post he held for twelve years.

Although Blackington functioned primarily in disaster service and public information operations, he held numerous board, exec. committee officer and committee assignments with both the Greater Concord and MA Bay Chapters. He saw active RC duty at the Worcester Tornado, the Eastern States Floods, the Northeast Storm Operation, Cape Cod Hurricanes, the Blizzard of '78, and the Boston Bellflower Street Fire and Chelsea Conflagrations.

He holds several field and chapter citations and was awarded the Clara Barton medal. He currently serves as secretary, New England unit, ARARC, and is the RC rep. to the Concord, MA Local Emergency Planning Committee.

CARL BREEDLOVE was born in San Jose CA on Nov. 27, 1923. He was a young Navy firefighter on Ford Island, Pearl Harbor, HI on Dec. 7, 1941, and served in the South Pacific campaigns, honorably discharged in 1945. He served in the CA Division of Forestry, Nevada City, CA; US Forestry, Reno, NV; US Navy, Hawthorne, NV and the USAF Hamilton AFB Marin. He also served more than 15 years as a volunteer in the San Francisco Fire Dept. Reserves. In 1969 he worked in newspaper distribution in San Francisco with the News, Call, Examiner and the Chronicle.

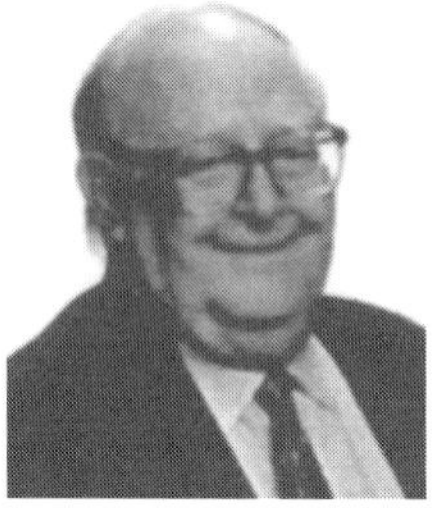

He provided disaster responses to San Francisco Fires through the Golden Gate Chapter, participated in the ARC Natl. Convention in San Francisco and attended conventions in San Antonio, TX; DC; Indianapolis, IN; Denver, CO; and Los Angeles. He is in Natl. DSHR as logistics coordinator, and has served on Natl. Disaster Operations in St. Louis, MO; Columbus, GA; Houston, TX; Kauai, HI; American Samoa and in numerous CA Quake Operations. Breedlove also was assigned to Natl. Fire operations in Oakland Hills, Redding and Ventura. He was one of San Francisco's first Disaster Action team leaders and is proud of his 25 years of volunteer service.

Breedlove has a son, Michael, and daughters, Deborah and Judy, and four grandchildren.

JOEL "JOE" K. BREITENHIRT was born in WV, graduated from Maryville College (TN) and attended graduate school at WA Univ. in St. Louis. College was interrupted by a five year stint of military service, while he served as an officer and a Naval Aviator in the Marine Corps.

Breitenhirt served his thirty year ARC career as follows: asst. field dir., Ft. Campbell, KY; Cam Rahn Bay, Vietnam; field dir., Redstone Arsenal, Huntsville, AL; exec. Chapter dir., Anderson, SC, Decatur, IL and Riverside, CA.

Retiring on Jan. 1, 1996, Joel and his wife, Patty, a RC service dir. for 15 years, have been traveling full-time in their fifth wheel across the US, Canada and Mexico. Both are Habitat supporters/volunteers, and Joel is an avid pool player.

ANNE WIESEN BROWN was born Nov. 27, 1926, in Medford, NJ. She graduated with her BS from the Univ. of NH in 1948 and with her MRE—ANTS, 1950.

Her ARC career took her to US Naval Hosp., Portsmouth, VA; Walter Reed AH, DC; USAH, Wuerzburg, Germany; 8th Field Hosp., Nha Trang, Vietnam; Malcolm Grow USAF Hosp., Andrews AFB, MD; USAH, Heidelberg, Germany; Walson Army Hosp., Ft. Dix, NJ; USNH, Bethesda, MD; Wright Patterson AFB; Osan AFB, Korea; Far East ARC HQ, Camp Zama, Japan; Mar. AFB, CA; USMC, Camp Pendleton, CA; ARC Europe HQ, Stuttgart, Germany.

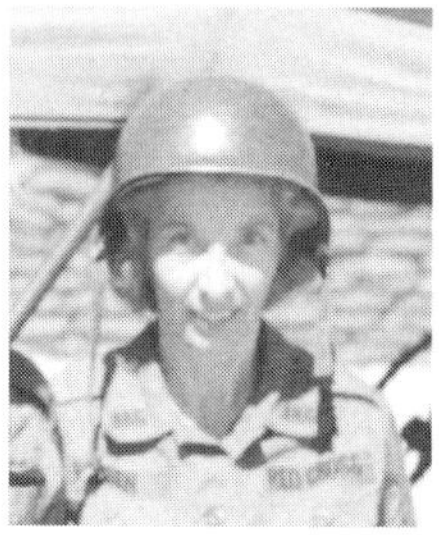

The most memorable experience she had was the night in Vietnam during the Tet offensive while spending the night under the bunk. She was able to discern the difference between incoming and outgoing mortar attacks. They spent the 48 hours assisting Army personnel anyway they could.

Brown received a medal for civilian service in Vietnam, 1967-68. She retired in 1988, married Dr. Richard D. Brown in Aug. 1995, and they have two stepsons and two granddaughters.

ROBERT G. BURGESS was born Sept. 12, 1938 in Salt Lake City, UT. He holds an AA from Mt. San Antonio Jr. College, Walnut, CA, 1969 and a BS, Cal Poly State Univ., Pomona, CA, 1973. He was assigned to asst. field dir.-Varo, Los Angeles, CA, 1973-76; asst. field dir.-Varo, Chicago, IL, 1977-79; field dir.I-Varo, Milwaukee, WI, 1979-81; field dir. III-Varo, Pittsburgh, PA, 1981-85; Allegheny Co. Chapter, Pittsburgh, PA, caseworker II, emergency social services, 1989-93.

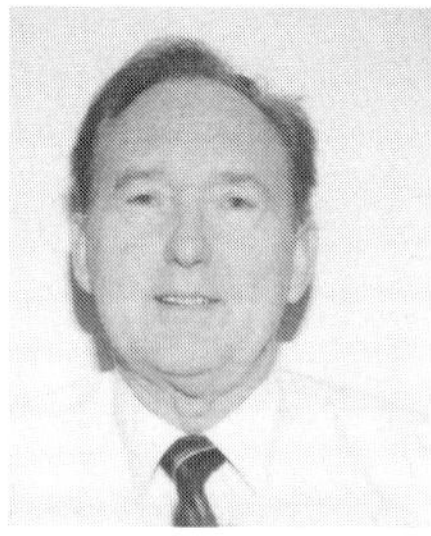

His most memorable experiences included disaster assignment at Oakland Community Shelter near San Francisco, CA Earthquake, 1989, as well as working as a family service technician, assisting families with emergency vouchers for food, clothing and shelter. His team was composed mainly of volunteers. He learned how important it is to give comfort and help to others in times of need.

Burgess received a certificate of gratitude from Pittsburgh Chapter chairman. He retired from the RC Oct. 1, 1993; retired from the US Navy Reserve, Sept. 12, 1998; and served in the active duty Navy Reserve Recruiting Office, Pittsburgh, PA, 1993-98.

He has a son, Garry, exec. chef, PA; a son, Kyle, high school English teacher, PA; and a daughter, Amy, student, Butler Community College, Butler, PA.

NARCE CALIVA, from Salinas, CA, was an Army lieutenant in Korea in 1953 when appointed, per 1949 Geneva Convention III/121, to the first UN Board of Inquiry Investigating POW mistreatment.

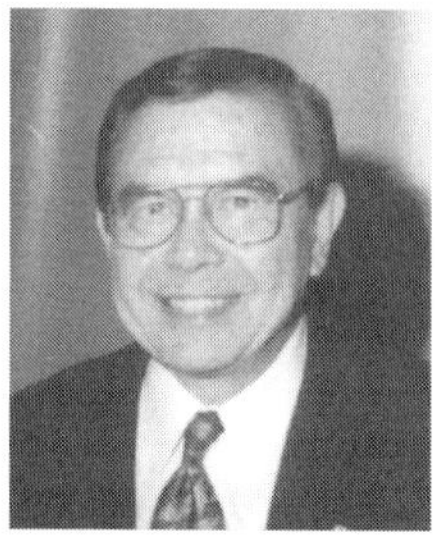

Employed as field dir. SMI, Mar. 1959. After asst. field dir./field dir. assignments in CA, Europe, and AZ, joined Service to Chapters, 1963, with territories at Yakima and Sacramento.

Assignments with the RC are as follows: 1966-1972 asst. dir., SMI, in Western, Vietnam, Far Eastern Areas, 1972 Western Area Training Dir., 1974 asst. mgr., SDC, 1978 mgr., SAF. 1981-1988 managing dir., Europe. He retired, HQ, Sept., 1989, and volunteered. VA/DC Field Service chairman since 1995.

ARC awards include: Tiffany, 1988; State Service Council Exemplary Service, 1997; Exceptional Volunteer, 1998.

Other affiliations: Psychological Consultants, Inc., Richmond, VA, 1989-1994; board certified in Behavioral Profiling by American Board of Forensic Handwriting Analysts; member, IGAS; fellow, American College of Forensic Examiners, 1994.

Caliva resides with wife, Leslie, in Spotsylvania Co., VA.

ENRIQUE J. CANAS, born Nov. 23, 1921, is a native of Alice, TX, and a graduate of FL Christian College, Ft. Lauderdale, where he majored in social work and personnel management. Canas retired from the US Arhis as an Officer. His military service included combat duty in Europe, WWII; the Korean conflict and Vietnam. He served as an enlisted serviceman, and infantry officer, personnel officer, asst. adjutant, and logistic supply officer.

Canas joined the RC career staff, immediately after his military retirement, Jan. 1961. His RC assignments included: Ft. Belvoir, VA, three months of induction training; asst. field dir., Ft. Dix, NJ; Far Eastern Area, one year, Third Marine Division. Okinawa; field dir., Wright-Patterson AFB, Dayton, OH; Far Eastern Area, Third Marine Division, Vietnam; field dir., Lowry AFB, Denver, CO; field dir. II, field dir. III, Travis AFB, CA; Long Beach Naval Station, CA.

Fluent in Spanish, he served during the summers of 1969-70, as a staff leader for the Friendship Latin America Projects of RC Youth, which sent Spanish speaking college students to Central and South American countries to teach health, and safety courses, and also to train local instructors to carry on such programs. He participated in various RC Disaster Preparedness and Disaster Operations.

In 1981, after 21 years, he retired. He enjoys good health, plays golf and is involved in the Sister City Program, Intl. People to People Program and various senior citizen activities. Canas resides with his family in the Olaloa Retirement Community, HI.

JOHN "JACK" H. CARROLL, JR. was born Jul. 1, 1928 in Philadelphia, PA. He obtained his BS degree from Villanova, 1949, and an MA from George Washington Univ., 1964.

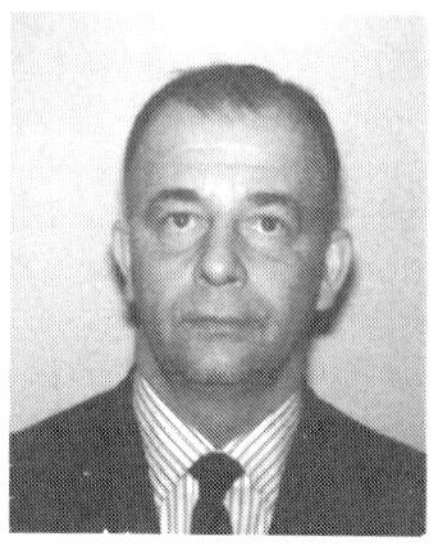

After retiring from the US Navy, 1971, he served as mgr. of Merrimack Valley, MA Chapter for 20 years. He retired in 1991. His most memorable experience was serving as delegate of the Intl. RC in Central and South America in the aftermath of disasters. He is the president of New England Unit of ARARC. Carroll divides time between hunting camp in Penna, and home in Andover, MA with wife, Dolores, three married sons, and five grandchildren.

CECILIA "CHRIS" G. CARY, born Dec. 25, 1907, graduated from high school in 1927 and became an RN in 1933. She joined the RC in 1936 while supervising at a hosp. in Wilkes Barre, PA. She did voluntary work with large classes of home nursing and baby care during the war, on her time off at work and in her home. She received a beautiful retirement part when she had lectured Home Nursing and Baby Care to Seniors of Akron City, Schools for almost 10 years. Cary enjoyed working for the RC after her husband passed away. The RC "was a wonderful organization to work for." Cary is now 90 years of age, retired, and has the RC drive her to the doctor. She is proud to be a RC Retiree.

JOHN B CATALDO, Italian born (1927), arrived in Walden, NY in 1935. He served in the Navy, 1944-46, and graduated from Columbia Univ., 1952. He served 32 years with the RC and was assigned as follows: asst. field dir., Ft. Belvoir, VA; Ft. Dix, NJ; Ft. Drum, NY; Ankara-Adana, Turkey; Patch Barracks, Boeblingen, Fulda, Wildflicken, Heilbron, Germany; Norfolk, VA; field dir., Plattsburgh AB, NY; Da Nang AB, Vietnam; Kaiserlatern, Germany; RD, Ft. George Meade, MD; Seoul, Korea; Ft. Dix, NJ; volunteer coordinator; Smansbach, Germany.

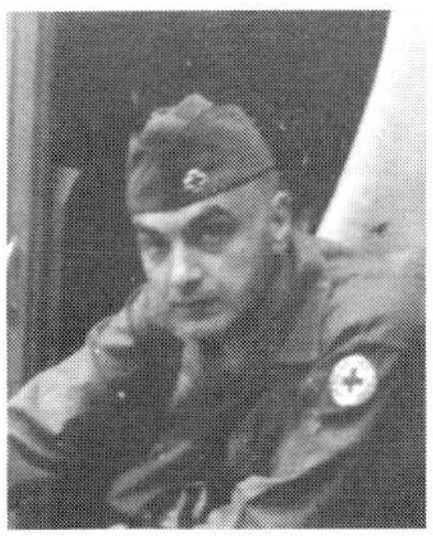

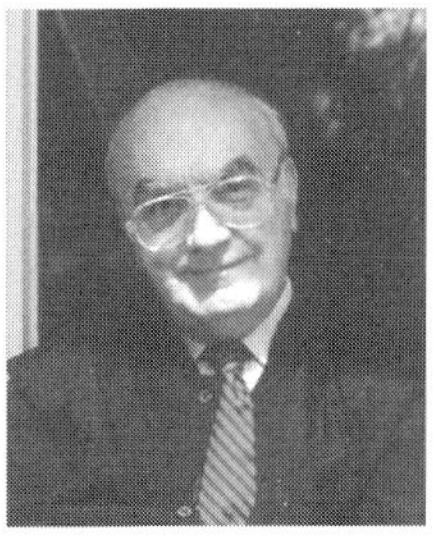

His memorable experiences include: opening recreation center, Adana, Turkey with Quin Smith, CD; incorporating all volunteer station staffing, USA/overseas, with dynamic ACS/natl. volunteer consultant, Jeanne Patton, HQ; energizing volunteer staffing/funding with Ruth Brock for 172 veteran hospitals; working with Jonie Brady, 1st Armored Div., Ansback, Germany, on special fund drives; the chaos of Vietnam, identifying killed colleague, losing soldier friends at the end of the war, viewing return MIowas on German TV.

Awards he received were the Tiffany Award, Certificate of Appreciation for patriotic civilian service, Order of the Purple Heart (Air Force, UN).

Cataldo retired in 1999 and resides in Columbia, MD with his wife, Annelise, also a former ARC employee (Patch Barracks, Stuttgart).

MARY LOUISE WELLER CHAPMAN joined the RC as a Clubmobile worker on Jul. 4, 1943, and spent a year in England and a year on the Continent. She then worked three years at the Chapter in Long Beach, CA, in Jr. RC and camps and hospitals.

In 1949 Chapman joined the San Francisco Chapter where she was dir. of Youth Services until 1980. During those years Mary Lou was a member of many Natl. RCY Committees, including the Natl. RCY Advisory Committee. Twice she represented ARC at Intl. meetings and conferences. In 1958 she was an adult leader for an RCY Study Visit to European countries, and in 1977 attended the Intl. RC Conference of Youth in Yugoslavia.

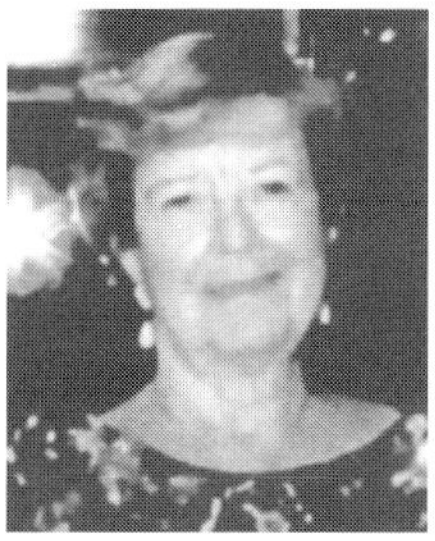

In Jan. 1980 Mary Lou became asst. mgr., Golden Gate Chapter. A Symposium on Intl. Humanitarian Law was held in 1981. Law professors from several countries, rep.s from the Internatl. Committee in Geneva, and experts in Human Rights as well as the Geneva Conventions and the Protocols attended.

At retirement in 1984 an Internatl. Student Fund called the Chapman/Holcombe Fund was established to honor Mary Lou and her colleague in RCY, Florence Holcombe. Each summer two to four students spend a month at the Chapter sharing RC program ideas and their culture with ARC youth.

NEIL M. CLARK joined the ARC in 1951 as an asst. field dir., Service to Military Installations. His first assignment was in Mason, CA, providing case work services to military personnel on troopships enroute to Korea. Clark served for 32 years in as an asst. field dir., field dir., district dir. and regional dir. His last assignment was as dir. for Northern Germany and England. He served a total of six overseas tours that included the Panama Canal Zone, Vietnam, AK, and three tours in Europe.

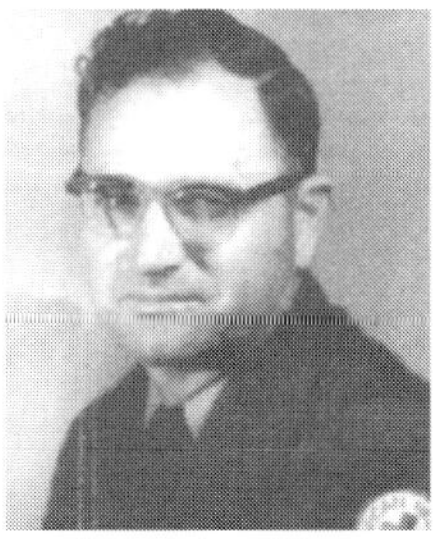

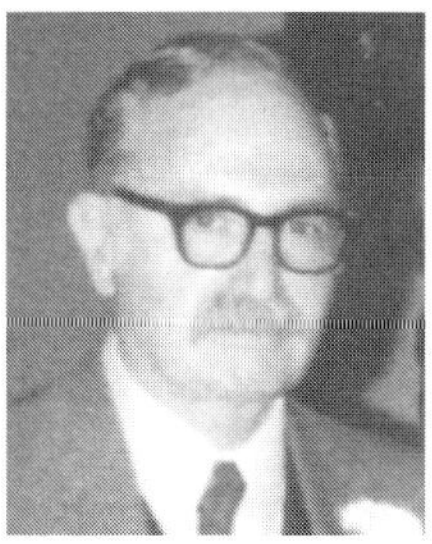

One of his most interesting assignments was as field dir. in Berlin, Germany, 1961-63, while the Berlin Wall was being erected.

Neil is an enthusiastic golfer. A couple of interesting golf games while in Berlin occurred in the fall of 1961 while playing as the partner of General Lucius Clay, President Kennedy's personal rep. in Berlin. Their opponents that day were General A. A. Watson, US commander, Berlin, and Colonel Charles Gingles, US hosp. commander, Berlin. As they preceded down the fairway, General Clay's aide came running to tell the general that the communist tanks that were at check point Charlie had chickened out and left.

Besides seven children, Clark has 10 grandchildren and 10 great grandchildren.

EDWARD F. COLBURN was born Mar. 11, 1913 in Buffalo, NY, and graduated from Ashland Univ., OH in 1937. He began service with the RC in Jan. 1943 at asst. field dir.-SMI (until 1953), where he was field dir. His many assignments included: Camp Young, Indio, CA; Walla Walla AFB, WA; Ft. Lewis, WA; Camp Stoneman, Pittsburg, CA; Korea, 2nd Inf. Div.; MT and CA. Colburn retired in April 1972 having served 35 years on staff and 14 years as a volunteer. He has two daughters and one son. His wife passed away in 1991, after 52 years of marriage. Colburn remarried in 1994. He resides in ID.

GAYLORD W. "RED" COLLE, "By Golly", began his RC career in 1936 as a member of the ANRC, Wichita KS, Sedgwick Co. Chapter's Water Safety Committee as a Water Safety instructor, and a First Aid instructor. Colle and his wife Billie were First Aid and Water Safety instructors for the Washington, DC Chapter, 1939-1945. He became asst. and then dir. of the Chapter's First Aid, Water Safety and Accident Prevention Programs, working with Mabel Boardman in the "Truck-Ambulance Corps." There Colle, along with Commodore Longfellow and others, worked to install First Aid training in government offices. They also conducted "Water Shows" at military bases and other places.

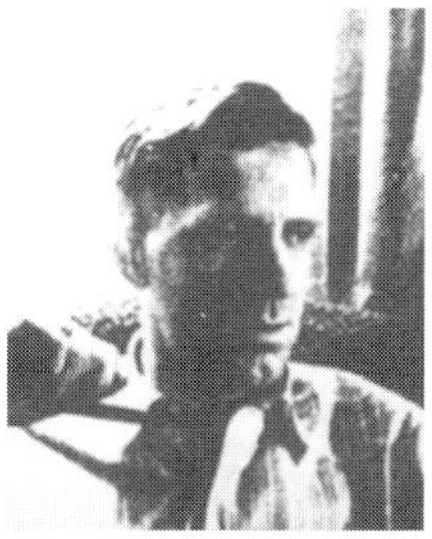

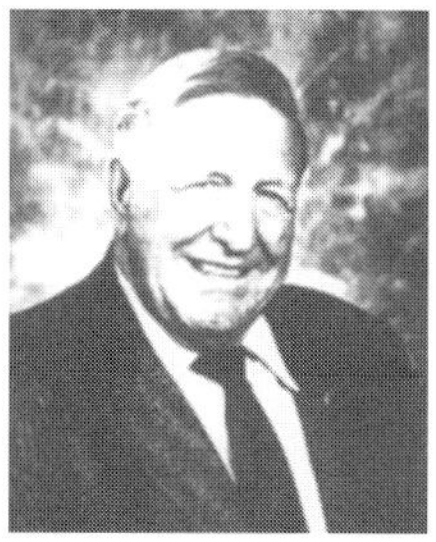

Other assignments included: dir., KS City, MO Chapter's First Aid, Water Safety, Small Craft and Accident Prevention Services; mgr. of the Rapid City, Black Hills Chapter, SD, West River Division; dir. of Disaster Services and admin. asst. to the mgr., Denver, CO Chapter, Rocky Mountain Division. He retired in 1980 and continued as a volunteer until 1986 when he completed 50 years of RC service. The most dramatic disaster he worked in during that time was the Big Thompson canyon and river flood. There were 139 deaths with nine still missing.

In 1995 Colle accepted a volunteer assignment to re-establish a Chapter in Ava, MO and Douglas Co. where he now resides. He would most like to be remembered for his pioneering contributions to RC.

HOWARD "HOWIE" E. CAMP, JR. was born Aug. 25, 1925 in San Antonio, TX. He obtained a BS in health and physical education in 1949 from LA State Univ.

Highlights of his RC career included: 1941-43, volunteer First Aid/Water Safety instructor, Pittsfield, MA; 1943-45, overseas military service, Theater Ribbon with five Bronze Stars and Good Conduct medal; 1957-61, dir., Safety and Disaster Services, Richmond, VA Chapter; 1962, asst. dir., Eastern Area; 1964, Eastern Area dir. of Safety Services, chairman, United Campaign; 1968, asst. regional mgr., New England Division Eastern Area; 1978, Eastern Area mgr. services to divisions and chapters (14 states, DC,

PR, Virgin Islands); 1983, mgr. services to divisions and chapter, Eastern Field office, ARC. Disasters: Hazel, Camille, Agnes and others. Natl. Aquatic Schools: Watikoh, Lutherlyn, Minnihaha, Ockanican, The Elms.

Camp married Janice Draper in 1955 and had two children and two grand children. He passed away April 15, 1994.

EUGENIA "SUSIE" P. CONSTABLE, born Dec. 1, 1920, was educated at the Univ. of NE, 1938-39. She worked at the Blood Research Center, Bethesda, MD, 1974-83 (clerk procurement and admin. asst.)

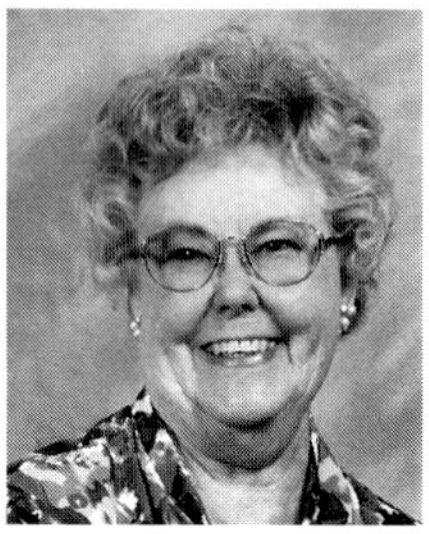

She is married to Erle M. Constable, and they have three children, Ronald L., engineer, Lockheed Martin; Barry K., deceased; and Ruth Nanette, business owner.

VIRGINIA BAKER CRAIN was born May 30, 1920 in West Liberty, IA, and educated at the Univ. of IA, 1943. Crain applied for a caseworker position with the RC, May 1945. Her first assignment was at Great Lakes Naval Hosp., to report Sept. 1, 1945. She likes to think the enemy knew she was coming since the war ceased in Aug. 1945.

After a year at Great Lakes, she transferred to Milwaukee, WI Chapter. Subsequent assignments included a casework position at Nashville, TN Chapter, dir. of Home Services at Macon, GA Chapter, then Midwestern area office as a Home Service rep.

Wanting to "get back to the troops" and hoping to go overseas, Crain transferred to Ft. Hood, TX in Aug., where she met an Army Officer who later became her husband. She then served at Air Force Hosp., Philippines; Camp Zama, Japan and Ft. Polk, LA. Her husband did not return from his second tour in Vietnam. She requested and was given a tour also in Vietnam, followed by a three year assignment at Letterman Hosp., then Germany for three years, and back to the US for one year at Travis AFB, one year at Ft, Ord, CA., then to WA State to cover five states as district dir. She returned to Europe as district dir. for West Germany, England, Belgium, Berlin and the Netherlands. Crain retired while in that position and continued as an instructor in social work classes. Twice she returned to full time positions, first at Naval Hosp. in Bremerton, WA and then at Yuma, AZ during Desert Storm. Also, with the help of many others she founded the ARARC in WA State that continues to be an active voice for RC Retirees.

LUZ M. ACOSTA-CROMER was born April 28, 1928, Puerto Plata, DR, Puerto Rico. She graduated from high school in May 1946, Arecibo, PR and in May 1948, finished 2 years of business school. She came to the States in 1948. In 1936 the RC in PR provided assistance to her family, and since then the RC has held a very dear place in her heart.

In 1949 she worked at Natl. HQ, DC in the typing pool. After several months she went to work with the Food and Agriculture Organization (FAO) regional office of United Nations in DC in the Spanish Translation Division. In 1954 she joined the Federal workforce and retired in Aug. 1985 as a GS-13.

In Oct. 1985 she again worked for the ARC at Arlington Co. Chapter, VA as a permanent, part-time admin. asst. Her supervisors were Mrs. Janice Murray (admin.) and Miss Anne Spence (public relations). She kept information on all donors' names, addresses and donations. She assisted in the writing of the Chapter's monthly newsletter; and served as a Spanish-English interpreter to disaster victims.

She retired in 1989 after marrying Jerry K. Cromer, Jr., and now works part-time as a Spanish-English interpreter/translator for Arlington Co. Public Schools; attends plays, concerts, movies, travels and entertains at home. Cromer has two daughters, one grandson, and three great grandchildren.

JEAN K. CROSLEY joined the ARC SRAO Program in 1953. After training at DC HQ and in Japan she arrived in Korea in Dec. 1953. She worked in the program in Korea for approximately 20 months.

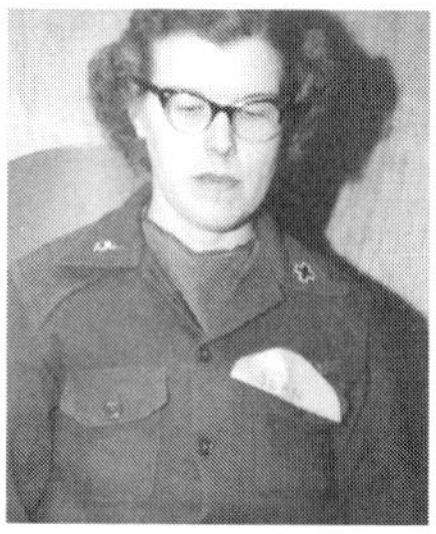

On returning to the United States she joined the Service at Military Installations (SMI) program. In that program she worked as an FOA and asst. field dir. at Ft. Lewis, WA; Camp Hanford, WA; Travis AFB, CA; Stuttgart, Germany and Portland AFB, OR. Because of her need to stay in Portland due to the illness of her parents she transferred to the Service to Military Families (SMF) program in the Chapter in Portland. She continued to work there for five years. She resigned from the RC in 1967 and returned to teaching. She had spent. a little over 13 years with the RC and thus has a vested interest in the retirement program.

Soon after retiring from teaching in 1983, she began volunteering in the RC Blood Program both at the center in Portland and at mobiles in Clark Co., WA. She continues as an active volunteer in the Blood Program. She organized and continues to work with a team of retired teachers who serve as volunteers at one mobile a month.

LUCIE DAVIDSON is Chicago born and a Univ. of IL graduate. She spent three years as a professional ice skater and teacher before an accident put an end to such endeavors. She was with RC for ten years and was assigned as follows: SRAO Korea, 1st Cavalry, ASCOM and Taegu (2/60-9/6 1); Hosp. Rec., Beaumont Army Hosp., El Paso, TX (9/61-3/62); SRAO Europe, Verdun, France and Adana, Turkey (4/62-4/64); Hosp. Rec., Fitzsimmons Army Hosp., Denver, CO (5/64-3/65); SRAO Korea, All Korea Program Dir., (3/65-3/67); Hosp. Rec, US Army Hosp. Camp Zama, Japan (4/67-4/68); Office of Volunteers, St. Louis, MO (5/68-5/70) and also served in Korea; AK and Selfridge AFB, MI. She retired Mar. 31, 1995 and moved back "home" to Chicago in June 1997. She keeps busy with writing (one novel published, the second in its final edit), working on a book with several other RC women about the Clubmobile days, volunteering at the YMCA, tap dancing, playing the guitar, photography and church activities. **See Red Cross Memories story, "Clubmobile Days at 1st Cavalry, Korea."*

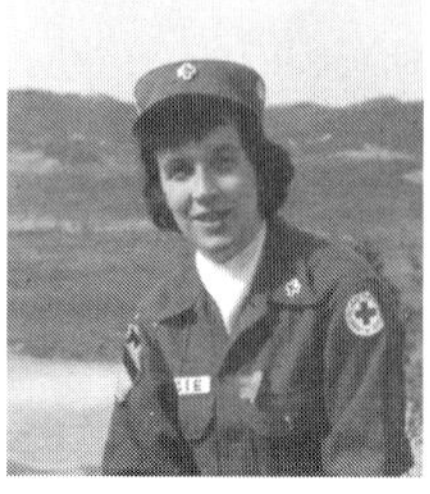

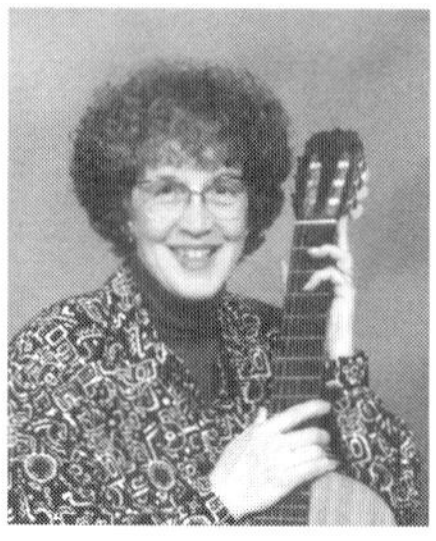

ELIZABETH "BETSY" REED DENMAN, began life Sept. 3, 1919 in Prospect, TN but was very soon removed to Fairfield, AL where she was reared. She received a BS in education from the Univ. of AL in 1948 and a M.Ed. with major in hosp. recreation in 1953 from the Univ. of MN.

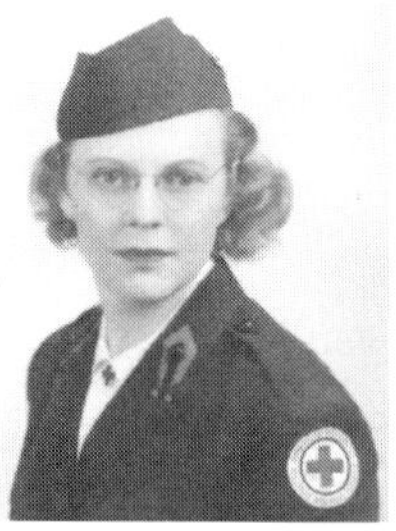

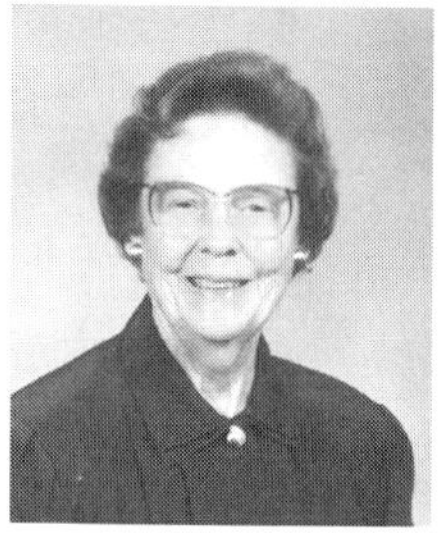

After brief tenure of teaching and as troop supervisor for Girl Scouts in Birmingham, AL she joined RC and boarded the train for DC on Dec. 25, 1943. After training at American Univ. and the hosp. at Ft. Belvoir, she was assigned as a staff aide to the Southwestern Pacific area and was stationed at the 363rd Sta. Hosp. at Ora Bay, New Guinea (3/44-1/45); Station Hosp., Morotai Island (1/45-5/45); a Gen. Hosp. in Manila, Philippines (5/45-12/45). This unit was set up in the grandstand of a horse racing track near Santo Tomas. Returning to the US in Dec. 1945, she was separated from RC until Oct. 1946, when she rejoined as a recreation worker and was stationed in Naples, Italy (10/46-5/47) and Udine, Italy (6/47-11/47); Lackland AFR, Hosp. San Antonio, TX (1/48-049); Army Navy Hosp., Hot Springs, AR (6/49-6/50); Warren AFT3 Hosp., Cheyenne, WY (6/56-7/51); Brooke Army Gen. Hosp., San Antonio, TX (7/ 51-8/52).

Denman took a year off for grad work at Univ. of MN and then worked at Fitzsimmons Gen. Hosp., Denver, CO. (9/53-5/55); Camp Zama Hosp. Japan (6/55-6/56) as recreation supervisor; Tachikawa AFB Hosp., Japan (6/56-1/57); 121 Evac. Hosp., Korea (1/57-3/58); Wichita Falls AFB Hosp.,(4/58-4/592); Lackland AFB Hosp. (4/59-2/60); Maxwell AFB Hosp., Montgomery, AL (2/60-10/60); Ft. Campbell Hosp. KY (10/60-6/61). At that time she resigned from RC and took the position of dir. of Adjunctive Therapy at Moccasin Bend

Psychiatric Hosp. in Chattanooga, TN until her retirement in 1981. At present, she lives in Louisville, KY, where among other activities, she works as a volunteer English teacher to recently arrived foreign residents. **See Red Cross Memories story, "VJ Night in Manila, PI."*

HAROLD D. DENNY joined the ARC on June 15, 1955 as an asst. field dir. He served in that capacity at stations in KY, NC, PR, France and Germany before being promoted to field dir. and assigned to Barksdale AFB, LA. In 1963, he left services to military installations to become a RC field rep. in TN, GA, AL, FL and MS.

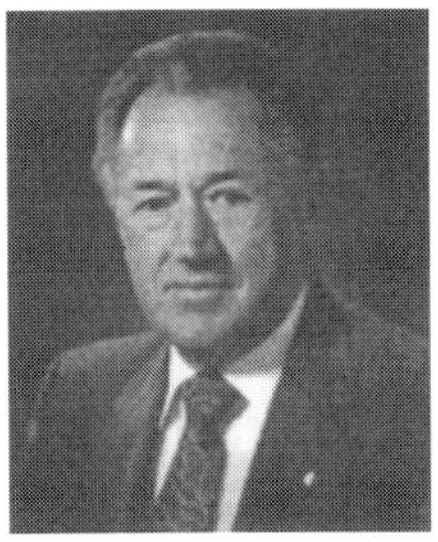

In 1967, he accepted a position with the Caddo Parish Chapter in Shreveport, LA as the asst. mgr. One year later he was promoted to mgr., a position he held until his retirement on May 30, 1989 after 34 years of service.

During Harold's service as a field rep. and Chapter mgr., his emphasis was on streamlining chapters and services. His efforts to reduce the number of marginal chapters resulted in merged operation for better delivery of services and fund raising at reduced costs.

The highlight of his career was the birth of a daughter in Wurzburg, Germany while serving as an asst. field dir., and the birth of two grandchildren while serving as mgr. of the Northwest LA Chapter in Shreveport, LA. He has served as vice pres. of ARARC.

KATHARINE "KAY" HARDESTY DESTLER was born Dec. 10, 1909 in Waco, TX. She obtained her BA at Tulane Univ. in 1930, her MS in 1932, and MSW in 1936. Her assignments included: volunteer social welfare aide, New London, 1941 51; exec. dir., 1954-59; dir., Svc. Military Families, Greater Hartford Chapter and CT Division, 1959-75; coordinator, Intl. Services, CT, 1975-93; natl. volunteer consultant.

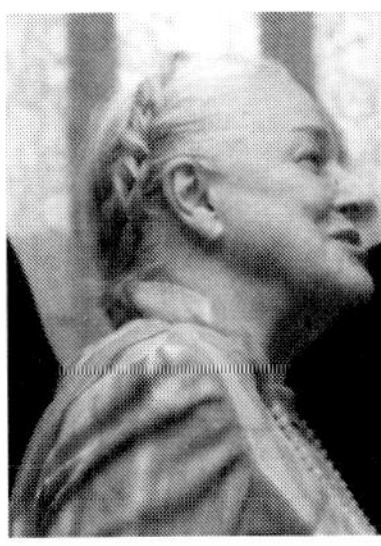

Pleasant memories include exchange visits, Tiansin, China RC and RC societies in Europe and Asia.

She was awarded the Clara Barton medal and Volunteer of the Year award medals from Greek, Spanish and Chinese Societies.

Destler is retired, married to Chester McA. Destler (since 1936) and has four children: Paul Lewis, Irving McA, Anne Destler Roberts and William Wallace Destler.

OLIVE M. DICKINSON, born Sept. 15, 1912 in Hartford, CT, received her BS in education from Teacher's College of CT. She served with the American Red Cross, 1943-77.

Her assignments included: hosp. rec. worker, Milne Bay and Hollandia; New Guinea; Leyte; Philippines; Brisbane, Australia (1943-46); Jr. rep. aboard *President Tyler*, "War Bride" ship sailing from NYC to Southampton, England and Bremmerhaben, Germany (1946-47); asst. field dir. and field dir., veteran hospitals, Lyons, NJ and Roanoke, VA (1947-52); natl. field rep., ARC Chapters in NJ and DE (1952-54); asst. dir., area office, Alexandria, VA (1954-57); exec. dir., New Britain, CT Chapter (1957-77). Special assignments: Disaster casework in CT, CA and PA.

Memorable was her first assignment in Milne Bay: Following an intense storm which flattened their native hut living quarters, they went quickly and anxiously to see about our RC hut only to find that destroyed as well, but they arrived just in time to see a native going into the jungle wearing our RC flag as a "lap-lap"! Christmas 1944, they had worked with patients in the nearby hosp. to have a "decorate your ward" contest to try to work up some Christmas spirit. By Christmas morning the humidity had done its work and all the crepe paper, ribbons and decorations had collapsed onto the patients' beds. Dejected they returned to their tent homes just in time to see them burn to the ground, sparked from a nearby fire. No one was injured but it left them with no belongings. This day was one of the most memorable Christmases of her life.

SUSAN "SUE" M. BLACKNEY DIKEMAN was born Mar. 14, 1918 in Saginaw, MI. She obtained her BA degree from MI State College in 1939. Her RC experience included: staff aide and asst. program dir., 1943-45, CBI Theater-India and Ceylon; exec. dir., 1950-70, Saginaw Co., MI Chapter; dir. of volunteers, 1977-83, St. Luke's Hosp., Saginaw, MI. She retired in 1983, enjoys life and is in good health. She married Ralph C. Dikeman in Oct. 1970. He passed away in 1976.

RICHARD V. DILLENBECK was born May 28, 1935 in Neptune, NJ and obtained his BA from the Univ. of Maine, 1957, and Mained at Boston Univ., 1974. Assignments included: asst. field dir., Fts. Belvoir, Eustis, Heilbronn, Heidelberg (1963-68); field dir., Long Binh (1970-71); field dir., Stuttgart, Germany (1971-73); field dir., Aberdeen Prov Gnd, USNA, Annapolis (1974-75); field dir. Camp Humphreys, Korea (1975-77); field dir., Ft. Belvoir, VA (1977-79); field dir., Heidelberg (1979-81); SD, Frankfurt (1981-83); SM, Ft. Bliss, TX (1983-86); SM, Munich/Augsburg/Schweinfurt (1986-94); SM, Ft. Gordon, GA (1994-96).

His memorable experiences included being rocketed in Vietnam, the Vietnamese Refugee Program, living in Germany for a total of 20 years, lengthy working relationship with Bavarian RC, providing First Aid at Oktoberfest, active Water Safety/First Aid/CPR instructor-trainer for 34 years, acquiring German as second language, and choosing to retire rather than to continue to work with current mgr. AFES Dillenbeck received the Tiffany award, 1991 and the Medal for Civ. Svc., Vietnam.

He is now retired and a mountain guide. He has a daughter Jane, born in 1963, and a son John, born in 1964.

ELEANOR "EL" C. DOW, born Nov. 15, 1933 in Brooklyn, NY. She graduated from Prospect Heights High School and from Hunter College, 1956 with an Art diploma.

She served with the RC at the in various capacities at the Monmouth Co. Chapter, now Jersey Coast Chapter: 1975-78, exec. secretary to dir.; 1977, Disaster training in Damage Assessment and Standardized Immediate Assistance; 1978, office mgr./accountant; 1978-1989, special events fund raising, designed events invitations/programs.

Disaster assignments gave her some interesting experiences. One she will not forget was during a hurricane. Some relatives called from the midwest about their 92 year old grandma who lived 1/2 block from the ocean. Eleanor called every RC shelter and could not find her. When the storm passed she called the lady, who said she knew that storm was coming, so at 6 a.m., she went to her friend's place, drank beer and played poker all day. "My kind of lady!"

Dow received several disaster certificates and a 10-year service pin. She took early retirement from the RC in Jul. 1989, and became a dental office mgr. She worked for a certified financial advisor, a dentist, and as the coordinator of volunteers. After 30 years of various careers Dow is officially retired, enjoying the Gulf of Mexico across the street from my condo, enjoying internatl. travel, and painting. She has one son, a journalist in the US Navy and a school teacher daughter in San Francisco, CA, an auto mechanic daughter in Oakland, CA, a third daughter with CBS TV in NYC and a fourth daughter who is a beautician in Holmdel, NJ.

EDITH "EDIE" A. DAY DRURY was born Sept. 6 in East Boston, MA and attended East Boston High School, Boston Clerical, Lincoln Prep (northeastern) Pre Nursing School, Newton-Wellesley Hosp. School of Nursing, and Broward Community College, FL.

Her employment included: secretary to asst. UP A+H Dept., MA Bonding and Insurance Company; RN, hospitals in FL and MA; admin. asst., two non-profit agencies; admin. asst. to mgr., Broward Co. Chapter, 1981.

Drury has one daughter, Carol Drury, RN, and two sons, Thomas J. Drury and Richard A. Drury, who are in construction. She enjoys reading, dancing, movies and shopping.

MARGARET "MAGGIE" GOOCH DUFFY joined the ARC because she was eager to assist US servicemen and wanted to have overseas experience. Duffy was serving at the Nashville, TN Chapter as dir. of home service when she was assigned overseas in military welfare service in the Far East and from 1943-51, and served in Australia, Philippines, Korea and Japan.

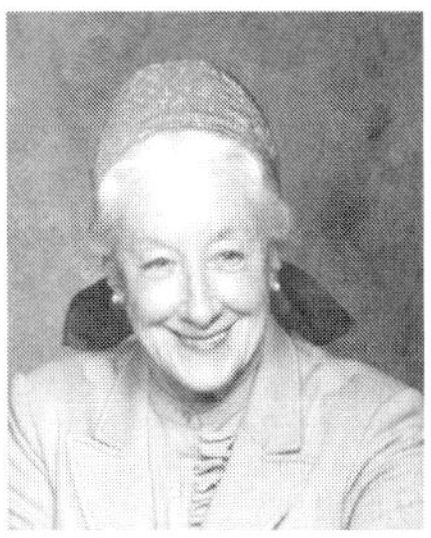

From 1947-50 she was one of a team of six ARC advisors assisting the Japanese RC to rebuild after WWII. This resulted in a lifelong interest in strengthening the bonds between US and Japanese citizens at the "Grass Roots" in the US. At the Embassy of Japan in DC in Nov. 1991 she received the "Order of the Precious Crown

Butterfly" conferred by his Imperial Majesty, the Emperor of Japan. The citation: "For her contribution in promoting volunteerism in Japan and in strengthening friendship between people of the US and Japan through various activities of the ARC."

Following her stint at Eglin AFB, FL she was sent to Europe as dir. of volunteers at the European Area HQ in Stuttgart, Germany from 1954-58. Following that she held positions in Eastern Area HQ and Natl. and retired in 1977 as natl. dir. of volunteer personnel. She has continued her RC affiliation as a volunteer consultant at Natl. HQ and the Nashville, TN Area Chapter with responsibility for the Japanese initiative promoting interest in involving Japanese corporate citizens in the US to participate as RC volunteers.

CLYDE EARNHARDT was born Feb. 23, 1923 in Charlotte, NC. He is retired ARC - USAF. Assignments included: Guadalcanal, 1943; Westpoint ACA, NY; Maxwell AFB, 1958. He was awarded the Humane Medal, a certificate of appreciation from Gov. George Wallace. He resides in Montgomery, AL with his wife.

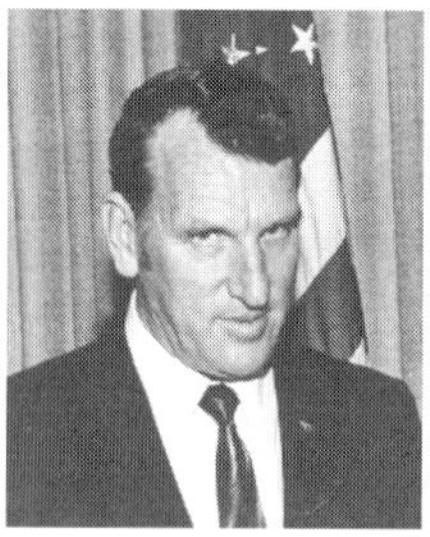

BOB L. EDWARDS attended high school in Sterling City, TX, graduating in 1945; TX Tech (BS, zoology), 1952; TX Tech and IA Univ. (grad work), 1961; GA Tech, 1964; and Jr. Colleges in San Angelo, TX and Clayton, GA.

Assignments included: Lubbock, TX, Atlanta, GA, Waco, TX, MN, WI, ND, AR, IA (1948-85). He has 37 memorable years in a service organization, knowing lives were saved with instructor courses. He received a fundraising award from the ARC.

Currently Edwards is retired, "RV-ing" in AZ, TX, and FL in the winter with wife, Glenda. They have four daughters and eight grandchildren.

HAZEL A. EGGLESTON was born Sept. 21, 1918 in Woodburn, OR. She became an RN at Emmanuel Hosp., obtaining her BS from Seattle Pacific Univ.

She served as staff head nurse, asst. dir., liaison DRD, Blood Services Nursing, and Bloodmobile in the Pacific Northwest. Her husband of 42 years passed away Dec. 10, 1996. She is currently retired, enjoying time to play after working 40 years.

ENOE DELIA ELIAS was born April 23, 1933 in El Paso, TX. She graduated from high school in 1952, and attended LACC, 1952-53 and Mission College, 1990-95.

Her assignments for the ARC included: volunteer nurse aide, 1973-74; part-time evening supervisor, Blood Program, 1976; senior clerk SMF/V and Disaster Services, 1976-86; admin. asst. I for SMF/V - Disaster Svc, LA, CA - San Fernando Valley District Office, 1987-89.

Memorable experiences: being bilingual (Spanish), working with different departments when needed and serving with Natl. during the 1971 and 1994 CA Earthquakes. A coworker and she were able to get transportation for a vet back east to see his dying mother as he had no resources. "I enjoyed working with the RC."

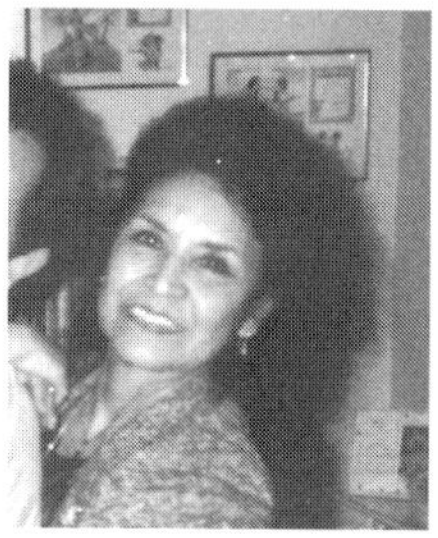

Elias currently freelances as a medical interpreter and resides with husband (Joe) of 43 years, who is retired from Hollywood Studios. They have a son, Conrad, contract electrician; a son, Mark, scenic artist; a son Adam, medical coordinator; a granddaughter, Deiandra, age 4; and two beautiful daughters-in-law, Laura and Lynda.

NEAL T. ENGLISH was born in Loveland, OH and is a graduate of the School of Journalism at OH State Univ. His experience with the RC included: community relations dir., Cincinnati Area RC; associate PR dir., Cincinnati Area United Appeal; asst. dir., Natl. Office of Public Information, ANRC, DC; natl. dir., OPI, DC.

English is now nearing completion of totally remodeling his 1965 house and grounds in Chesopeian Colony, VA Beach, and on the bike trail at the resort boardwalk, and is enjoying all VA Beach offers. He is currently retired after operating English Remodeling for a number of years in Arlington, VA. He is married to Grace Bradford and they have two sons, Jeffrey Neal, architect in NYC and Mark Bradford, engineer in Arlington, VA. **See Red Cross Memories story, "How I Lent President Kennedy My Hands."*

HELEN L. ETTLIN was born May 11, 1928 in Boise, ID. She graduated from high school in 1946, nurse's training in 1949, and obtained a BSN in 1971.

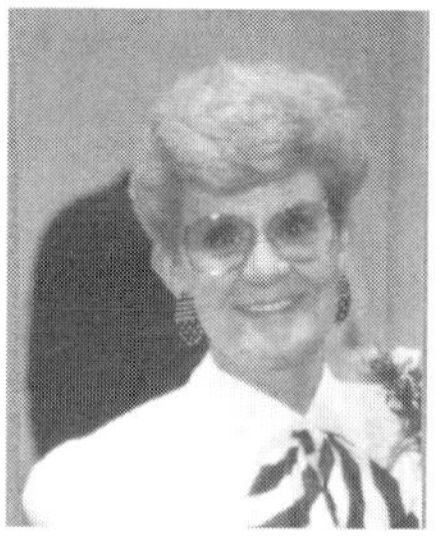

RC assignments are as follows: asst. dir. of education and safety, Tacoma-Pierce Co. Chapter, WA (1965-71); dir. of education and safety (1971-76); asst. chapter mgr. (1976-88). She received the Tiffany Award in 1988.

She is currently retired — work/FEMA; secretary, Evergreen State Unit, ARARC; lifetime member of Commodore Longfellow Society. Her husband, Robert, is also retired, and their family consists of daughters Rheta; Karen Russell (and her son Jeremy); Lisa Porter (and her husband Mark Porter and son Robert). **See Red Cross Memories story, "From Disaster Exercise to True Trauma."*

BYRON WILLIAM EVANS was born on Nov. 28, 1913 in Detroit, MI. His mother, Blanche, was born in England. His father, Thaddeus, born in Youngstown, OH was the son of a Welsh immigrant. Byron's grandfather, father, and he are poets, a Welsh legacy. When Byron was five years old, the family moved to Cleveland, OH, his home until 1939. During the intervening years, Byron graduated from Cleveland Heights High in 1932 and Western Reserve Univ. in 1937, with a teaching credential. Unable to find a teaching position, he received training as a recreational and occupational therapist at the Menninger Clinic, Topeka, KS.

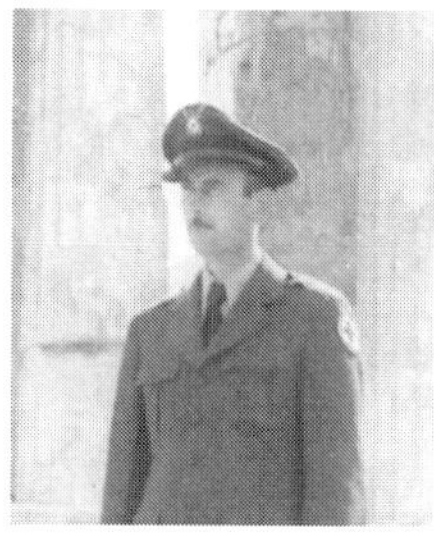

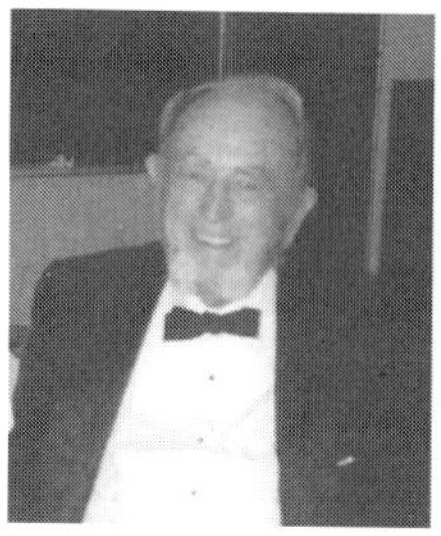

From 1940-42, he was employed by a psychiatric hosp. With the advent of WWII, the ARC appointed him to provide social services to members of the armed forces and their families. He continued employment with the RC (interrupted by graduate study at the Univ. of CA for a Master's in social work) for 36 years. A variety of assignments were served in CA, NE, Kwajelein, Germany, France, Greece, Turkey, and finally Natl. HQ, DC.

He is retired, serving church and community in encouraging the hiring of older workers and their value as leadership volunteers. He and his wife Myrtle live in Dallas, TX. They have four children, ten grandchildren, and seven great-grandchildren. He has two sisters, Lois and Elizabeth, both living. **See Red Cross Memories story, "Serving Troops in Greece and Turkey."*

MARGARET EVELYN THOMAS EWING was born Mar. 13, 1899 in Riverside, CA. She graduated from LA State Normal College in 1919. Her RC activities included: volunteer wartime service, WWI, 1916-17; motor corps, disaster relief, blood recruitment, asst. dir. of San Fernando Valley Chapter, 1945-82.

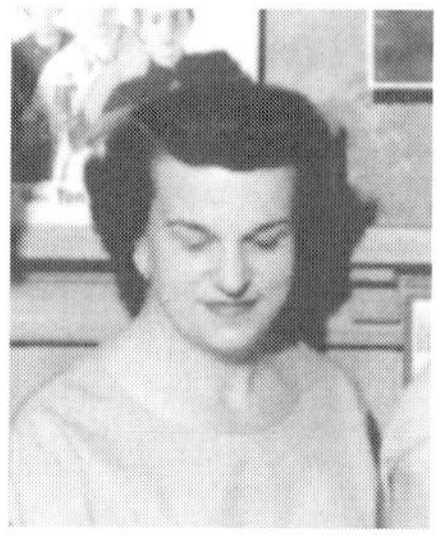

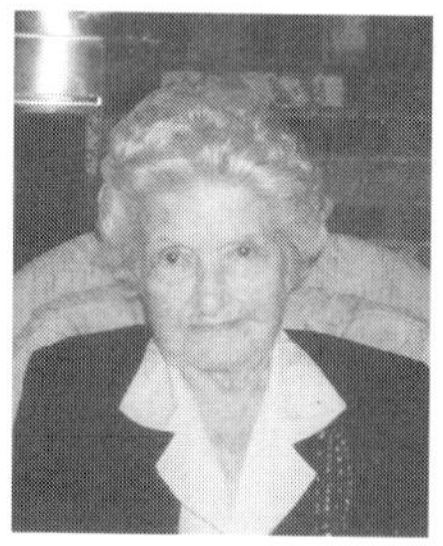

Margaret married John Finis Ewing in 1922. Her family consists of one daughter, Margaret Jeanne Broadwater, son-in-law Eugene Sharp Broadwater, and grandsons David Eugene and Douglas Austin Broadwater. Margaret Ewing celebrated her 100th birthday in 1999.

WALLACE "WALLY" K. EWING was born Sept. 11, 1932 in Grand Rapids, MI. He received his BA and MA from MI State, and also finished his PhD. He served as exec. dir., Ottawa Co. Chapter, MI from Oct. 1986-Oct. 1995. His memorable experiences were raising money and surviving AIDS threat to blood supply.

Wally is currently retired, researching and writing a local history, and residing in Grand Haven, MI. He has two married daughters and 10 grandchildren.

DOYE L. BURKETT FANNIN, was born in TX. She attended high school in Stephenville and Brownwood, TX; and one semester, in 1941, at John Tarelton Jr. College, in Stephenville. She is a 1968 graduate of Heald Business College, San Francisco, CA.

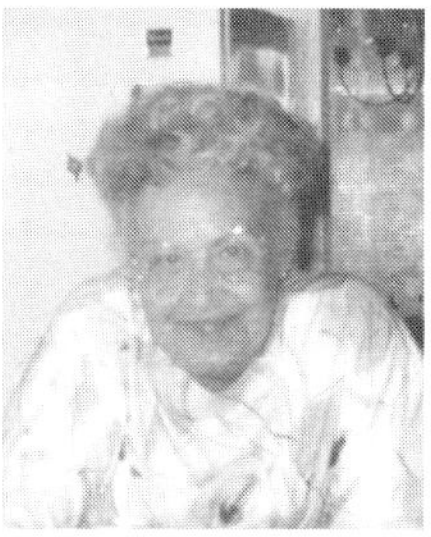

In 1941, Doye married, then US Army Staff Sergeant Robert Fannin. They have three children; Dolores, Robert, Jr., and Darryl. The daughter married, and lives in FL. The sons married, and live in CA.

While stationed with her spouse, at Ft. Lewis, WA, Doye worked as a volunteer in the RC field dir.'s office. In Oct. 1956, the field dir. hired her, on the Natl. payroll, as a clerk stenographer II. She left there June 28, 1963, when her spouse retired as major from the Army, and moved to CA.

After a one year hiatus from employment, Doye returned to work for RC, in 1964. She continued that employment for the next twenty years and six months, interrupted only by leaves of absence for serious illness, and family emergencies.

From June 29, 1964, until Mar. 25, 1973, Doye worked at the following RC Field Stations, progressing from CS III, to admin. asst., to field office asst.: Ft. MacArthur, CA (twice), VA Regional Office, San Francisco, CA, and Long Beach Naval, Station, Long Beach, CA.

On Mar. 26, 1973, she received a promotion to asst. field dir., and held assignments in that position until April 26, 1977, at the following stations: Ft. Carson, CO, 11th Naval District HQ, San Diego, CA, 32nd St. Naval Station, San Diego, CA, and Miramar Naval Air Station, Miramar, CA.

After her promotion to field dir./station dir., on May 14, 1977, Doye served, in succession, at the following stations, until Dec. 31, 1984: USMC Air Station, Yunw, AZ, 19th Support Command Taegu, South Korea, Miramar Naval Air Station, Miramar, CA, Mar. AFB, CA, and Seventh Army Training Command, Grafenwoehr, Germany.

In her last five assignments, as field dir./station dir., Doye held responsibility for the operation/direction, under RC policies, of all RC programs, at those stations.

In the course of her RC career, Doye performed special assignments, as a case worker, with the RC Disaster Relief Service. She provided assistance to victims of a hurricane (TX) an earthquake (CA) and refugees of the war in Vietnam (US Marine Corps Base, Camp Pendleton, CA).

Doye received many plaudits, and expressions of appreciation, for her work with the military communities. The most prized of her awards is the Seventh Army Training Command Scroll of Appreciation, with Helping Hand Medallion. The Command presented the award to her, on Aug. 24, 1984, "For outstanding contributions toward the betterment of the Seventh Army Training Command Military Community."

At the time of her retirement, Doye had more than 26 years, on the payroll of the ANRC. She retired Jan. 1, 1985. In retirement she busies herself with family genealogy research (has one self-published book, based on that research) gardening, and, with the affairs of her church. Doye lives in Copperas Cove, TX, with her spouse. **See Red Cross Memories story, "Custody Assistance."*

EVELYN LIFSEY FAY, born Sept. 28, 1915, in Ft. Valley, GA, graduated from high school in 1932. Her RC assignments included: volunteer Genessee Lapeer Chapter, 1942-45; ETO Club Program in France and Germany, 1945-46; club dir. in Germany, 1949-82; dir. of Youth Services, Genessee-Lapeer Chapter, Flint, MI, 1958; one of three adults with 23 high school students on an eight-week RC study in Europe.

Fay received a 40-year certificate from ANRC and a Congressional Certificate of Merit. She is currently retired and resides in MI.

JUANITA JUNE FEKEN, born June 6, 1917, in Joplin, MO, has always loved helping people. She served from 1983-85 with project help, from 1985-95 with AFES and Disasters. She retired in Oct. 1998 due to a heart attack. Feken has received the RC Clock Exceptional Volunteer Plaque for 43 years of service as a volunteer and on staff. She is currently retired, is a widow and has three daughters, eight grandchildren and 25 great grandchildren.

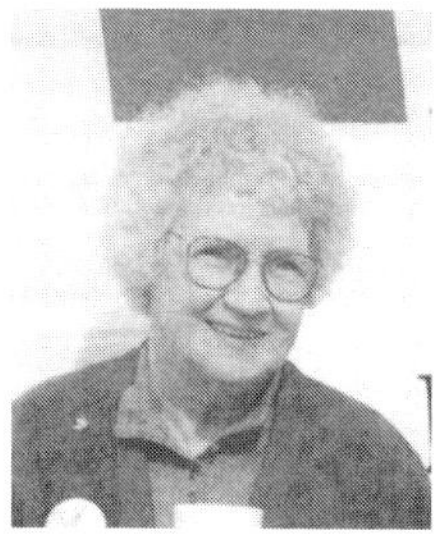

MARGARET "PEGGY" HENRY FLEMING, born in Milwaukee, WI, on Mar. 10, 1920, holds a BA, BSouth Carolina, and MA. She served from 1943-46 as recreation dir. in England and France; Clubmobile Group F in Belgium, Luxembourg; and as dir., 28th Division, Rest Center, Luxembourg. She was at the latter on Dec. 16, 1944 when the town and RC Club were captured by the Nazis (start of the Bulge). She escaped at night to Bastogne with two local girls who worked in the club. She served as club dir. in Holland and Germany, and was discharged Oct. 1945, receiving the Bronze Star signed by Truman, three battle stars. Fleming served as Jr. RC Field Representative in PA, OH, and IN. She was an active volunteer for 50 years in Columbus, OH Chapter, a board member from 1981-98 with the Blood Program volunteers, Intl. Committee and MV and CS Advisory Committee. Fleming received the RC Chairman's Award, RC Intl. Award, Stecker Intl. Service Award (RC) and Marquis Who's Who of American Women.

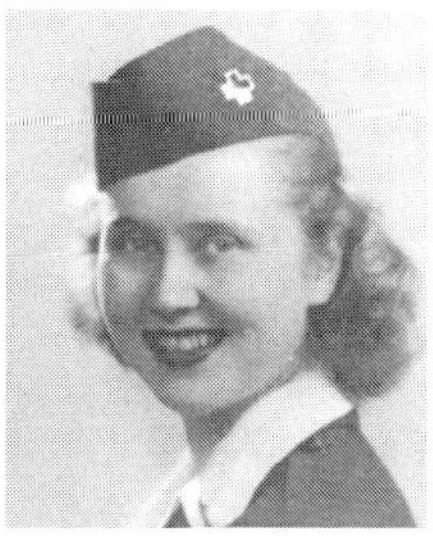

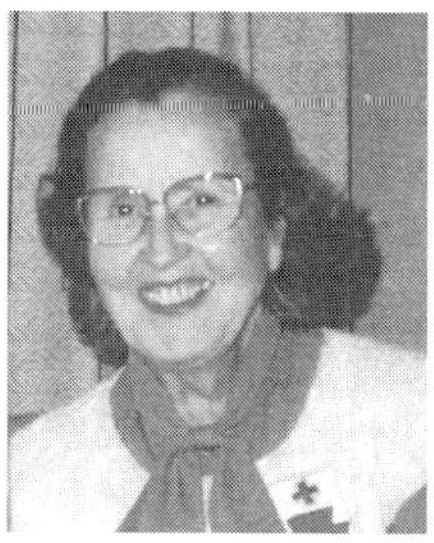

During her return veterans' tour in Belgium and Luxembourg in fall 1994, she located both girls she had helped to rescue — 50 years later! She is currently a retired co-owner of Fleming's Bookstore and travels (88 countries). She has been married for 52 years to Fred Fleming, with whom she went to high school. They had their first date in England. They have one daughter, Patricia.

JAMES B. FOLEY, born in West Sommerville, MA on June 2, 1913, graduated from Tufts Univ. in 1938 with an AB degree and from Boston College School of Social Work in 1940 with an MS degree. He began his RC career June 20, 1941, as a special asst. in Foreign War Relief. His assignments included: special rep., Portugal; field rep., Civilian War Relief in Eritrea and Ethiopia, Lebanon, Palestine, Iran, British East Africa, the Belgian Congo, and Italy; asst. dir., Middle East operations; deputy dir., Balkan relief operations; dir., RC Civilian Relief, Mediterranean Theater; asst. administrator, Disaster Services, National HQ; asst. mgr., SAF&V, Eastern Area HQ, Alexandria, VA; deputy mgr., VA and Southeastern Area HQ, Atlanta; asst. to senior vice president and asst. to the exec. vice president, National HQ; vice president, National HQ.

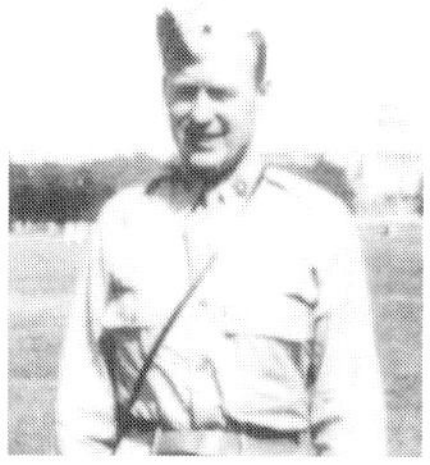

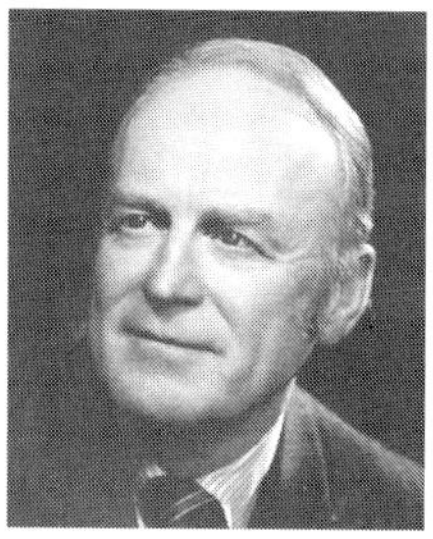

Foley was decorated by several RC Societies and foreign governments. He received a Department of Defense Public Service Award. Foley passed away Aug. 26, 1993. He is survived by his wife, Genevieve, three sons and two granddaughters.

MELVIN H. FREDRICKSEN, was born in Nekoosa, WI on Oct. 21, 1924, and raised in IL. He obtained a GED and after military retirement, taught school for a year. He then became the city mgr. for a year, entering RC service in 1965. Trained at Ft. Sill, OK, he was sent to the 2nd Infantry Division in Korea. After his year's assignment in Korea, he was transferred to Itazuki AFB covering Itazuki, Hakata, and Yamada, Japan. His wife joined him in 1967. He was promoted to field dir.1, and transferred to Ft. Leavenworth, KS in 1969. He was promoted to field dir.2, TRF in 1970 to 2nd Bgd., 101 Abn. Div. at Phu Bai, Vietnam. Served one year TRF to Chanute AFB in IL and in Nov. 1971 was assigned as RC field rep. to cover 30 counties in Southern MO. In Jul., 1972, he went to Wilkes Barre for Disaster Work. In 1973 he was hired as GP2 Chapter mgr. in Springfield,

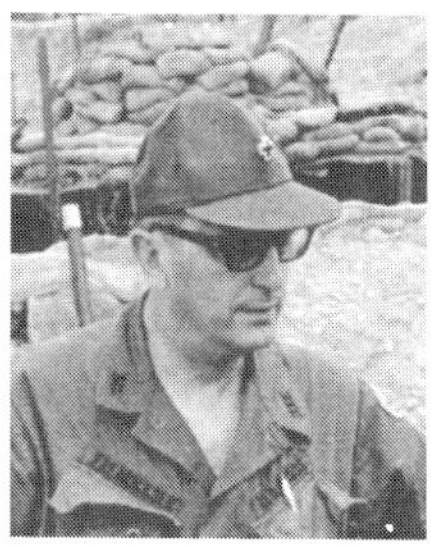

MO. He retired from RC in 1975 due to ill health, and served as a volunteer on the RC Board in Lawton, OK in 1979, and served on the Lawton City Council for 10 years. **See Red Cross Memories story, "Field Director in Phu Bai, Vietnam."*

RUTH FURSE, born in WA Co., PA on Jul. 31, 1913, graduated from high school in 1932, nurse's training in 1940, and attended college in 1948. She went through phlebotomist training in Chicago in 1945, and served with the RC until 1972. She is currently retired, and has one adopted daughter and three grandchildren. **See Red Cross Memories story, "Blood Bank."*

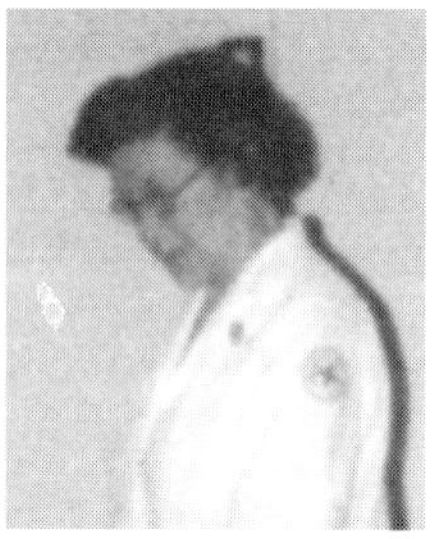

PHILIP GADDIS joined the Army Air Force as WWII was winding down and fell in love with the airplane. He said he spent most of the rest of his life in one. He was honorably discharged in 1947, and graduated from Eureka College. After working as a reporter and editor at the Woodford Co. Journal, in 1953, he began a career with the ARC that would lead him to service on four continents.

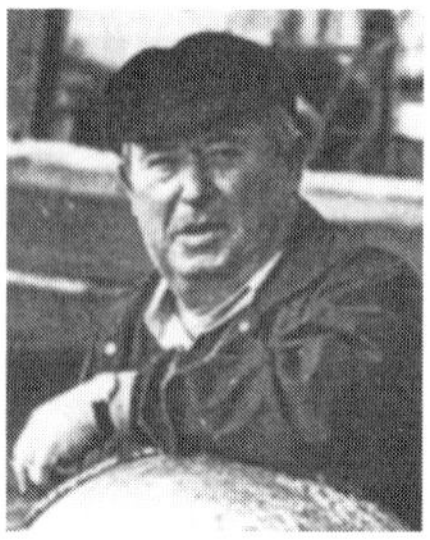

He spent the first nine years in SAF&V assisting American servicemen and families, and in 1962 joined the RC Office of Public Affairs and Communications using his talent for communications and writing. For the next three and a half decades Gaddis practiced and perfected his skill of helping people struck down by natural disasters. Gaddis was cited for outstanding humanitarian service by the League of RC Societies and Intl. Committee of the RC. He retired from the RC OPA in 1988.

Gaddis died in his sleep Sept. 29, 1997. He is survived by his wife, daughter and three grandchildren.

DEXTER D. GALUSHA had a RC career of 37 years all over the country. He was Safety Services asst. mgr. in the Boston Chapter, dir. of financial development in Los Angeles, and division mgr. for 10 years in Eastern NY. In 1998 he was elected president of the Association of ARARC, bringing a wealth of experience and vast resources of personal contacts to serve in this capacity.

JACK PHILIP GARVER, born April 6, 1919 in Mobridge, SC, was educated at UCLA, receiving his BA in 1947, and USouth Carolina, receiving his MA in 1950. His RC assignments included: Naval. Amphibious. Base, Little Creek, VA, 1953-54; Augsburg and Frankfurt, Germany, 1955; VA and NYC (as field dir.I), 1957-58; Osan, Korea, 1959; Japan, 1960; Pioneer field dir., Vietnam and Yokota, Japan, 1962; field dir.2, Ft. Jay, NY, 1964; field dir.3, McGuire AFB, NJ, 1965; Asst. Dir., Alexandria, VA HQ, 1967; Yong San, Korea, 1977; National HQ, 1979. He retired in 1984, having served 31 years on staff, then served nine years as a volunteer.

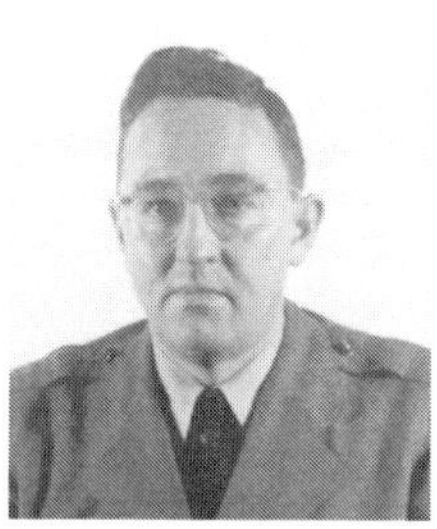

His memorable experiences were opening and closing field dir. stations, most notably opening Vietnam in 1962, special assignment in 1956 to evacuation of Americans from Holy Land War Zone, pride in serving US Military overseas (eight tours), serving on numerous installations. Garver received commendations as natl. staff and as a volunteer at National HQ, DC. He has a framed commendation letter presentation by Ms. Dole at 1990 ceremony at Marble Palace. He is currently retired, but active from time to time on various committees. He resides in VA with his wife of 35 years, Hisako, whom he married in Tokyo, Japan. They have a daughter, Nora.

PATRICK FRANCIS GILBO, holding a BA from Roosevelt Univ. (Chicago) where he majored in internatl. and regional studies, and a MS in education from the Univ. of S. CA, began his career with the ARC in Sept. 1969. A former wire service bureau chief (United Press Intl.) and Univ. of RI public affairs officer, he presently directs the society's public inquiry center and oversees research and preservation activities connected with its vast holding of historical documents and artifacts.

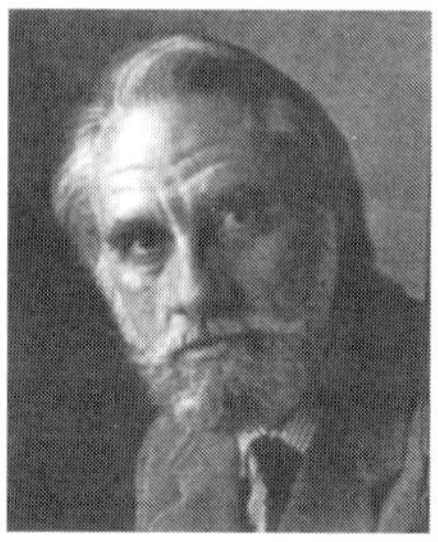

Considered the ARC' resident historian, he published his first book, *The ARC - the First Century*, in 1981 as the society's centennial celebration showpiece. A second book, *The ARC*, was published as part of a series for high schools. His latest book, entitled, *A Triumph of Spirit*, commemorates the 75th anniversary of the Geneva-based Intl. Federation of RC and Red Crescent Societies.

Gilbo has served as asst. field dir. at military installations in Korea and Germany, natl. field rep. to chapters in New England, and dir. of public affairs in Europe. His past positions at National HQ include asst. dir. for centennial activities and asst. dir. for public information. A winner of the organization's Tiffany Award for employee excellence in 1990, he has served in his present position since 1987.

Gilbo, a native of Detroit, MI, is married to Rosalind F. Gordon of Cambridge, MA, a teacher. He has three children, a daughter, Heather; a son, Christopher; and a stepdaughter, Jennifer.

KATHLEEN "KAYE" GILBRIDE, born Feb. 16, 1918 in Houghton, SD, graduated from high school in 1932. She served with the RC in DC starting in 1949; Japan, 1950-52; Korea, 1953-54; Japan and the US, 1955; France and Germany, 1959; Berlin, Germany, 1960; NATO, Italy, 1961; Ft. Hood, TX, 1963; USAF Academy, Co. Springs, CO, 1964; Korea, 1967; Philippines, 1968; Canon AFB, NM, 1970; USMC Recruit Depot, San Diego, CA, 1971; USMB, Philippines, 1973; Castle AFB, CA, 1975 and Mathew AFB, CA, 1977. She retired in 1981.

She says all assignments were memorable, particularly AF Academy and MC Recruitment Depot. She received commendations from military units. Gilbride is currently retired.

SHARON LEVERSON GIMA was born in Minneapolis, MN, and was educated at Moorhead State (1959) and Univ. of MN (1967). Assignments included: Beaumont Hosp., recreation supervisor, El Paso, TX, 1967-68; Vietnam, 1968-69; Lackland, TX, 1969-70; Ft. Sill, OK, 1970-71; Okinawa, Japan, 1971-73; St. Cloud, MN Chapter (as **Sharon Abbott**), 1977-84; Presidio of SF, 1985-87; El Paso, TX, 1987-88; Ft. Polk, 1988-89; Blytheville, AR, 1989-90 and Okinawa, 1990-95.

All Vietnam experiences were memorable starting with her "forgotten" arrival, being issued an M14, and spending the first night under a desk at Tan Son Nhut Airport. Gima received a Vietnam Ribbon and the Clara Barton Award. She is currently a dir. with Navy Marine Corps Relief Society, Okinawa Auxiliary. She resides with husband, Shinsho Gima of Okinawa with one dog and two cats, and has two daughters, two sons-in-law, and three grandchildren in the States.

RALPH E. GODE holds a BS in management from Hofstra College (1951). He began his RC career as dir. of Safety Services, North Shore Chapter, Flushing, NY, also serving as asst. dir. of Safety Services, NY Chapter (now ARC, Greater NY.) His memorable experiences include working with police and firemen at scenes of disasters. As a boy scout he was inspired by Capt. Chas. Scully (NYC) and eventually came to fill his shoes as a "RC pro." He received the 500 Hours Volunteer Service Medal, the Clara Barton Society, citation for work in 1955 floods, Silver Bearer and the Golden Triangle. He is currently retired from the NYS Dept. of Health Immunization Program (19 years) and EMS Development (8 years). He was married to Florence for 54 years before she passed away, and has a daughter Karen (25-year RC volunteer) and sons, Brian and David.

EDGAR C. "BUD" GOOD, JR., joined the staff of the ARC in 1967 as editor of two monthly magazines read by young Americans in more than 600,000 elementary, secondary and college classrooms. The ARC Youth News and Journal presented information about RC principles and service programs in which children and youth could become involved.

In 1970, Good became deputy natl. dir. of public relations. President George M. Elsey named Good as his exec. asst. in 1975. Three years later, Good became dir. of communication resources. In 1984, he was appointed the first vice president of corporate communication of the American Red Cross, by President Richard F. Schubert. For the next decade, he directed those responsible for the public image, communication among RC units, and production of all communication products used by the corporation.

His achievements include the adoption in 1975 of television as a primary means of communication for the ARC, the creation of unprecedented levels of public awareness and support for RC during the 1970s and 80s, efforts between 1987 and 1992 to enable all elements of the Intl. RC Movement to speak with a single, coordinated voice, and startup of the organization's first satellite-based business television system in 1989. He retired in 1994.

GRACE JAMISON GORDON, born Dec. 19, 1917 in Helena, AR, entered RC service as a telephone operator in Los Angeles, CA on Sept. 9, 1980. Prior to her RC service she attended cosmetology school, accounting school, and worked for H&R Block and in real estate. Her memorable RC experiences included working nights whenever a disaster hit. If it was a fire, a fireman would call and want a catering truck with sandwiches and hot coffee. The ARC would put the fire victims up in a motel and give them an order for clothes and groceries. "Long live the ARC, the people's friend."

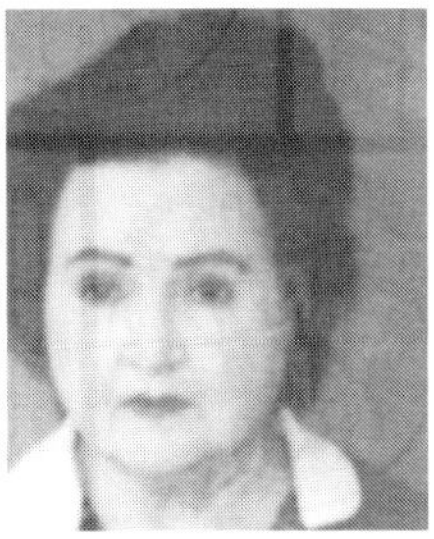

HELEN M. GRANDCOLAS was born June 30, 1916, Belleville, IL. ARC employment began Jan. 1946 Midwestern Area Office, St. Louis, MO as volunteer services correspondent following assignment during WWII as a USO club dir. in Alexandria, LA. Other ARC assignments in a 32 1/2 year career included: Personnel Services (1/46-8/46); general field rep., IL and MI (8/46-8/52); asst. field dir.-SMI Scott AFB, IL (8/52-8/53); Hosp. field dir.SNM, Scott AFB (8/53-6/55); personnel asst. II and III MWA (6/551/58); temporary asst. training dir. MWA (1/58-7/58); personnel asst. III MWA (7/58-9/59); dir. personnel, Far Eastern Area Office, Japan (9/59-10/61); asst. dir., Personnel Recruitment MWA (10/61-6/66); area dir., Personnel, MWA (6/66-6/78).

Following retirement in 1978, he has traveled extensively natl.ly and internatl.ly, an African Safari in 1989 being one of the many highlights. He maintains a home and garden, serves with a number of community organizations, plays golf and bridge, attends concerts and seminars and continues to give programs on travels and historical topics relating to his home area. Grandcolas has written articles for St. Clair Co. Society Journal. He received two special awards from IL College at Jacksonville, IL, his Alma Mater: 1985, Distinguished Citizen and 1987, Honorary Doctorate of Laws. Grandcolas completed his MBA at St. Louis Univ. in 1959.

His fondest memories of his career are of the people with whom he worked and associated. Those friendships continue until this time.

MYRTLE F. GRAVER, born in Dobbs Ferry, NY on Mar. 31, 1918. She graduated from Packard School in 1937. She served as a RC volunteer from 1942-45; dir. of youth services, 1957 and dir. of volunteers, 1970. Her memorable experience was participating in the Youth Council Trn. (Yearly planning and week at conference.) Also she enjoyed working with wonderful volunteers. She has been awarded the Betty Walsh Award and Volunteer of the Year. Graver retired in Mar. 1964, is the widow of Albert F. Graver, and has two sons, five grandsons and one granddaughter.

DANIEL "DAN" GREEN entered RC service in 1940 as GFR in OH, and later in NJ. He resigned to enlist in the Air Force in 1942. Green was S-2 (Intelligence Officer), in Jorhat, Assam, India for a year. He flew over the "HUMP," over Burma into China, 35 times. Back in the States he was chief of Special Services. Air Transport Command, and discharged as major.

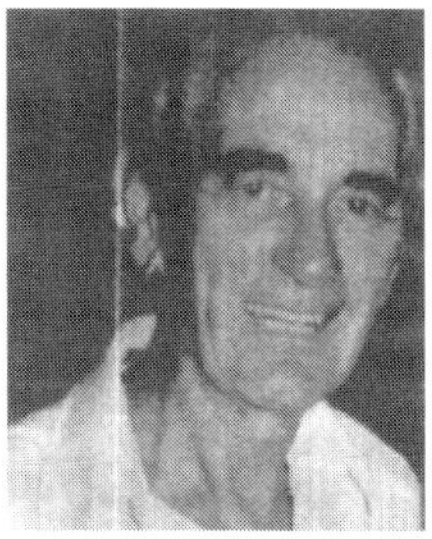

Green rejoined the RC in 1945 as administrator, Social Services, NY Chapter. He became asst. exec. dir., and finally exec. dir. Before he resigned in 1963. He then served as exec. dir. of the Children's Aid Society and exec. dir., Graham-Windsor Society. He served on The Board of the ARARC from its inception, and on the Retiree Advisory Counsel for three years, helping to devise the existing plan for pensions and benefits.

At the age of 82, he began a new career as a poet. At 88, he had published four volumes of poetry, and his poems appeared over a thousand times in literary magazines. He and Leona, his wife, have traveled to China, India, Nepal, Galapagos, Someo, East Africa, the Seycholles, and close to Antarctica.

TIBOR J. GREENWALT, MD. Was born in Budapest, Hungary, Jan. 23, 1914. He received his MD from NY Univ., 1937. He served as dir. of the Natl. RC Blood Services, Jan. 1967-Sept. 1978. He was awarded a plaque at his retirement ceremony, signed by Dr. Frank Stanton, chairman of the Board of Governors and George M. Elsey, president of the ARC. He established the outstanding rare donor registry in the world with an internatl. network. In Sept., 1979 he left RC Blood Services to assume the dir.ship of the Hoxworh Blood Center of the Univ. of Cincinnati. After retiring from that post he has remained as deputy dir. for research. He is also an emeritus professor of internal medicine and continues an active research career in transfusion medicine.

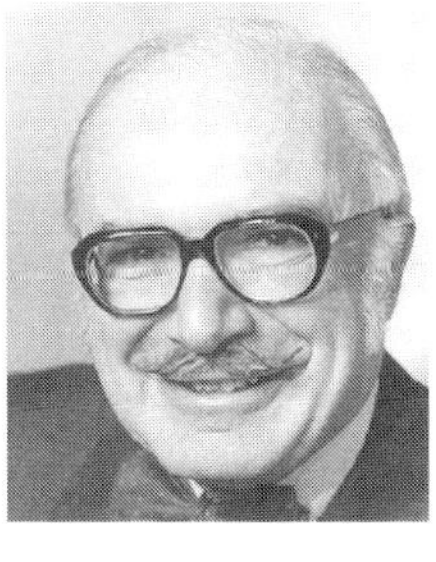

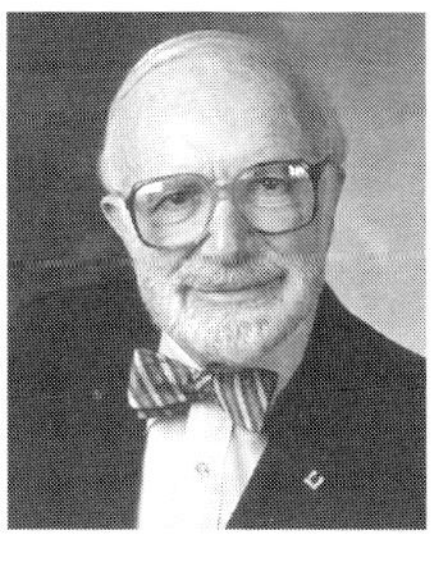

He received the first Charles R. Drew Award, and was elected to Senior Membership in the Institute of Medicine of the Natl. Academy of Sciences. At present he is the only Blood Banker (Transfusion Medicine specialist) to achieve this distinction.

CAROLINE SCHNABEL GUYTHERIE born in San Francisco, CA and raised in Richmond, joined the RC in 1959. Schnabel studied at CA State Univ. at San Francisco. In her early years with the ARC, she initiated a program at Richmond Hosp. where students served as volunteers helping to make patients comfortable and to assist with their daily needs. As part of her duties as admin. asst. in the Richmond office, Guytherie was also the liaison between the RC and the community in fostering good will and mutual cooperation between health agencies and the RC. She retired after 24 years with the Richmond, CA office of the ARC.

Guytherie got much pleasure from working with the ARC Teacher Advisors. A most rewarding experience was the week-long Leadership Training Center held each summer with youth from the five Bay Area Chapters at a camp site.

She currently enjoys swimming, volunteering at the hosp., and playing with her great-grandson. She is learning about remodeling a house. She has a daughter, Arlene Moran and two grandchildren, Gretcher and Josh.

ERNA M. GUY took RC Volunteer Training as Nurse's Aide and Gray Lady in 1956, and worked two years at Fitzsimmons Army Hosp., CO. She then served three terms as record and volunteer chairman at RAF Station Wethersfield, England, Homestead AFB, FL and Bitburg AB, Germany.

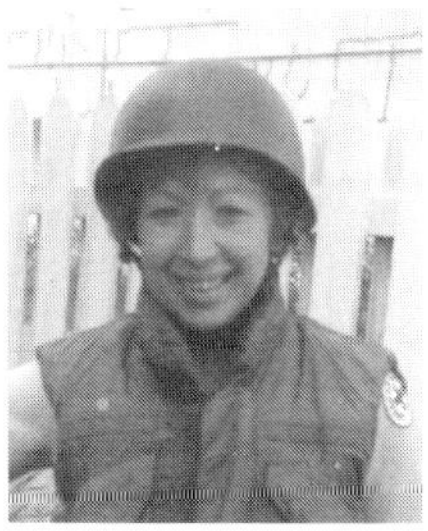

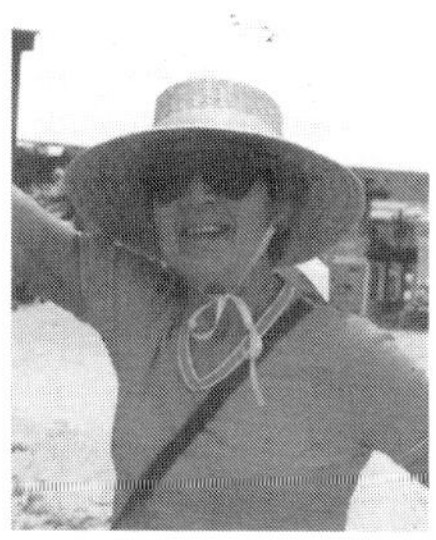

After the sudden death of her husband on active duty she became natl. staff member, SAF-V, her first duty tour being at Robins AFB, GA. She was sent to Tan Son Nhut AB, MACV; Redstone Arsenal, Huntsville, AL; Basic WAC Training Center, Ft. McClellan, AL; U-Tapao, Royal Thai Navy Airfield, Bangkok; Cambodian Baby Airlift and the Refugee Camp; Germany; Marine Corps Air Ground Training Center, 29 Palms, CA; Leighton Barracks, Wuerzburg, Germany. Then she retired as station mgr. II, Nov. 1985, moving to Santa Monica to be near the long hoped-for first grandchild.

Guy currently volunteers at the Kaiser Clinic and Senior Center, chauffeuring her granddaughters from school to music and sports activities and helping elderly neighbors. She finds time to roam the world, visiting her daughter at such foreign service posts as Kazakhstan and Belarus, frequently stopping on the way to see dear old "RCers."

RUTH H. HALLER's RC experience from 1950-85 included Japan, Korea, France, Germany, Turkey, Italy, Mare Island (NS), NAS Alameda, San Francisco and Washington, DC. She studied at UC Berkeley, CA. After attending college, she had the choice through an employment agency to work for either the American Can Company or the ARC. An innate desire to help others led her to choose the ARC and with this choice a whole world, a rewarding career and adventurous life opened up to her. She took lessons in CPR and had the opportunity to use her knowledge when a family, going on vacation, left in her care a goldfish named Charlie. One day upon coming home from work, she saw to her horror that Charlie was gasping and floating on his side. She rushed for a bowl of fresh water and dunked Charlie. Suddenly CPR flashed into her mind, and as a last resort, she gently squeezed and released his tiny sides several times in the palm of her hand. A large bubble emerged from his mouth and after a few minutes of gentle squeezing, Charlie appeared to have recovered. A happy child was able to return to a healthy fish, thanks to the ARC and CPR.

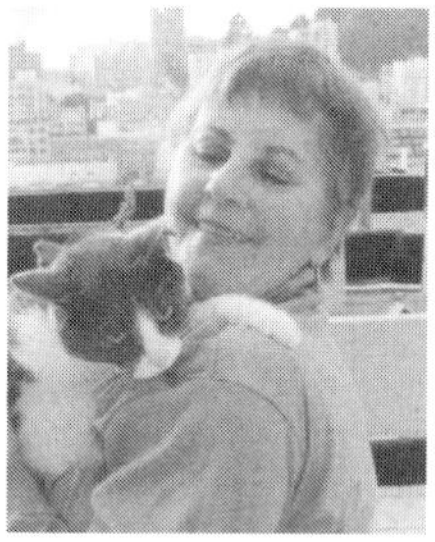

JOHN K. HAMRICK, born Sept. 30, 1926 in Cedartown, GA, was educated at Berry Boys High School and received his AB degree from Mercer Univ., Macon, GA. His 27-year tenure with the RC included: asst. field dir., Ft. McPherson, GA; asst. field dir., Hanau, Germany; field dir., Orleans, France; field dir., England AFB, LA; field rep., AL; field rep., NC; asst. AD, RC Youth, Atlanta, GA; Chapter mgr., San Bernardino, CA; RC advisor, Defense Civil Preparedness Agency, Denver, CO; asst. Division mgr., Nashville, TN. His memorable experiences with the RC include serving as field dir. in Germany in France; area dir. with RC Youth in Atlanta, GA; overseeing work at the Thompson Flood, Estes Park, CO. He is currently retired, is a widower since his wife Irene passed away, and has two children, John and Carla.

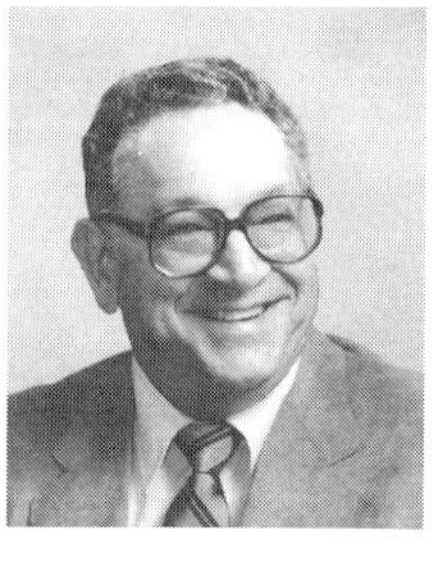

JESSE V. HAWS was born in Vernal, UT and graduated of UT State Univ., 1950. He worked in the retail business before and after WWII in UT, ID and WA. He left this occupation to join ARC as asst. field dir. at Ft. Lewis, WA, 1956-1958. He served as field rep. in UT and NV, 1961-65, and was mgr. of the Weber Co. Chapter, Ogden, UT, 1965-68. He was in the Western Area as a Disaster rep. where he stayed until June 1971, going back to field service in ID and western WY until his retirement in Oct. 1983.
He has served on many disaster operations through the years, including hurricanes Carla, Camille, Celia, floods in MT and OR and the Teton Dam Break.

While at Ft. Lewis he helped a serviceman, who was on leave, get out of a murder charge. To get money to return to Ft. Lewis he had his local chapter send a TWIX for a loan. He stopped just out of Ft. Lewis at a restaurant. The waitress thought she recognized him as the murderer, and a few days later he was arrested. His only alibi was the TWIX. He came to the Ft. Lewis for help. Haws was on duty at the time. The time and date stamped on the TWIX proved he was not in the area at the time of the murder.

Haws has been married 52 years to his wife LoraLee Reid. They have 4 adopted children and 17 grandchildren.

DOROTHY "DOTTIE" MARIE HENEBERRY was born Oct. 2, 1919 in Bethany, IL. She graduated from Bethany, IL High School in 1937 and attended Brown's Business College, Decatur, IL, 1937-38. Her RC assignments from 1945-83 included: secretary to asst. dir., Jr. RC; secretary to associate dir. and dir., Blood Program; admin. secretary to exec. VP, admin. secretary to VP, Admin.; admin. asst. to chairman and president, ARC.

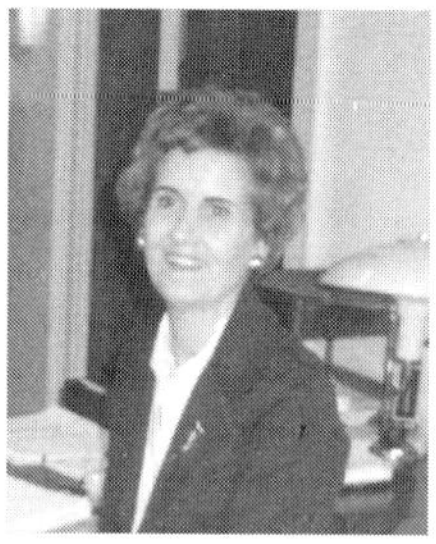

Her memorable experiences were working for many interesting bosses, and her pride and joy is her 50-year Service Pin with a small ruby earned after 37 1/2 years as a paid staff member and volunteering in the Convention Management Office, 1984-96. She is currently enjoying retirement and keeps busy. She has served on the first Retiree Advisory Council, 3 years and as secretary, ARARC, Greater WA and Baltimore, and has been a member of the ARARC since 1983. She is active at St. Thomas Apostle Church, serving as treasurer, and enjoys traveling. She is also a member of the Quebec House Health Club.

LESTER E. HILL was born in Boonville, MO on Nov. 22, 1928. He attended Central College, MO, and obtained a BA in social science; Univ. of MT, graduate studies in psychology and VA Commonwealth Univ., graduate studies in literature and creative writing.

His ARC service spanned 40 years (1953-90), with service as asst. field dir., MO, OK and Korea; field dir. in Kyushu, Japan, 101st Airborne RCT; Fuchu, Japan, Far East Air Forces; OK, Tinker AFB; CO, US Air Force Academy; England, Lakenheath AFB; Germany, HQ 4th Armored Division; MN Naval Air Station, St. Paul, MN; Ft. Riley, KS. He served as asst. dir. in Midwestern Area HQ, St. Louis, MO and Siagon, Vietnam and acting dir. In Vietnam and Midwestern Area HQ, St. Louis, MO. With RC Youth Services, he served as dir., Midwestern Area HQ. In management, he served as exec. dir., Pioneer Valley Chapter, Springfield, MA; division mgr./exec. dir./CEO, Richmond, VA (VA Capital Division) His final position with the ARC was chief exec. officer, VA Capital Chapter, Richmond, VA.

Hill is currently a board member, ARC Retiree Council, ARC Overseas Association, Art Space Advisory Council (past president) and the Hollows Golf Club. He is married and has 3 children. He retired in 1990.

ALICE D. HIXSON's 20-year association with the ARC began in 1966 as a hosp. volunteer. From 1968-77 she performed case work and social work duties for the Wyandotte Co. Chapter, KS City, KS.

Having experienced military life with her Army husband in Japan after WWII, Hixson relished assisting veterans and their families through the ARC, especially helping get discharges upgraded and disability benefits approved. Her favorite memories include an elderly man applying for benefits based on his father's death in the Civil War, working with a Korean War veteran who had been a POW in China, and hearing a Vietnam veteran's eyewitness account of the Fall of Saigon. "It was just a fascinating job every single day!"

Although she retired from the chapter office in 1977, Hixson continued as a hosp. volunteer for nine more years. Now widowed, she enjoys visiting with her two sons and four grandchildren.

JEANNETTE F. HOSLER paid $1.00 when she joined the RC in Nov. 1919. She was 15 years old and living in a suburb of Philadelphia.

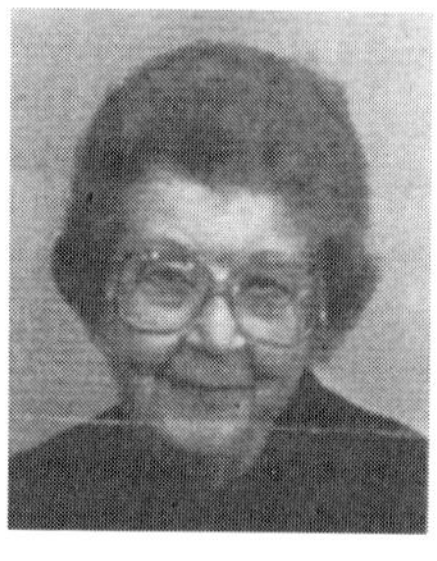

In 1941, Hosler and her husband moved to NY and she became a volunteer at the Naussau Co. Chapter. She began her 18-year career as a staff member teaching a course in what she called "Glamour" two days a week. She was a nutritionist and the course focused on weight loss. In 1955-56, she was chief of emergency feeding for Nassau Co. Civil Defense. She was sent to Ft. Dix to be trained in feeding large numbers of people. When she returned, she used this knowledge to train other Nassau Co. volunteers.

As a volunteer, Hosler was president of the Hempstead Branch and vice-president of the Locust Valley Branch. She appeared on television to announce a fund raiser for the NC Chapter in Nassau Co.

She received a 70-year pin and a letter from President Bush congratulating her on her service. In 1994, she was honored by the Locust Valley Branch of the RC with a pin from the Nassau Co. Chapter, and a letter from RC president, Elizabeth Dole. She currently has retired in Nazareth, PA, where she plans to volunteer for the RC.

AILI L. IMARISIO was born in MI, and obtained a BS in business education and economics from Northern MI Univ. in 1941. A certified teacher, Imarisio began service with the RC in 1949. Assignments from 1949-60 included: work with services to military, Tokyo, Camp Drake, Japan; Aschaffenburg, Heidelburg, Wurzburg, Germany; Ft. Hamilton and Brooklyn Army Term, NYC; services to military and Hungarian refugees and Dorian ship disaster in Brooklyn, NY. Some of her most memorable experiences were: Yokohama amidst the Cherry Blossom Festival and being greeted by girl's band in white silk, contemporary music and a banquet; seeing Gen. Douglas MacArthur in his shiny black, flag-decked limo stopping all traffic, pedicabs, rickshaws and pedestrians; climbing Mt. Fuji, peering into the deep, dark sulfuric hole; and visiting the flat, treeless Hiroshima.

Imarisio is currently retired, active in ARC Overseas Assn., Chicago Medical Society Alliance and American Assn. Univ. Women. Her husband John is a retired physician of nuclear medicine and medical school instructor.

RUTH M. JACOBS was born on Mar. 26, 1910 in Saluda, SC. She became an RN in 1932 and graduated from Catholic Univ. in 1950. Her RC services from 1941-71 included volunteer work and dir.ship in the nursing and health program, Pinellas Co., St. Petersburg, FL. She remembers the Centennial Celebration and helping during Hurricane Betsy, New Orleans, 1965. She received awards in 1988 and 1990. She is married and has four children, nine grandchildren and seven great grandchildren.

DR. GRAHAM JAMIESON has been a leader and distinguished scientist at the ARC.

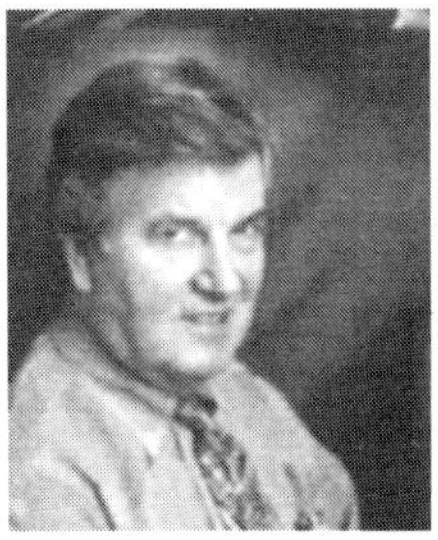

Jamieson was born, raised, and educated in New Zealand where he received both BS and MS degrees from the Univ. of Otago. He received his PhD in organic chemistry at the Univ. of London, Lister Institute of Preventive Medicine in 1954. An additional degree, the DSc in organic chemistry and biochemistry, was conferred in 1972 by the Univ. of London.

He joined the ARC as a research biochemist in 1961. In 1964, Jamieson became a senior scientist and the asst. research dir. He became research dir. in 1969 and organized the Annual RC Scientific Symposium on Transfusion Medicine. Under his guidance, the research and development programs work achieved natl. and internatl. recognition and respect.

Jamieson relinquished his position as dir. in 1984 to return his full attention to his research. In 1997, the Intl. Society on Thrombosis and Haemostasis selected Dr. Jamieson to receive the Shirley Johnson Award, and he became a fellow of the American Association for the Advancement of Science.

PATRICIA "PAT" M. JERMON joined the ARC in 1949. Her assignment was the Tokyo Army Hosp. (later United Nations Hosp.) after the outbreak of the Korean War in June 1950. In addition to recreation programs and social services the ARC staff took turns meeting convoys of new casualties after 11:00 p.m., serving coffee and cookies. In late 1951, Jermon was assigned to the Yokosuka Naval Hosp. Annex near Kyoto. Here convalescing Marines waited to return to Korea. She helped with office work and recreation, including dancing and horseback riding lessons.

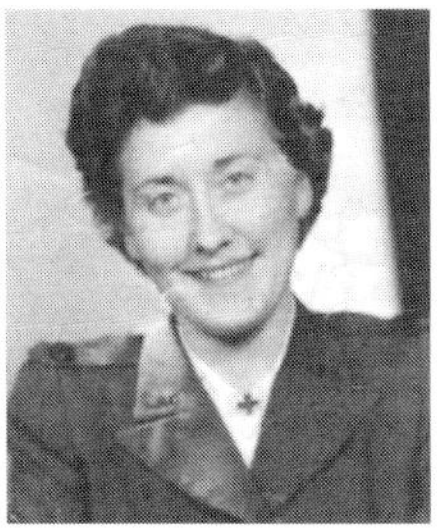

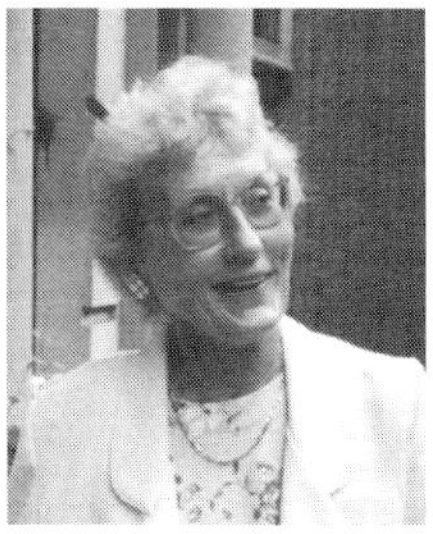

Later, she served as CSII at the 5th General Hosp., Bad Cannstadt, Germany; Service to Military Installations at Ft Hamilton, NY; Griffiths AFB, NY; USNAS Pstuxent River, MD and Ft. Meade, MD. She received a Civil Service Award from the commanding general at Ft. Holabird where she manned a one person annex for the field dir. at Ft. Meade.

In 1965, she took the position of Service to Military Families dir., Prince George's Chapter, MD. In 1968, she completed her MA in sociology, and took over the Disaster Services for the Chapter and participated in Natl. Disasters. Before her retirement in 1984, Jermon was asst. casework supervisor on Natl. Disasters. Jermon is now living in Dunedin, FL, near Clearwater, where she helps neighbors with transportation to important appointments.

LAWRENCE L. JONES was born Dec. 17, 1941 in Spring Hope, NC. He was educated at Spaulding High School, Spring Hope, 1959; NCA&T State Univ., Greensboro (BS, applied sociology, 1963); East Carolina Univ., Greenville, 1975; Webster Univ., St. Louis, MO (MA, human resource development, 1989).

He joined the RC in 1966, and his many assignments from 1966-96 included: Camp LaJeune, NC (asst. field dir.); Camp Ranh Bay, Vietnam (asst. field dir.); Ft. Bragg, NC (asst. field dir.); Quang Tri, Vietnam (asst. field dir.); SEAO, Atlanta, GA (disaster rep); Cherry Point Marine Air Station, Havelock, NC (asst. field dir.); Neu Ulm, Germany (asst. field dir.); Myrtle Beach AFB, SC(field dir.); KY Division, Louisville, KY (field service rep); MWFO, St. Louis, MO and Chicago, IL (field service mgr.).

Jones has one son, Nikolaus Ainsley Jones.

MARGARET TRUITT JOYAL, born Oct. 4,1917, entered RC service in 1945. She had three overseas tours: Germany (1949-50), Japan (1954/56), and France (1961/63). Her assignments were: US Naval Hosp., Bainuridge, MD; US Army Hosp. Frankfurt, Germany; US Army Hosp., Ft. Dix, NJ; US Army Hosp., West Point, NY; Walter Reed Army Hosp.; US Air Force Hosp., Nagoya, Japan; US Air Force Hosp., Orleans, France; US Naval Hosp., Bethesda, MD and US Naval Hosp., Portsmouth, VA. **See Red Cross Memories story, "Hollywood Celebrities and the Cherry Blossom Dance."*

JOHN T. KANE joined the RC in Feb. 1956. He was in the Navy during the Korean War and the RC job sounded interesting since he was anxious to travel. The RC more than gave him both of these for the next fifteen years. He was assigned as an asst. field dir. in Service to Military Installations. His duty stations were: 1956-58, Carswell AFB, TX; 1958, James Connally AFB, TX; 1958-59, Pagarii, Korea; 1959, Inchon, Korea and 1959-60, Kadena, Okinawa.

His assignment to Okinawa became particularly important and memorable to me. He met this "cute little Army librarian" from NY and they were married Jul. 1, 1960 at the Ft. Buckner Chapel. In May 1961, he was promoted to field dir. and reassigned to Altus AFB, OK. In June 1962, he transferred to the accounting office at Natl. HQ. He served in disasters in Crescent CA, Hurricane Camille and Hurricane Betsy.

When he left RC in 1970, he was an asst. natl. dir. of Accounting and Auditing. Before he left, he had become a CPA and a partner in a major accounting firm. He is ready to retire after almost thirty very satisfying years.

MARY KARABAICH, a native of Seattle, spent close to 25 years in communications roles with the Seattle-King Co. Chapter and former Pacific Northwest Division. She started as public information dir. Earlier she was a hosp. recreation worker with SMH, assigned to hospitals in San Diego, Oakland, Bremerton and Ft. Lewis. She earned a bachelor's degree in journalism and a master's in communications from the Univ. of WA. Her thesis was "A History of Official Organ Publication by the ANRC." She had experience as a writer/publicity rep. with a major airline and as a weekly newspaper reporter/writer. Bicycle touring has been her retirement career since mid - 1988.

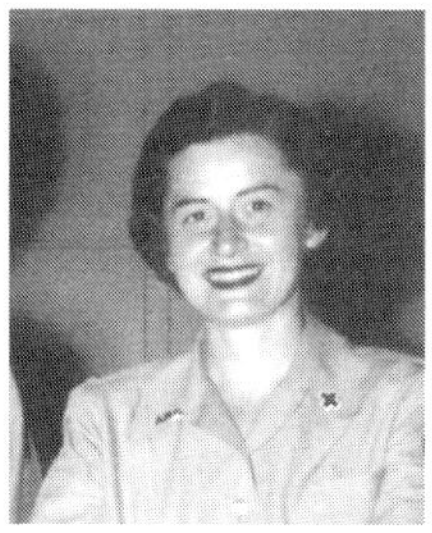

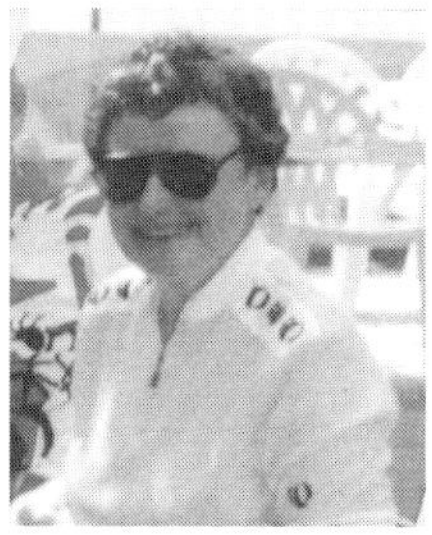

She has been on many tours in the US and abroad and is a volunteer ride leader with two Seattle area bicycle clubs. Her next scheduled tour abroad is in June of 2000 and is in France's Dordogne region.

JOHN KASSAB, was born on Jul. 31, 1921 in Houtzdale, PA. He graduated from high school, 1939. Army Air Corps in Pilot Training 1942, graduating Oct. 1943. He flew B-24 Liberators, first mission being D Day, June 6th 1944 in Europe. He flew 35 missions, plus 10 extra non combat missions, supplying General Patton's troops with fuel for armored equipment. After numerous assignments in USAF he retired from the Air Force and joined ARC as asst. field dir, NAS Pensacola, FL for one year. He then went to Da Nang, Vietnam with 1st Marine Division for six months. He was transferred to Da Nang Navy Facility as field dir. with Seabees Organization. He returned to the US in Dec. 1967, field dir. Camp La Jeune, NC;

He accepted a position with Mobile Regional Blood Center as Dir. Blood Donor recruitment and then Administrator of Mobile Regional Blood Program; Dir. Safety Services until Aug. 1983. He retired Aug. 1983 and have been doing volunteer work with ARC plus hosp. auxiliary. He still works and has accumulated in excess 10,000 hours volunteer services to date.

Kassab received the Clara Barton award, Vietnam Civilian Service Medal and numerous commendations from the local RC chapter.

He has been married to Nita for approximately 54 years, and they have two children and five grandchildren.

HILBERT FRYE KEISKER, was born on May 31, 1904, in St. Louis, MO on May 31, 1904. His first contact with the RC was as a volunteer office boy one day per week, SW Division office, St. Louis in the summer of 1918. He was loaned out to the RC for St. Louis tornado operation in Sept. of 1927 to early 1928. He was employed in the Midwest Area Oct. 8, 1928 as a field rep., and promoted in 1928 to staff asst. to the mgr. Keisker retired on May 31, 1969. He enjoyed all positions, most experiences and most of all the fellow staff members and volunteers.

ESTHER COXE KELLY was born in Bennettsville, SCand graduated from Columbia College in Columbus, SC.

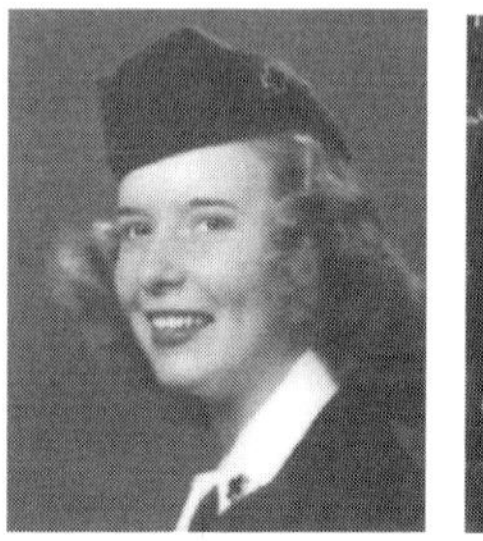

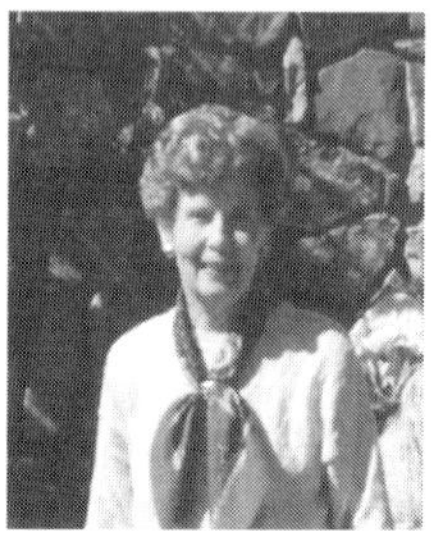

She reported to the American Univ. in Washington, DC in Jul., 1945 for training to be a RC Hosp. worker. Her first assignment was at the US Naval Hosp. in New Orleans, LA. When the hosp. closed she was sent to South Eastern Area Office in Atlanta, GA for more training to be a Home Service worker in the Cumberland Co. Chapter, Fayetteville, NC. Later she returned to SC to work in the Central SC Chapter in Columbia. her service totaled 35 years and spanned three wars, WWII, Korean and the Vietnam War. She retired from the Central SC Chapter as dir., Emergency Community Services on Jan. 1, 1987.

Retirement is wonderful! She is the mother of two children and active in volunteer work and church work. She is an avid sports fan and loves to travel.

MIRA B. KENNEDY was born in Pesotum, IL, Sept. 28, 1907. As a graduate of the Univ. of IL in 1931 (her first year's tuition in 1925 was $25.00) and a member of the Acadamy of Certified Social Workers, she was hired by the ARC Chicago Chapter in Oct., 1937. There she worked for thirteen years. When her husband accepted a position in Columbus, OH in 1950 she left to join him there.

After two years of direct contact with clients, families, servicemen and completing guardianship reports for the VA, she was given responsibility for the supervision of 12 to 15 social workers.

The need for more workers grew with the threat of war. The staff quickly grew to 5000 workers in the Chicago area. She was made dir., Casework Services. She traveled to each area office for conferences and case discussions.

One of the highlights of service was the Christmas giving plan. Caseworkers elected families in greatest need and had the parent or relative complete a wish list for each child. Volunteers then made or bought one item from each list so that the parent of relative could come for the gifts and have the joy of giving them to their children.

Kennedy kept busy in Columbus volunteering for several agencies through the years.

MARTHA KILLEBREW'S hometown was Seattle, WA and she was born in 1921. She graduated from UC Berkeley in 1942 and got her Masters from Harvard Graduate School in business in 1944. She was the executive dir. of Alameda CA Chapter for 22 years. She is now retired, but came in contact with the RC again when her two homes burned to the ground in the 1991 Oakland/Berkeley firestorm. She said she received the royal treatment. She stated, "It was tremendously helpful and heartwarming, from the "other side" of the line.

LEO "LEE" C. KIRK, born Sept. 3, 1922 in Louisville, MS, and graduated in 1952 from Univ. of MS, Oxford, MS.

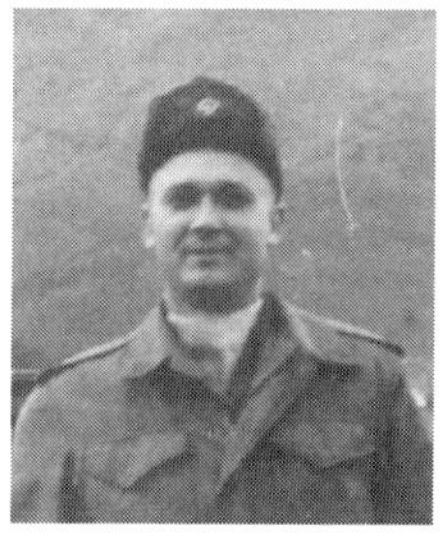

After training in Atlanta, he was assigned at Ft. Benning, GA; Korea; Japan; Philippines; Turkey; Vietnam; Columbus, MS; Permasens, Germany; Bremerhaben, Germany; Ft. Campbell, Ky. After retiring he volunteered with the local Chapter in the Blood Program. He resides in Huntsville, AL.

Turkey was memorable because the base was raided periodically and one had to be escorted off base. One was not allowed to wear any kind of identification off base. In Vietnam his office was bombed. All overseas tours were interesting because he was able to see many countries and meet many people.

Kirk is married to Charleen, and they have two daughters, one son in-law, one grandson and one granddaughter.

JILL PITTS KNAPPENBERGER graduated from Stephens College with an AA, 1938 and Univ. of IL with a BS, 1950. She served with the extension staff until she married Champaign attorney, T. Gaillard Knappenberger (1/3/53).

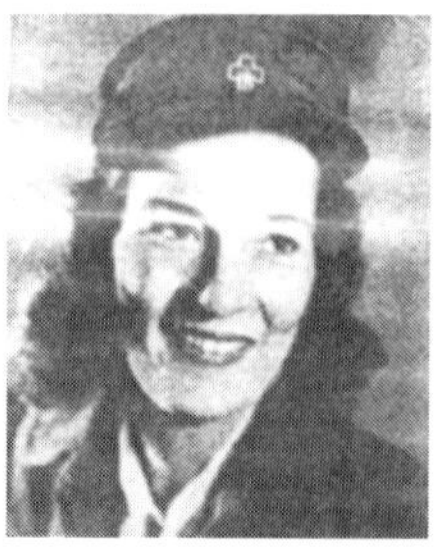

In Nov. 1943, she graduated from ARC school at American Univ., DC, and sent to ETO in the largest convoy to leave the States. She served coffee, donuts and sweets, candy, gum, and cigarettes to new troops landing at Grenoch and Gourock, Scotland, and Liverpool, England. She was assigned to a Clubmobile on the largest B-17 base in England, and her superior rating in the driving course brought her back to London to teach the new girls 1st echelon maintenance, double clutching, changing 55# tires, etc. on the 2-1/2 ton GMC trucks. The enemy was constantly bombarding them. She landed on Utah Beach and was assigned to 8th Corps. She worked through Normandy, Brittany; the Brest Peninsula; Bastogne, Belgium; Vielsalm. At Vielsalm, the 106th Inf. was immediately cut off and surrounded by the enemy. She was among the only Clubmobile girls actually caught in the Battle of the Bulge. After seven days with constant shelling and gunfire, no radio communication and little food and ammunition, they were 'escorted' out by a POW interrogation team. She operated a donut dug-out in the bombed Belgium barracks in Bastogne, and crossed the Moselle and Rhine Rivers. She saw the horror of Ordnff and Buckenwald concentration camps at their liberation. For six weeks, she operated a donut club at Mailly le Camp, France until returniing to the States in Aug. 1945, when she was discharged from the ARC.

FLORENCE KOHOUT In 1968 she became an ARC volunteer for the Lane Co. Chapter, Eugene, OR in the department known then as Service to Military Families & Disaster Services. In 1970 she joined the staff and retired in 1984.

She took many disaster training classes but had never gone on a natl. disaster. After her retirement, and the death of her husband, she went back to volunteer status and has served on many natl. disasters in the Family Service Function.

She keeps busy with volunteer projects in her home town as a hosp. volunteer, St. Vincent de Paul and service on the RC Disaster Committee. She enjoys golfing, gardening and card playing.

Her family consists of twin daughters and two sons-in-law, a son and daughter-in-law, two grandchildren and one step grandson.

CHARLOTTE KILBOURN EASTER KRESS was born on Mar. 20, 1920, in Chicago, IL, and received her BA from Reed College in Portland, OR in 1944 and MS from the Univ. of MT in 1977.

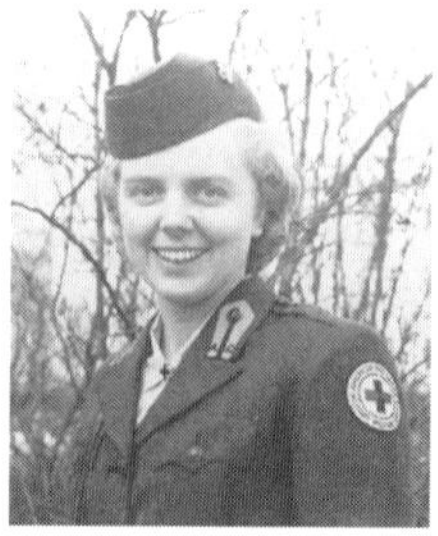

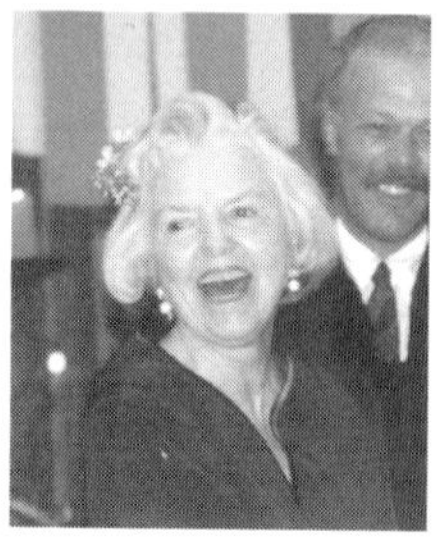

From Feb., 1945 to Jan. 1946 she was a recreation hostess for the Air Force Angleterre Hotel. In 1946 she was a hostess on trains delivering families to servicemen in Germany who were with the Army of Occupation. She was a supervisor, Volunteers McGuire VA Hosp., Richmond, VA; served with Disaster Services, KS City, MO flood; with SMF, Richmond, VA Chapter; and was a Gray Lady (volunteer) and SMF volunteer in different chapters. Her last assignment was from 1980-87 on the staff of St. Louis RC Chapter for SMF and Natl. Disaster work. Kress is now retired.

She married Bob Easter in June 1947, and they reared three children and divorced in 1978. She is now married to a retired Missoula, MT doctor, Jack Kress. She has lived in Missoula for 28 years.

JUANITA "NITA" FRANKS LANGER is NM born and a graduate with a BS in 1926. She also did graduate studies in 1934. Her first assignment was in WA early Feb., 1944 and assigned to the 62nd Hosp. as asst. field dir. At the end of the war she was assigned to Camp Lucky Strike. She crossed the English Channel in an Indian boat that lasted three days with a lot of bombing.

She is 96 years old and still drives her own car. She is retired, but still volunteers. Franks resides in NM.

HERBERT C. LARSON, born in Tacoma, WA on Jan. 8, 1911, received his BA in 1933 and had one year of his MSW. He served 24 years with the ANRC, primarily with the Services to the Armed Forces and Veterans (SAF&V), but in his later years, as a senior official. He often was sent to coordinate major disaster relief efforts. One of these disasters was the massive Alaskan Earthquake of 1964. Weeks afterward there were still frequent aftershocks and the inhabitants were fearful of possible damage from those shocks. While eating lunch in the BOQ about a week after the initial shock, a tall officer came into the BOQ, and as he walked to his table, he happened to hit a cord that hung from one of the light switches. The cord started swaying. Within minutes, the place was cleared of personnel; everyone had run out, apprehensive of the collapse of the BOQ! Despite that daily fear, Larson was very impressed with the courage, fortitude and sense of humor of the residents as demonstrated by the hand printed sign on one of the homes that had slid 50 to 100 feet over a collapsed embankment. It read: "I knew times were bad, but I never expected to sink this low!" Larson served from 1950 to 1974. He was stationed in Tacoma, WA, Ogden, UT, Korea, Japan, CA, and at Natl. HQ. Larson passed away in 1978.

VIRGILENA "VIRGIE" RICHARDSON LEE was born in Saluda, SC. She was with the ARC for 24 years and was assigned as follows: DC Chapter Blood Program as a sterilization clerk from 1957 to 1967. She also volunteered at Walter Reed Army Hosp. for senior citizens. She wanted to become a disaster worker, but was never accepted. She transferred to Natl. HQ in 1968 as a clerical supervisor. She states, " She had many wonderful experiences while working with the ARC." She also raised three beautiful children, two boys and one girl. She still works with the US Environmental Protection Agency in Washington, DC.

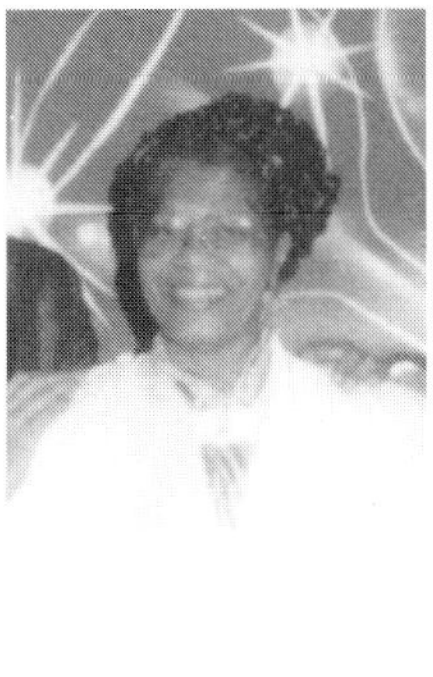

HELEN "PENNY" MITCHELL LEHMAN was born in Farmington, ME on June 9, 1939. She was educated at the Univ. of ME and graduated in the class of 1962. He ARC history began in May, 1967 when she was assigned to Valley Forge General Hosp. as a social worker. From 1970-95, she was employed by Los Angeles Chapter, initially as a social worker and then appointed supervisor of Emergency Services. In 1994 she was appointed Field Dir., Department of Veterans Affair and took an early retirement in Jul. 1995. Currently she is a social worker with Jewish Family Services of Los Angeles, Protective Services Program. She is married to Bernie Lehman. She says that the RC was a wonderful career.

ELMA M. LESLIE-PETROFF has made her home in FL, but was born in Grass Lake, MI on Feb. 20, 1921. She began her volunteer service with the Jackson Co., MI Chapter in 1942 during WWII. She continued with the chapter in various assignments and was elected Chairman of Volunteers in 1963. She served on the Board of Dirs. until 1971. She retired after 42 years of RC Service at Chapter level. She joined the Natl. Disaster Reserves and gave immediate assistance on 15 natl. operations.

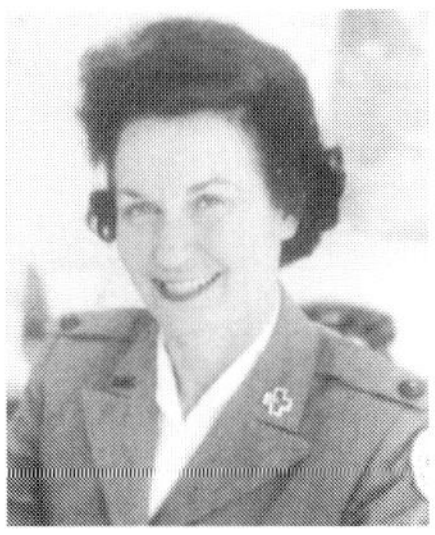

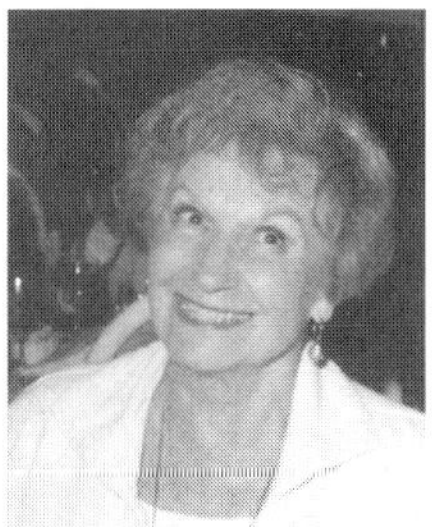

She was awarded many times over her career in the ARC. She is presently busy with travel and writing her first book.

GLADYS L. LONGORIA was born in Van Alstyne, TX on May 3, 1916. She received her BS degree in 1936 and an MS degree in 1948 from the Univ. of North TX, Denton, TX. She began her career with ARC in 1945 until June, 1947 as a caseworker in Loredo, TX Chapter. In June of 1947 until June, 1978 she was a caseworker & dir., SMF&V Austin, TX. In early 1979 until Aug., 1983 she was a Natl. Reserve worker. In Jul. 1978 to Jul., 1996 a volunteer with the Centex Chapter, Austin, TX. She had a special Assignment in 1973 as a Capital Area Division dir. for the Project Find Program initiated by US White House Conference of Aging.

Gladys is retired. Her husband died May 24, 1984, but she has four wonderful children, two sons and two daughters. She also has five

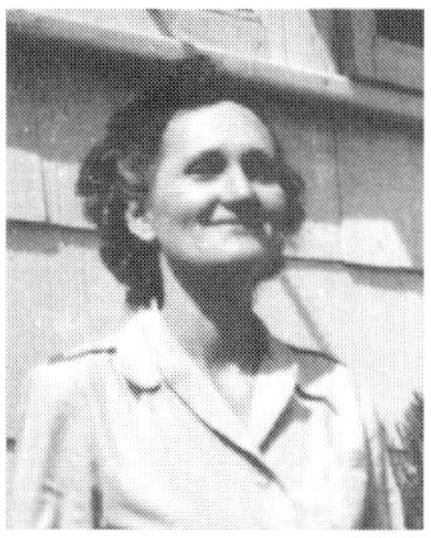

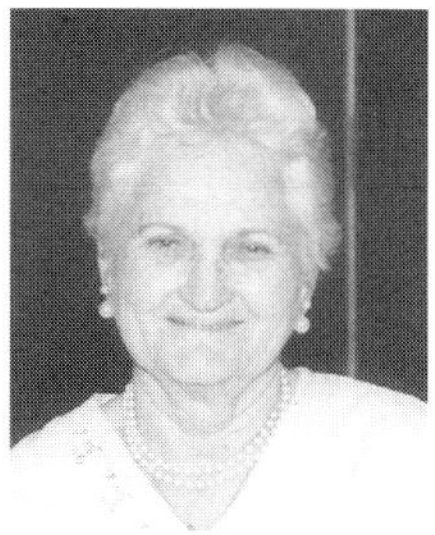

grandchildren and four great-grandchildren. She received many awards and certificates for her service and even had a day named in her honor: "Gladys Longoria Day," June 17, 1978. **See Red Cross Memories story, "Working wiht Military Families."*

CHARLES "CHUCK" A. LUDWIG was born in Edgewood, PA on Jul. 5, 1925. He received his BA in 1948 and his Masters in Music in 1949. He was a Field Representative in MO, KS, ND and SD. He was on disaster in TX, MS, TN and Korea. He spent one year in Korea working with the Korean RC. He is retired and married to Betty Bryan. They live in Kimberling City, MO.

PEARL DUTY MALLORY was born on Feb. 3, 1922 in Washington Co., VA. On May 8, 1942, she became a caseworker and night duty worker at the Princess Anne Co. Chapter of the American Red Cross, now Tidewater Chapter. Through her years with the ARC, Mallory has accumulated a wealth of experience and knowledge. During WWII, she helped foreign born war brides settle into their new home here in America. The Korean and Vietnam Wars gave she new challenges such as increasing drug problems and deserters. She has shared many joys and sadness with many people.

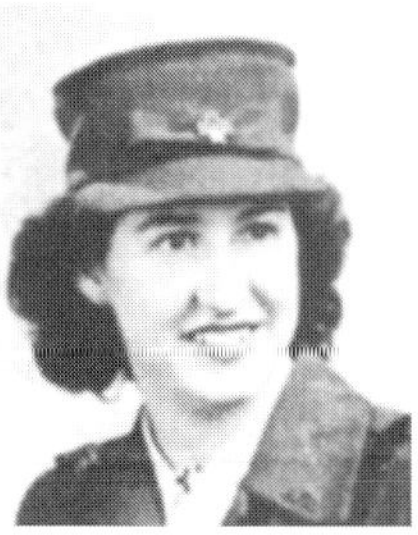

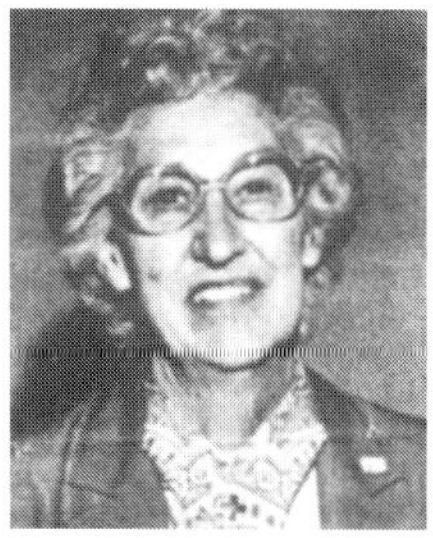

Mallory is respected and admired throughout the RC for her dedication and her love of humanity. She has been on duty with the ARC for over 43 years. She is retired now and lives in VA with her husband and has two step-children and grandchildren.

CLEO "CLECIE" MAE MARSHALL was born on June 26, 1927, in McClean, TX. She graduated from McLean High School in 1944. Marshall worked for the Coryell Co. Chapter, Gatesville, TX, from 1973 to 1988. She served as secretary, bookkeeper, and interim executive secretary. After retirement

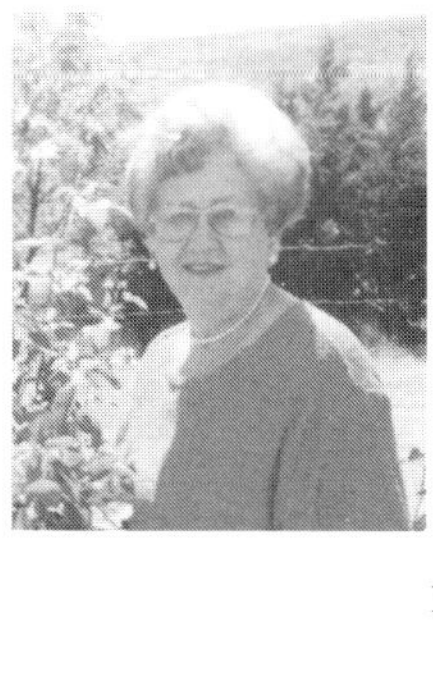

she and her husband volunteered. She has received many awards and recognition for her help in the ARC. She has three children, five grandchildren and one great-grandchild.

ALICE MACBRIDE WARING MCBRIDE joined the staff of the Syracuse and Onondaga Co. Chapter of the ARC as General Office Secretary in May 1941.

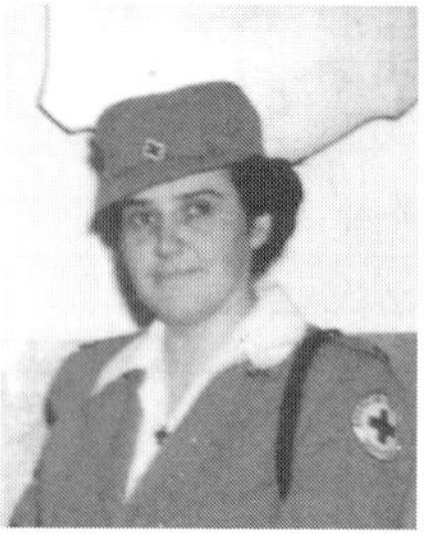

On Dec. 1, 1941, she was assigned the position of Home Service secretary. This position included an inquiry service locating relatives and friends from whom there had been no word. This was a satisfying endeavor.

Mrs. Mae Huntington Cross, dir., Jr. RC, Syracuse and Onondaga Co. chose McBride as asst. dir. At Cross' death, McBride was appointed dir.

She served the Chapter in this capacity for approximately 20 years.

She truly enjoyed serving as a staff member for Jr. RC. Training Centers at Hood College in MD and Wellesley College in MA. I also directed several Chapter Jr. RC. Centers at Manlius Military School in Manlius, NY.

She will always be grateful to her minister, Dr. Ellsworth C. Reamon, then Chapter Chairman for the Syracuse and Onondaga Co. Chapter, who led her to her RC "fun job."

MARION R. MCCONNELL started as a volunteer in Blood Services in 1950. She served on the board of the Berkley, CA Chapter, first as Chairman of Volunteers and then as Chapter Chairman twice.

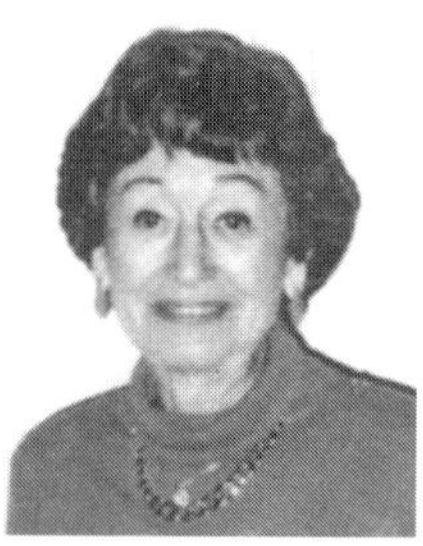

Marion became involved in Disaster Services in the Western Region and was the first coordinator of Volunteers in the country, helping to write the Manual for coordinators throughout the US. She served as coordinator in many large disasters and when the five Bay Area chapters merged into one she was a leader in this project and became the first Bay Area Chairman of Programs where she served for three years. She served on the first Bay Area Board for several years.

Marion received the Cynthia Wedel Award in recognition of distinguished Volunteer Service at the Natl. Convention in 1996.

She still serves on Alameda Co. Board of Dirs. and as a Disaster liaison volunteer in her community, as well as many committees dealing with disaster and/or blood. She is looking forward to receiving her fifty year pin of service to the RC.

FRANK A. MCGURK was born in NY City, NY on Sept. 29, 1912. He received his BA from Marshall Univ. in 1935. His most memorable experience was his retirement ceremony on Oct. 1, 1977. In addition to the usual, he got to thank the volunteers for helping to achieve the dream of a textbook chapter. That is what the Baton Rouge Chapter had become, with over 4,000 volunteers.

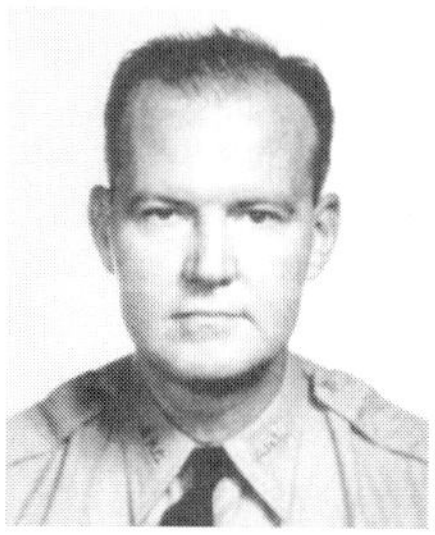

He served at the Natl. HQ; SE Area and in AL from 1941 to 1950. He was then appointed Field Dir., SMI 1950-1960 and Chapter Mgr., Baton Rouge, LA, 1961-1977. He states that with the exception of the year 1945 in an area office he enjoyed all of his various jobs.

DOROTHY ZIMMERMAN MCLAUGHLIN, born and raised in Omaha, NE, and graduated from the Univ. of NE in 1931 with a Bachelors degree and received a Masters degree from Columbia Univ. in 1937.

She was associated with the RC for almost 50 years in various capacities. From 1927 to 1942 she taught First Aid and Water Safety on a volunteer basis. In 1942, she was assigned to England. After various assignments, she became asst. club dir. for a GI Service Club (Milestone) in London where she stayed until she returned to the States in 1945.

In 1944 in Plymouth, England, she married Clarence McLaughlin then a lieutenant in the US Army. He later became a major.

In 1945 she returned from England and was assigned to ARC Natl. HQ as dir. of the Returnee Unit and a disaster worker on call. In 1946, she left Natl. HQ for a social work job in Maine, but remained on call until retirement on Oct. 1, 1973. During this time she had served on disasters all over the US and Guam.

She keeps very busy with the Lions Auxiliary Association of Republican Women, traveling with the Friendship Force and is a life member of the American Legion Auxiliary.

ANGELO F. MENNA was born in Philadelphia, PA on Sept. 21, 1913. He received his BA from Temple Univ. in 1933 and a Masters in education in 1943.

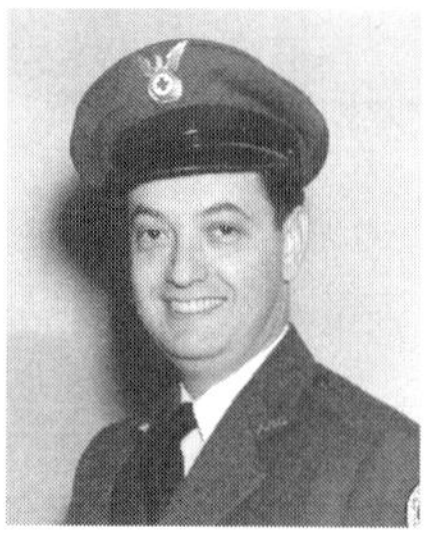

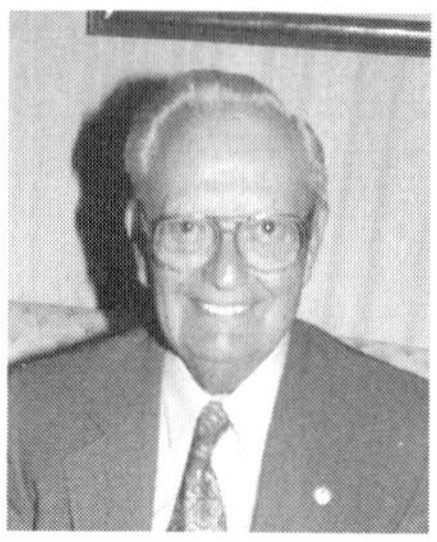

He married Natalie "Sis" Menna in 1938 and is presently retired. Before the ARC, he taught high school in Ambler, PA.

During his service to the ARC from 1943 to 1981, he served as: field dir., Roberts Field, Liberia; field dir., Philadelphia Naval Base; dir. field service, asst. exec. and exec. dir., Southeastern PA Chapter.

He received many awards during his service including the Clara Barton Award, Presidential Citation for 39 years, several certificates of appreciation and his 55 yr. pin for continuance staff and volunteer service. He also succeeded in raising the funds to build a new Chapter HQ in 1972.

MADELINE MERRIMAN was born in Minneapolis, MN. She received her BA in education from the Univ. of MN.

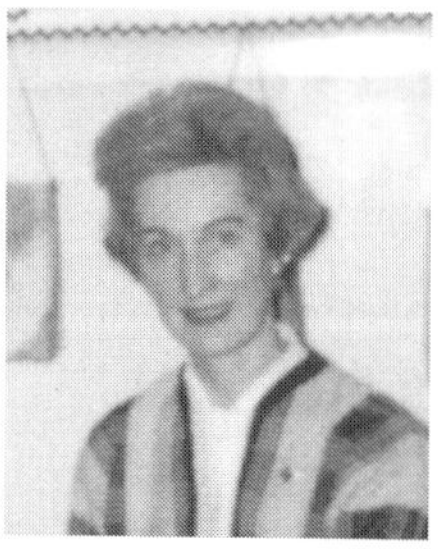

Her RC career began in the late 1940s as a youth program volunteer. She then became the MN RC Chapter Jr. Dir. in the 50s and 60s, as well as Northwest Division staff during the 70s. She was a volunteer in human resource development and continues today as a volunteer on the MN State RC Advisory Council.

Her awards and recognitions include: the Clara Barton award for meritorious volunteer leadership; Leader with the ARC Youth Study to Europe in 1956; ARC Natl. Instructor and Trainer in human resource development; and consultant to the state of MN Human Resources Volunteer Programs.

She is the treasurer of the Upper Midwest RC Retirees Unit and active in many church and civic groups.

BEULAH I. MILES was born in Nacogdoches, TX Sept. 9, 1922. She became a registered nurse in 1943, receiving her BSN in 1949 and MSN in 1972.

She served with the ARC in over 75 disasters between 1950 and 1970. Her positions included nursing rep., nursing supervisor and nursing dir. Her primary assignment being that of nursing field rep. with the field HQ in Nacoghoches, TX. She also served on the Intl. RC team in Austria in 1957 following the Hungarian Revolution.

She says that all her experiences were memorable but there are some that stand out in her mind. When her assignment in Austria was coming to an end, the Hungarian refugees surprised her with an acapella rendition of "The Eyes of Texas". Needless to say, she cried.

She received a special certificate for service from the League of RC Societies following the Hungarian Revolution.

Today she keeps busy working with feeding the hungry, visiting her friends and participating in many church activities.

THOMAS "TOMMY" D. MILLER graduated with a BS in physical education from Normal College of the American Gymnastics Union in indianapolis, IN in June 1936. Miller began his work with the ARC in 1944 in Columbus, OH. He has served as dir. of Safety Services in several different locations such as: Erie, PA; South Bend, IN; and Miami, FL.

He has received many awards that include the Golden Whale in 1974, the Silver Whale in 1974, and the Wally Van Claussen Small Craft Award in 1976.

Thomas is currently residing in Miami, FL with his wife.

WAYNE MEREDITH MILLER was born in Harmony, PA. Miller holds a BA from Geneva College, 1942; a MDiv from McCormick Seminary, 1945; a ThD from Iliff/American Bible College, 1950. He also attended Austin Seminary and the Univ. of TX.

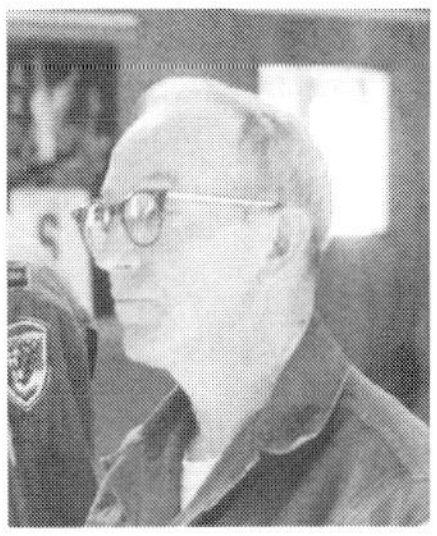

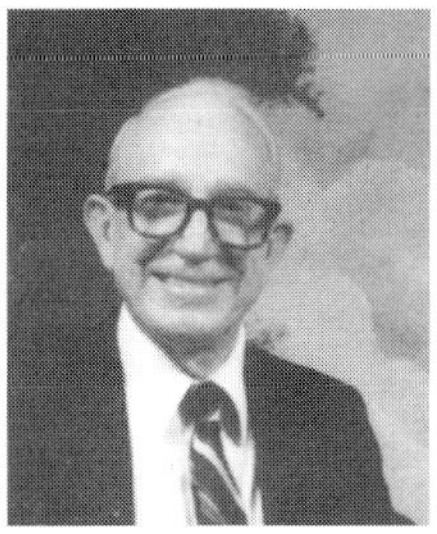

His assignments with the RC from 1969-1984 included: Smoky Hill AFB, KS; United Kingdom; Sheppard AFB, TX; Phouc Vinh, Vietnam; Tay Ninh; Phu Cat AFB; Pearl Harbor; Ft. Shafter; Wheeler AFB; Hickman AFB, HI; Ft. Riley, KS and Ft. Hood, TX.

Miller's most memorable experiences were in Tay Ninh, Vietnam. One day he found his bunker demolished by mortar rounds. The postal clerk had been killed on the post office/RC doorstep. A Filipino RC worker invited him to use quarters at Philippines Civic Action Group. The first night of his arrival exploding mortars were heard everywhere. A few days later a RC meeting was interrupted by rocket fire. Temporarily blinded, they crawled to the rear of the building. One member, a veteran of the Bataan "death march," experienced a flash-back and was seriously impaired. Every ambulance in the camp was damaged or totally destroyed.

He received the following RC awards: Commendation, Intl. Relations; commendation, dir. of operations, South East Asia Area HQ; and Civilian Medal.

Currently, he is an English and philosophy instructor at Central TX College (20 years). He resides in TX with his wife Juanita Tee Co, a Chinese linguist. He has three children: Angelica Maria De Geer, Swedish Baroness; Philip Meredith Miller, composer/instructor, Rice Univ.; Wayne Cimafranda Miller, Pre-Med Univ. of TX. His son-in-law, Baron Marcus De Geer is a medical doctor. His grandchildren are Sebastian, Christoper, Emelie and Jonathan.

MARY MINAMOTO was born in Olympia, WA. She attended Henager Business College and worked for David H. Oliver, attorney, in Salt Lake during WWII and returned to Portland, OR when the military curfew against all persons of Japanese ancestry was lifted in 1945.

Mary served as registrar as well as receptionist for the Chapter and teletypist for all ARC offices within 100 miles radius of Portland. She helped recruit volunteers, blood donors and solicited financial support. She was the first NISEI (American born of Japanese ancestry) to be sent abroad by the ANRC. She was assigned to office admin. in Tokyo, Japan and then was transferred to the Tokyo field office and Yokohama field office. She also accompanied FDs as interpreterto Japanese homes and hospitals to obtain Health Welfare reports on the Japanese war brides and children fathered by GIs. She had served a total of 36 years on Aug. 1, 1979.

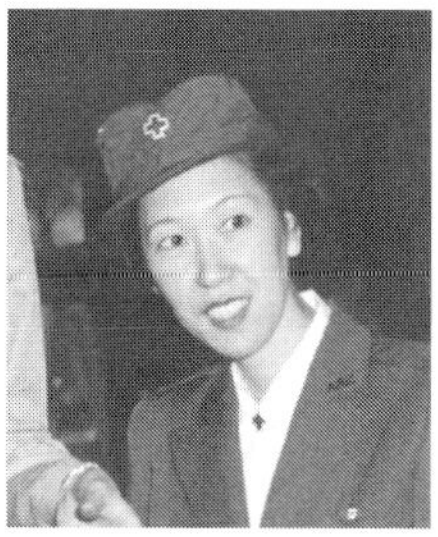

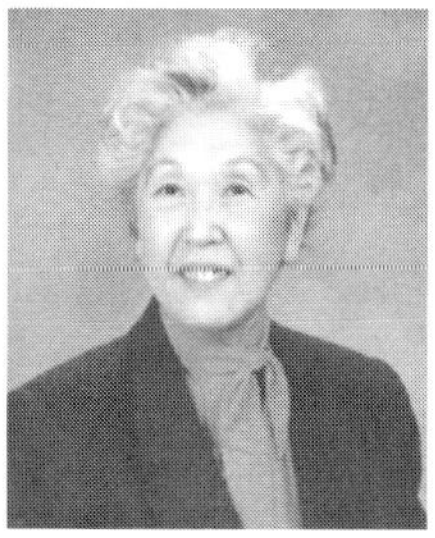

She now lives in Portland, OR. and is actively involved as exec. board member of Osteoporosis Support Group of Providence Portland Medical Center.

EDMOND J. "ED" MONGEON was born on Feb. 20, 1915 in Lisbon, Maine. Ed reported to Natl. HQ on Jan. 2, 1942, and this was the beginning of his 37 years with the ARC professionally. He served as a natl. field rep and asst. dir. Safety Services in Alexandria, VA; dir., Safety Services in Pittsfield, MA, St. Louis, MO, and Stuttgart, Germany.

Mongeon reflected on one of his career highlights which was his European Tour of Duty from 1975-1978. Approaching 60 years of age, he opted to take the position overseas of dir. of Health and Safety for European Area with HQ in Stuttgart, Germany. He said that those four years were a God-send! They provided a chance to, once again, work directly with instructors and instructor-trainer candidates in the field, see a great deal of Europe, and represent the ARC at Intl. RC conferences on First Aid and/or water safety.

He has received many awards including the following: Intl. Swimming Hall of Fame; Distinguished Natl. Safety Council; CNCalifornia Top Honor Award; Golden Whale Award; RI Aquatic Hall of Fame.

After retiring in 1978, he continued as a volunteer in Safety Services for Fairfax Co., VA Chapter from 1979-1982. He passed away Feb. 25, 2000

RICHARD MOORE was born in 1927 in Hollywood, CA. He received a BS from the Univ. of MO in 1949; his PhD from the Univ. of Rochester in 1955; a DSc, from George WA Univ. in 1970.

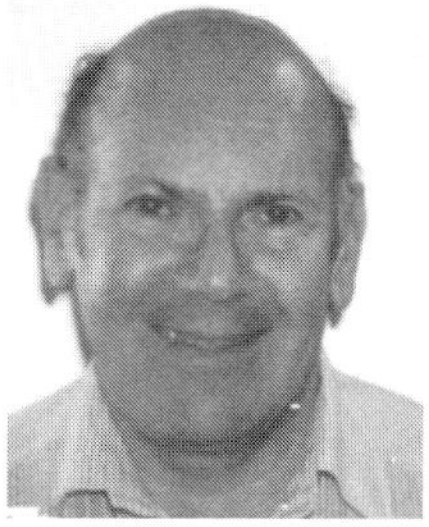

He worked in the Blood Program Research Laboratory, HQ, from 1960 to 1969. Reflecting back on one of his most memorable experiences. He remembers the biological research they did to develop a method, which stored blood cells at the temperature of liquid nitrogen (-170 degrees C). This research was very meaningful and exciting to him.

The awards he received were the following: Fellow, American Association for Advancement of Science and Fellow, American Heart Association.

He is currently living in ID where he is a scientist for the US Department of Energy. He was married in 1969 to Lillian Hagedorn and they have two children, Don and Ann.

ANNE KING MOYE graduated from the Baptist College of Charleston in 1979 with a BA. She began her work with the ARC in Feb. 1968 and continued until Nov. of 1995. She worked for the Carolina Low Country Chapter as the dir. of Volunteers and Youth Services.

Some of her most memorable experiences were disaster assignments. In Aug. of 1969 Hurricane Camille had touched down on the Gulf Coast and she was there for three weeks. In 1979 it was Hurricane David and in Sept. of 1989 it was Hurricane Hugo in Charleston, SC.

She received a 25 year service pin and a Natl. Certificate of Appreciation.

Ms. Moye is currently retired and residing in Isle of Palms, SC. She has two children and five grandchildren. She now volunteers with the local RC Chapter and Blood Services.

GARLAND B. MURRAY was born in 1921 in Greensboro, NC. He attended Guilford College from 1938-1941 and then Springfield College from 1941 to 1943.

Mr. Murray served as Safety Services dir. for Greensboro RC Chapter and the exec. dir. from 1973-86.

His awards include: member, Commodore Longfellow Society of Life Saving Hall of Fame; "Father of the Year" award, 1966, Greensboro Merchants Association.

He retired after 39 years of service all with the Greensboro RC Chapter. He has been married for 55 years to his wife Elizabeth. They have five children and seven grandchildren.

DONALD "DON" GROSE NORTHEY was born in Columbia, SC in May 1914. He attended Belmont Abbey College in NC, 1929-33; Univ. GA Evening College, Atlanta, 1941; Tulane Univ., New Orleans, LA, 1943; Cleveland College, Cleveland, OH, 1945-46; and Lasalle Extension Univ., 1957-65.

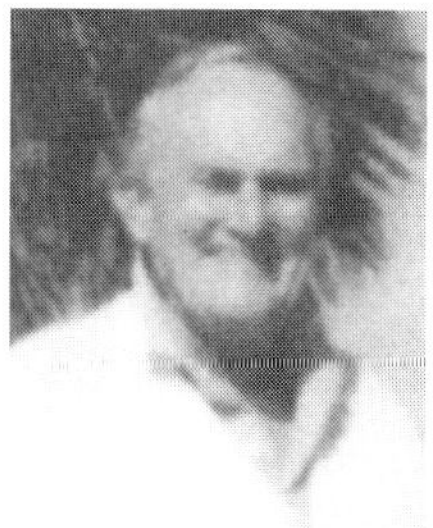

Northey served as a RC volunteer for 10 years before he joined the career ranks in 1941 as a Safety Programs field rep. in the Eastern and Southeastern areas. During his career he served as dir. of Safety Programs in New Orleans, LA; Cleveland, OH; and Dade Co., FL chapters, and as dir. of Disaster Services in the latter two chapters. He has been asst. mgr. in the Dade Co. Chapter and the mgr. of the central FL Chapter. He had many other assignments as well. In 1973 he moved north to the Eastern area to serve as deputy mgr. He served in capacities on domestic major disasters; worked on the Cuban Relief Operation; and in 1969 spent 4 months in Nigeria assigned to the RC Nigerian-Biafran Relief Operation. He retired as deputy mgr. of the Eastern Area in 1976.

His most memorable experience was the memory of the wonderful and talented volunteers and staff with whom he worked in many places, countless hours, which became years, which became a lifetime.

Among the many awards he received are: the Intl. Order Of The Golden Whale and The Conite Intl. De La Croix-Rouge Geneva Switzerland, for service relief operation Nigerian/ Biafran war.

Today Northey is a volunteer for the Association of ARC Volunteers and he is doing some foreign traveling.

KENNETH MEREDITH O'CONNOR was born in Lacross, WI. He graduated from the Univ. of WI with a BS in 1922 and did his graduate work at WA Univ. in St. Louis, MO from 1950-52.

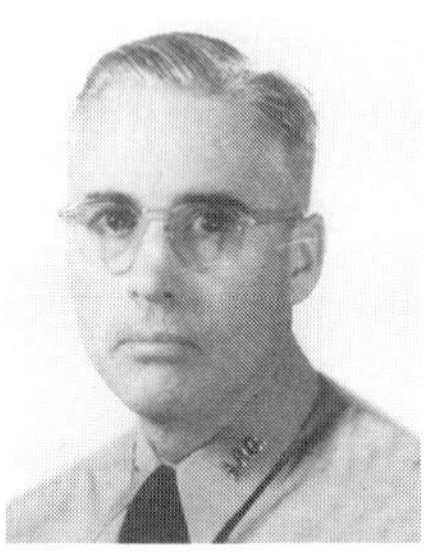

His assignments consisted of the following positions and locations: asst. field dir., Camp Services, DC; field supervisor, regional dir., asst. dir., and field dir. of the Military and Naval Welfare Service; general field rep., Chapter Service, exec. dir. of the Dane Co. Chapter in Madison, WI and the Division Mgr. of Madison, WI.

He is currently retired and is still residing in Madison, WI. He was married to Lillian Schneider O'Connor from 1940-96. They have one child and two grandchildren.

MARY D. O'GEARY was born in Onondaga Co., NY. She received her CVA in 1993.

She was the dir. of Safety Services, 1980-83; dir. of CUS and Youth, 1983-86; dir. of Youth Services, 1986; and has been a disaster volunteer from 1990 to present.

Some of her memorable experiences were establishing LTC in Aug. 1985, assisting in setup of LTC in 1988 (Bahamas), and receiving the Geo. Elsey award in Seattle Natl. Convention.

Awards received were the following: S.S. Del. of Authority 4/82; Silver Beaver (BSA) 2/86; CVA 3/93, and the Spirit of Excellence 9/96.

She is currently retired and a community educator at All Children's Hosp. in St. Petersburg, FL. She has been married for 44 years to her husband Bill. They have two children and four grandchildren.

WALTER H. O'KEFFE was born in 1923. He attended the South Suburban Community College for two years.

His assignments were the following: Mid-America Chapter, Chicago, IL; Disaster Dir., 1970-1983; RC Liaison, FEMA, Region 5, Chicago, IL, 1984-1987.

He said that serving the RC was one of the most rewarding times of his life. Working with some of the finest people and serving families in need made him proud to be part of the organization.

O'Keffe is currently a volunteer in Senior Life Program at Memorial Hosp. in Harvey, IL. He is a chaplain for the VFW Post 9964, South Holland, IL. He is also a member of 1st, 2nd and 3rd Division Marine Corps Associations. He resides with his wife Dorothy.

EDITH OLSON was born Aug. 1, 1989 at Vaughn, WA, of Swedish immigrant parents. Edith graduated from Tacoma High School and from Bellingham Teachers College. She taught elementary grades for several years at Vaughn, Albany and the Aleutian Islands. She graduated from Stanford Univ. in CA with an RN degree in 1928. She took a position with the ARC and worked with RC chapters in various western states. In 1933 she took a leave of absence and traveled through the Panama Canal to Europe to find relatives and see the countries. She earned a Masters in public health nursing at Columbia Univ. in NY. She worked in San Francisco during WWII. In 1946 she sailed for India from NY City and then traveled by air over the Burma Hump to China. She worked at Peking and Shanghai, looking after the health of RC workers there. Later she worked for the Intl. RC helping to reopen RC hospitals in Japan, Korea, Siam and other Asian countries. She was recognized for her accomplishments by the Empress of Japan and the Queen of Siam. Before retirement, in 1965, she was the RC nursing rep. for the State of FL. She resides with a niece in IA.

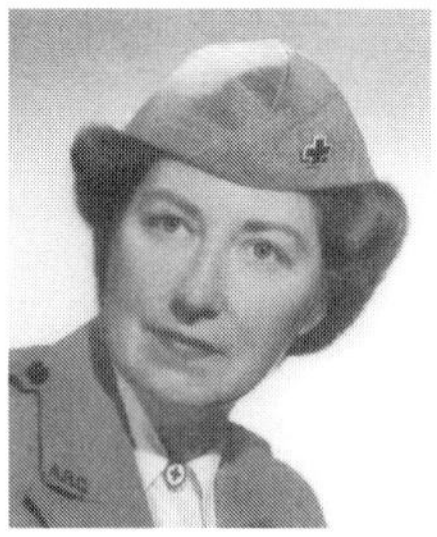

ELIZABETH A. OLSON, a native of Milwaukee, WI, began her RC career in 1943 as a graduate student in community organization and psychiatric social work at the Univ. of Chicago. She was assigned to the Chicago Chapter, ARC, in service to the military and their families.

After receiving an MA, she became a field consultant for service to military families in Midwestern Area; area dir., Midwestern Area; area dir. of Training and Career Development. In the later 60s and early 70s she was loaned, as the first training officer, to the League of RC and Red Crescent Societies in Geneva, Switzerland. There she launched a series of regional institutes for developing societies, focusing on program and management development. On her return to the US, she served as asst. natl. dir. of Disaster Services and natl. dir. of Training.

Since her retirement in 1980, Olson has continued active in programs, committee and board work of the World Federalists, Society for Intl. Development, the Asia Society and the United Nations Association. At the community volunteer level, she is involved in programs for the elderly and for the homeless. She lives in a retirement community in Falls Church, VA.

BARBARA ANN MACE OTAKI, born Dec. 1, 1930, Exeter, NE, graduated from the Univ. of NE, Lincoln, Feb. 1959.

Assignments with the RC included: SRAO Korea, 1st Cavalry. Div. 19th Field Artillery (2/59-2/60); secretary to asst. dir. of Personnel, Far Eastern Area HQ, Camp Zama, Japan (2/60-2/65); Chapter correspondent and secretary to asst. mgr., Western Area HQ, San Francisco (6/68-4/74); admin. asst., Personnel, Los Angeles Chapter (4/74-5/77); secretary to Chapter mgr., Orange Co. Chapter, Santa Ana, CA (7/77-7/79).

Her memorable experiences: Probably the first day at my assignment at 1st Cavalry. Div. in Korea stands out as a most unforgettable experience while working for the ARC. Three of us girls out of the group that arrived in Korea in Feb. of 1959 were assigned to 1st Cavalry. After a week of orientation in Seoul, we were flown to 1st Cavalry. in a small plane. Greeting us at the end of the runway were several soldiers and women dressed in Army fatigues standing behind a large banner welcoming us to the First Team. As we got out of the plane, we were approached by three soldiers carrying MI rifles. Each of us girls was escorted by a rifle toting GI to open jeeps and swiftly driven to a large community recreational center where we sat around talking and having a fun, relaxed time. Several hours later we all left the center and were driven to our billet at 19th Field Artillery. Although we had gone through two weeks orientation at Natl. HQ in DC and one week in Seoul, my first day on assignment was not what I had expected. I was to learn later that we had arrived during one of the many surprise mock alerts that were staged in Korea to help prepare us in the event the North Koreans crossed the border which was not too far from our unit. It wasn't until our second day that we were able to understand what our job was really all about.

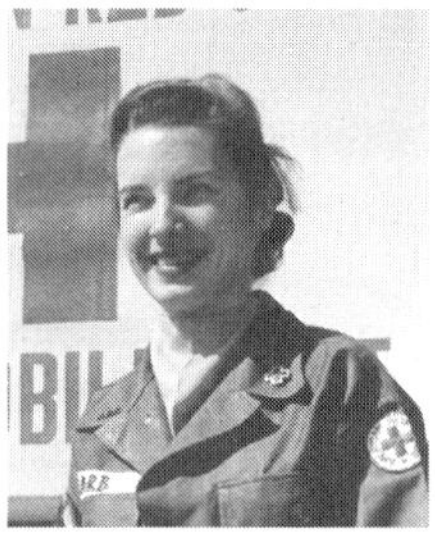

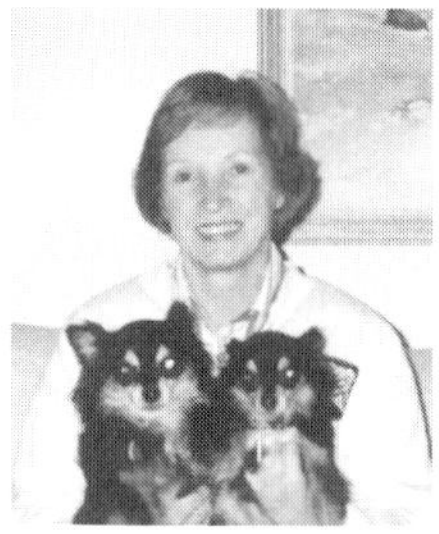

She is currently retired, and resides with her husband, Hirohisa Otaki in Mission Viejo, CA.

GERALD NORRIS PAGE was born in Anaheim, CA on Aug. 18, 1916. He graduated from the Univ. of CA in 1941, and received his certificate in social services, UCLA extension in 1968. His RC assignments included: asst. field dir. Catalina Island, CA, 1942; asst. field dir. Naval Station, Alleutian Islands (Adak), 1943; Ft. Richardson, AK, 1944-45, 1965-66; Camp Pendleton, CA Marine Base, 1945; Army AFB, Las Vegas, NV, 1945; El Toro Marine Base, Santa Ana, CA, 1946; Edwards AFB, Mojave, CA, 1948; Kobe and Sasebo, Japan, 1950-51; Korea, 1950-51; Camp Cook, CA, 1951-53; Ft. McArthur, San Pedro, CA, 1954; US Naval Station, Long Beach, CA, 1955-56; AFB Bordeaux, France, 1956-57; Karlsruhe, Germany, 1957-60; El Toro Marine Base, CA, 1960-65, 1967-71 and AK, 1965-66. He also assisted in several disasters.

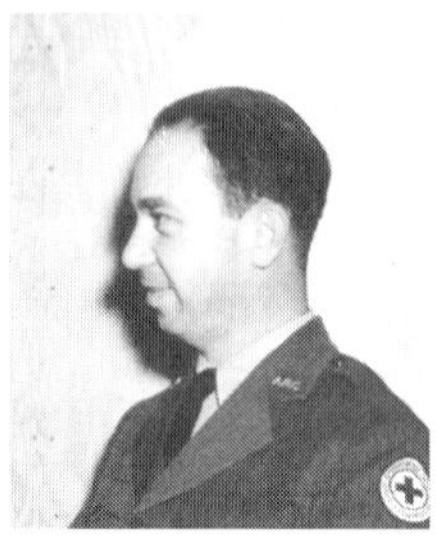

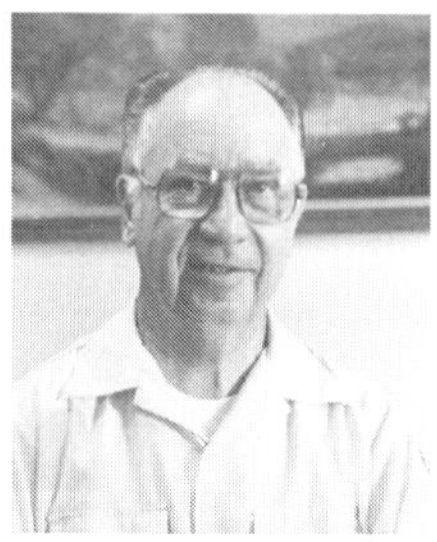

Page received the Presidential Medal of Freedom; RC Overseas Certificate; Army Certificate of Appreciation; Faithful Service Certificate, Karlesruhe, Germany and Certificate for 40 years with the RC, 1982.

Page retired Jan. 1, 1982, and passed away Sept. 9, 1998. He is survived by his wife, Henrietta; daughter, Mari Elizabeth; son, Gerald Norris, Jr. and three grandchildren.

PATRICIA M. PARENT joined the ARC in 1974 in Los Angeles, CA. She lived and worked in the San Fernando Valley but was also assigned all over the LA and surrounding areas in the county on Blood Mobiles. She is still in contact with some of her nurse friends.

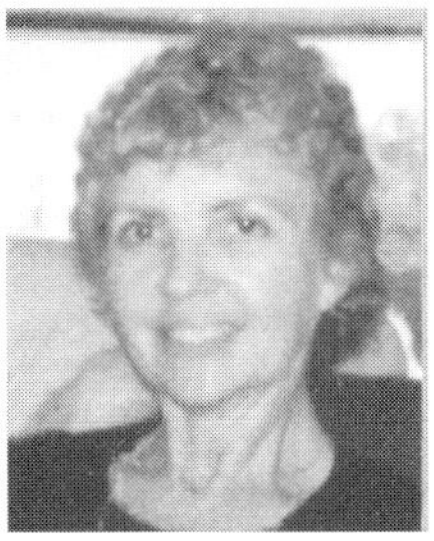

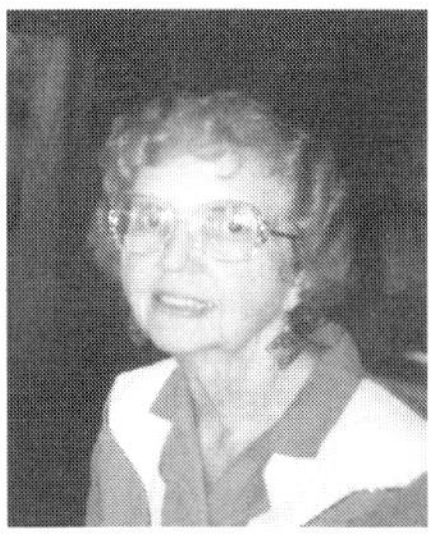

She was an RN and after moving to FL in 1980, earned a BA in psychology from St. Leo's College in Tampa. She joined the RC in Daytona Beach, FL and retired from there in 1988. Since then, she has nursed in a doctor's office on a part-time basis. She is now retired and enjoying traveling, bridge, exercise and visiting family.

Her husband of twenty-five years died in 1977. They had six children, one of whom died of lung cancer. She has a son, a daughter and son-in-law in San Francisco, and three granddaughters. She also has a daughter and grandson in St. Louis, and a daughter in Daytona Beach.

Parent's fondest memories are those of her time spent in LA with the friends she made there.

HENRY COLE PARKER was born Mar. 15, 1914 in Halifax Co., VA. Graduating from high school in 1932 and from Richmond Univ. in 1936, he married Minnie Jennings on Sept. 22, 1942. He served in WWII from 1941-45.

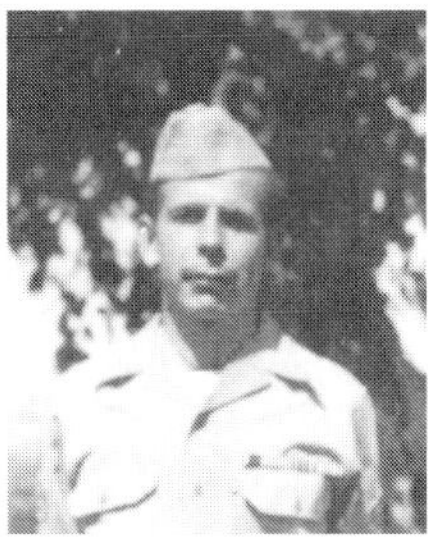

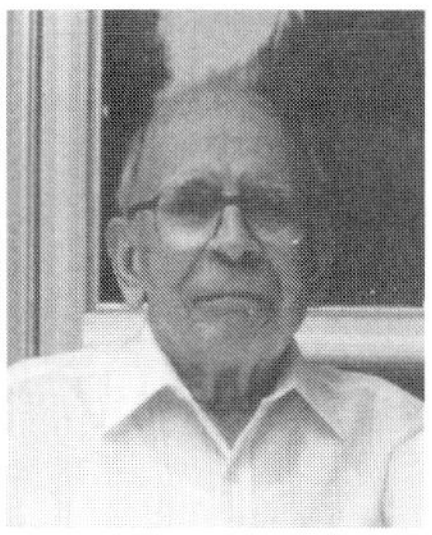

Some of his assignments with the RC were: Veteran's Admin., 1945; Winston Salem, 1950; Nashville, TN (field dir.). Parker loved his work with the RC. He retired in Mar. 1979, but stayed in Nashville until Jan. 1995. He has one grandchild, Colin Lloyd McArthur, and resides with his wife Minnie in VA.

DWIGHT "PAT" E. PATRICK was born on June 12, 1925 in Macon Co., IL. He graduated from high school on May 13, 1943.

His RC assignments included: volunteering, Macon Co., IL, dir. of labor participation, Midwestern Area; 14 major disasters (worked with wife, Jean). He received the Tiffany Award and several awards from Midwestern states for programs performed for their membership. Currently, Patrick is retired, working with Veterans programs and Macon Chapter Blood Program. He is president of the St. Louis Retirees. He resides in IL with wife, Jean, and they have four children: Karen, Ron, Cynthia, and Mark and five grandchildren, three step grandchildren, two great grandchildren and three step great grandchildren.

ROBERT "BOB" J. PAVILONIS was born on June 7, 1931 in Youngstown, OH. He attended Youngstown College, now Youngstown Univ., and obtained a liberal arts degree in pre-law and math. He participated in Army ROTC program and joined the military. His RC assignments from 1962-97 included: Ft. Belvoir, VA; Ft. Knox, KY; Pease AFB, NH; Camp Howze, Korea; Bangkok, Thailand; Korea, Thailand; Ft. Lee, VA; Camp SD Butler, Okinawa; US Naval Station, Boston, MA; Ft. Buckner, Okinawa; Andrews AFB Hosp., MD; Natl. Cap Area of United Way; OH HQ, Alexandria, VA; Charleston AFB, SC; US Naval Base, Chas, SC; Ft. Belvoir, VA.

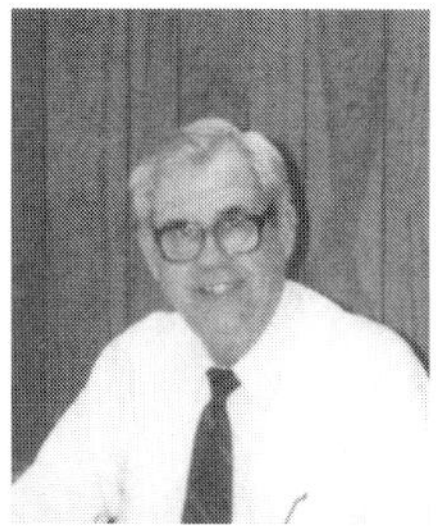

Pavilonis retired April 1, 1997 after serving the ARC over 34 years. He resides with his wife Mildred in Alexandria, VA. They have three grown children, John, Andrew and Susan.

DONALD PEAK is a retired Chapter mgr., whose career began in 1953, as an asst. field dir. for Military Families at Ft. Bliss, TX and at White Sands Proving Ground, NM. At White Sands he lunched with German rocket scientists confined there. In Korea he served as an asst. field dir. with the 1st Marine Division. He transferred to the 3rd Marine Division at Camp Fuji, Japan. While serving at Camp Fuji he married Joy Saalfrank, a Special Services librarian serving the troops at Camp Fuji.

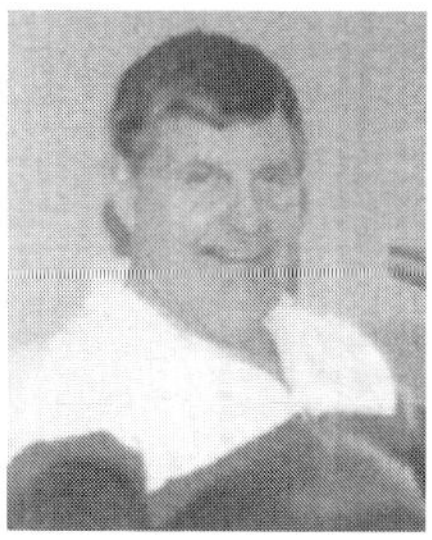

Upon returning to the United States Donald became a field rep. in the Midwestern Area, serving the Rio Grande Valley, TX Chapters. He became Chapter mgr. of the Galveston, TX RC Chapter in 1958 and remained there during Hurricane Carla (Sept. 1961). In 1967 he accepted the management of the Washtenaw Co. RC Chapter at Ann Arbor, MI where he served until 1980. He returned to Galveston and was rehired as the Chapter mgr., serving during Hurricane Alicia (Aug. 1983).

He is a graduate of Drury College and WA Univ., St. Louis, holding a Master's in sociology/anthropology. He is a history buff, an old house restorer, a writer of historical adventure fiction as well as editing the Galveston East End Historic District News. He resides with his wife, Joy, and has a son, William, and daughter, Catherine. They also have three grandchildren, Christopher, Joe and Sheryl.

JAMES H. PERT graduated from Dartmouth College, AB, 1946, and Cornell Univ. Medical College, MD, 1951.

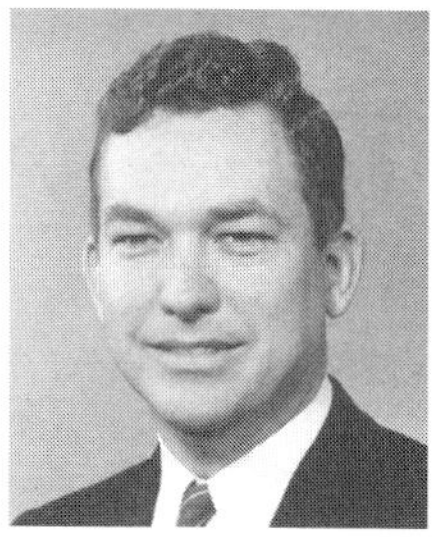

His positions with RC included: Research dir., 1958-68, Natl. HQ, DC, and Research Laboratory, Bethesda, MD. He started Blood Research Program at HQ and established branch laboratories at NYU for clotting and platelet research and at LA for blood immunology. The central WA-Bethesda Research Lab provided reference products such as thrombin, plasmin and antihemophilic factor (AHF) to NIH and WHO. Started Virgin IslandsG program with DOD to treat complications of vaccinations, about 800 cases a year, leading to stopping routine vaccinations against smallpox. Pert worked to change the Heart and Lung Institute of NIH to Heart, Lung and Blood Institute, started first natl. technologist training program, matching funds for regional centers, and Natl. Rare Donor File, developed liquid-nitrogen freezing method for red cells and first method for making platelet concentrates so NCI could treat leukemia and make component therapy practical. He has given numerous medical/scientific lectures and has written for publications. Research mostly funded by grants, about $1.5 million in his last year at ANRC.

He has been married 51 years to Trudy Thompson and their children are Caren Pearson, James C. Pert, MD, Hilary Stecklein, MD, Ellen Saltsman. They have 11 grandchildren.

WILLIAM J. PHILLIPS, born in Akron OH and educated at the Univ. of Akron and Temple Univ., volunteered in First Aid and Water Safety, Akron, OH. In 1951 he joined the staff of the RC as asst. dir. of Safety Services, SE PA Chapter at Philadelphia, PA. In 1954 he became dir. of Safety and Disaster Services, Richmond VA, and in 1957, the dir. Disaster Services Boston, MA. He was appointed in 1962 as asst. regional mgr., Eastern Area in Alexandria VA with responsibility for activities of chapters in VA, MD and DC. Subsequently his territory was changed to Maine, NH, VT, MA and RI.

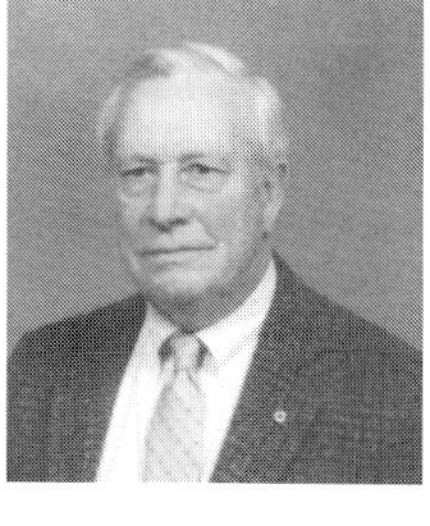

In 1968 he became special asst. to the natl. dir. of fund raising, then asst. dir. of Disaster at Natl. and had many disaster assignments including Hurricane Hazel; Hurricane Camille; KY, VA, WV floods and others. In 1972 he was appointed Natl. Government liaison officer with responsibility of coordinating RC interests and activities with their governmental counterparts both legislative and program.

He retired early in 1984 but is still an active volunteer and was president for a period of time of the natl. Cross Retiree Association. He served in the Navy during WWII as a fighter pilot and remained in the Reserves after the war. He was recalled to active duty during the Pueblo crisis in Jan. 1968 and later retired as a Lt. Commander.

He is married and has five sons, 10 grandchildren, and two great grandchildren.

MILDRED "MILLIE" B. POWELL was born in Elliott, IA on Mar. 10, 1912. She holds a BSM which she obtained from Drake Univ., Des Moines, IA, 1938. She began service with the ARC in Mar. 1944, and her assignments included: Santa Fe, NM; Abilene, TX; Norman, OK; Battle Creek, MI; San Antonio, TX; El Paso, TX; Hot Springs, AR; Corpus Christi, TX; Philadelphia, PA; Wichita Falls, TX; Great Lakes, IL; Tokyo, Japan; Camp Sakai, Japan; Yuokohama, Japan; Wiesbaden, Germany; Ascom City, Korea; Chateauroux, France and Denver, CO. She also served as a disaster worker in TX.

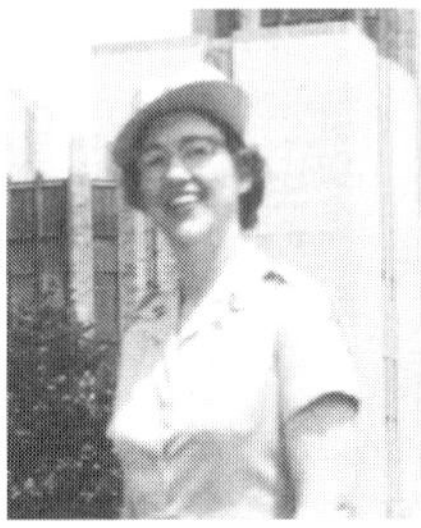

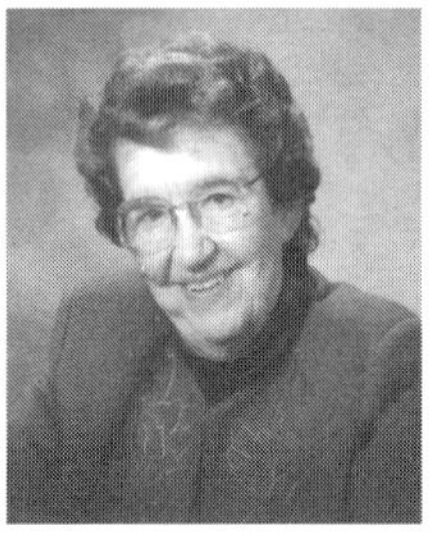

With a title suggestion from a WAC, she composed a song by which she became known as the "Rice Paddy Daddy gal." And she sang it everywhere. Her music enabled her to have many unique experiences. She had a program on Armed Forces Network in Tokyo where she played on Mrs. MacArthur's piano. During a tour of a cathedral in France, speaking French to a custodian, she procured a key to the huge organ and played a number.

She retired in 1975. Her family includes seven nieces, two nephews and their children.

ANN WOESSNER PRIEM was born in Southington, CT in 1923, and grew up as a "PK," preacher's kid in small towns. She taught school (PE) for six years before joining the RC. She holds a BA from Syracuse Univ. and an MS from Springfield College. She became a RC recreation worker in 1951, serving at Murphy Army Hosp., MA from 1952-55; at three military hospitals in Germany; 121st Evac. Hosp., Korea; USNH, Yokosaka, Japan; USNH, Saigon; 6th Convalescent Center, Cam Then Bay, RVN; US Army Tripler Hosp., Honolulu, HI.

During her 26 years as a recreation worker, she was faced with several interesting challenges during disasters, where she set up activities for children who were disaster victims and were living in temporary RC shelters. While stationed in HI, she met and married Carroll "Buck" Priem, a retired army colonel. He is now deceased.

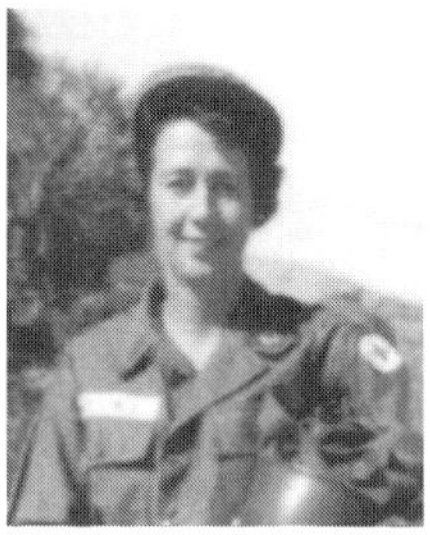

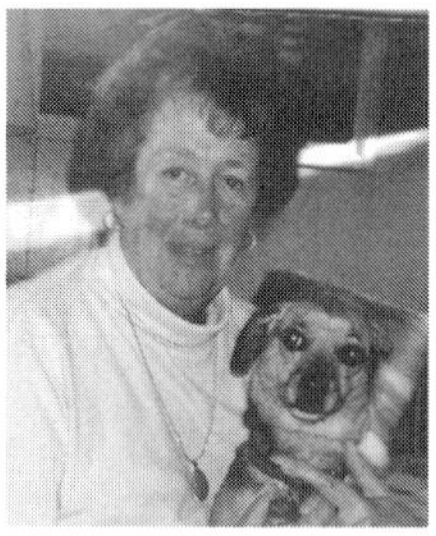

She is currently retired, and lives overlooking Monterey Bay in Butterfly Town, USA, Pacific Grove, CA. Her hobbies include golf and volunteering at church, thrift shop and the Monterey Bay Aquarium at the information desk. Her experience with the RC, being stationed around the world is a real asset in dealing with people from other countries who visit the Aquarium.

CHARLES "CHARLIE" A. PROHASKA was born in Brentwood, NM on Dec. 22, 1922. He joined the ARC in 1972 as chief engineer of the Frank Stanton Production Center at Baileys Crossroads, VA after a 20 year career in radio and television broadcasting. He located the AV Center building and toured the facility with Dr. Frank Stanton and President George Elsey when they approved the plan to build an Audio Video Production Center. Prohaska personally designed the studio facility and installed the television cameras, video tape recorders and other electronic equipment. He was responsible for training the producers and dir.s who were to operate the facility.

When mobile equipment was added, Prohaska supervised the establishment of TV studios and recording crews to provide TV coverage of the annual ARC Conventions in LA, Atlanta and other cities.

When he retired in 1986 after 14 years, Prohaska volunteered as a liaison asst. with the Convention Office and assisted at conventions in Orlando, San Diego and Houston. He volunteered his expertise to install the Satellite downlink for the Tidewater Regional Blood Center in Norfolk, VA. He now lives in VA Beach with his wife Lil.

THELMA GIBSON-RADDEN, founder of the Gray Ladies, was born and educated in Oakland, CA. Ninety-five-year-old Radden, remembering segregated quarters for "colored" nurses in nursing school, exemplifies what she teaches, "If you want to achieve something, you pull yourself up and you do it."

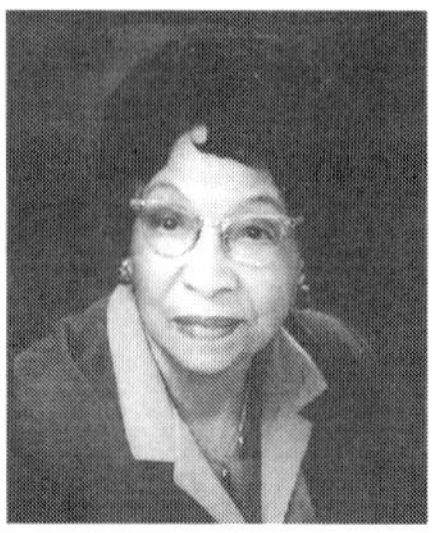

Radden became the asst. dir. of RC Nursing Services and served for 21 years in Detroit, MI. She wrote and taught special courses where she saw need, such as in home services for school-aged, single parents.

In 1941 Radden established and trained the Gray Ladies, the first African American volunteer branch of nursing for the RC. Radden trained the "Ladies" at Detroit Metropolitan Hosp., then known as the "colored hospital."

Radden, a fourth generation descendant of a Pioneer CA family, moved back to CA in 1975. She is actively involved in a multitude of volunteer efforts and shows no indication of slowing down.

RUTH F. RAFNER, born in Cleveland, OH, Aug. 14, 1922. She graduated from Bowling Green State Univ., OH with a Bachelor's degree in sociology and psychology. She has a heritage in humanitarian service in that her father and brother are both WWII veterans, and her mother, a volunteer RC Motor Corps driver. RC service began during WWII in 1943 as a casework aide in Service to Military Families. Employed with Dayton Area Chapter, OH, serving three counties, she remembers very emotional times attending draft board gatherings at 5:00 a.m. and witnessing families bidding good-bye to their men as they departed for military service.

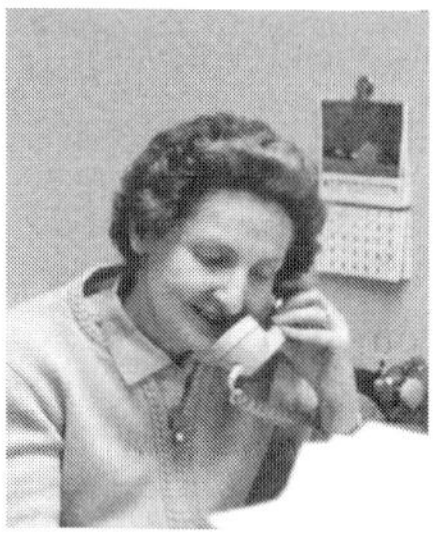

Rafner was married in 1946 and assisted her husband, Alter, in business for 15 years. In 1960, she rejoined the staff of Dayton Area Chapter as a caseworker and remained for 24 years, making a total of 27 years of RC service. During the dir.'s illness, she became acting dir. for a time. She also provided assistance at a number of area disasters including the Eaton, OH tornado in 1961, the Spring Valley, OH and the Clinton Co., OH floods as well as the Xenia, OH tornado in 1974. In addition, she provided casework assistance for a great number of Vietnam veterans and became a specialist in all phases of veteran's services. She retired in 1984, and is very gratified she could serve so many people. Rafner is a member of the Natl. Association of Social Workers and the American Association of Univ. Women. She resides in Dayton, OH and volunteers in the nursing home where her husband resides.

DOROTHY EWING RAINE was born Feb. 2, 1918 in San Francisco. She holds a BA from the Univ. of CA at Berkley (1939) and an MS from Western Reserve Cleveland (1946). Her RC assignments include: Camp Young Desert Training Center; 107th General Hosp., England; Baxter General Hosp., Spokane, WA; Naval Hosp., ID; Naval Hosp., Vancouver, WA; Brooke Army Medical Center, San Antonio; Naval Hosp. and Naval Station, Corpus Christi, TX. She served as social worker and field dir. She remembers living and working in tent hospitals in the CA desert on her first assignment, welcoming POWs back to American Hosp. in England following VE Day and watching Naval Hosp. in Corpus Christi be destroyed by Hurricane Celia.

Raine is now retired and a community volunteer. She is married to C.M. Raine (since 1946) and they have two children, W. Woody Raine and Patricia Raine Price. They also have three grandchildren.

ELLA MARIE HUNTER RAST, born Dec. 22, 1929, American Falls ID, and educated at American Falls High School, 1948; Emmanuel Nursing School, 1951 and Linfield College, 1977. Her service with the RC was from 1983-1993 as staff nurse, Blood Services with OR Trail Chapter, Portland, OR. Her memorable experience was being a traveling nurse and covering 54,000 square miles with Blood Donor Services.

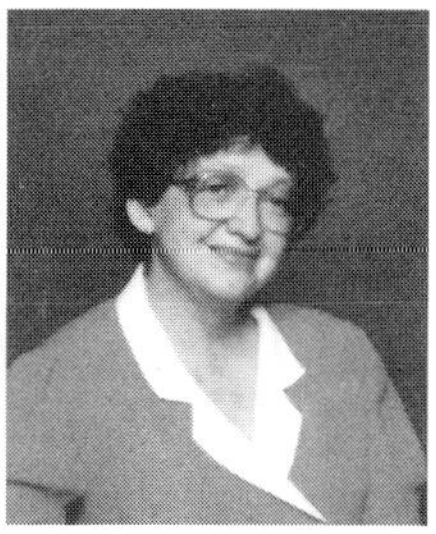

In 1997, she wrote and had published a historical biography, *I Remember That Good Yet.*, the German-Russian-American immigrant story spanning both continents.

Rast retired in 1993, and is currently president of the Pocatello Art Center, actively painting in water color and oils as well as continuing to write. She has two children and six grandchildren.

ELEANOR PERRY REIF was born in Craftsbury, VT on Dec. 17, 1918. She graduated from Penn Avenue High School, Cumberland, MD, 1936, and Western MD College, MD, 1940. Her RC hosp. recreation worker experience included: Forest Glen, MD, 1944; Camp Patrick Henry, VA, 1945; Ft. Knox, KY, 1946; Bethesda Naval Hosp., MD, 1947-49. Prior to ARC, she taught high school home economics and then was a home economist for the Junket Food Company. She is now active in church and community affairs. She volunteers for Meals on Wheels, RC Blood Drives and at a health care center. She is a Girl Scout life member, and a life member of the American Association of Univ. Women.

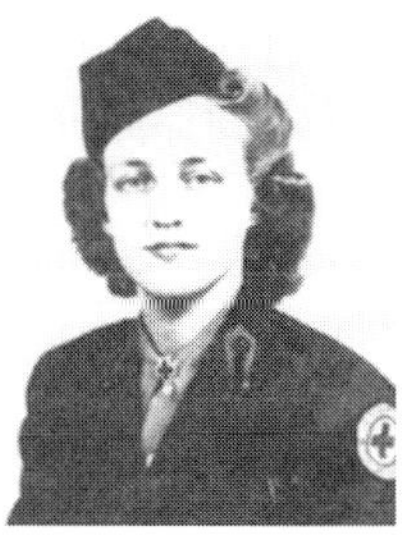

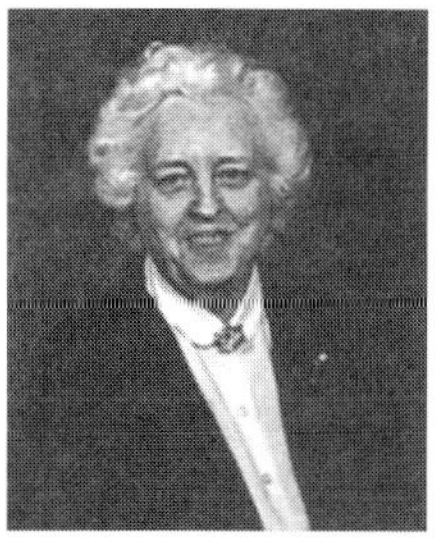

Reif has one daughter and three grandchildren, and is the widow of Gerald Reif, who a few years after marriage was also employed by the ARC as field dir., serving at Camp Atterburg, IN; Ft. Meade, MD; Brooklyn Naval Yard, NY; Sampson AFB, NY; McGuire AFB, NJ; Portsmouth Shipyard, NH; Quantico Marine Base, VA; DC; Germany; England and Panama.

LUDMILLA "LOU" FERENZ RICE was born Nov. 2, 1921 in Yonkers, NY. She graduated from Yonkers High School in 1939, and attended St. Luke's Hosp. School of Nursing from 1940-43; Rio Hondo College, Whittier, CA, 1950 and Univ. of AL, Tuscaloosa, AL, 1946-47. Her RC assignments included: LA RC Blood Services, 1974-85 and volunteering at Van Nuys Chapter, 1985-92. Rice joined the Army Nurse Corps in 1944; received ground flight training in 1945, Randolph Field, San Antonio, TX, attended the School of Aviation Medicine, 1945 and joined the Civil Air Patrol as an observer. Her most exciting experiences were in the South Pacific where she was involved in picking up the wounded and flying them stateside. Awards she received were the American Campaign Medal, Asiatic Pacific Campaign Medal, the WWII Victory Medal, the Meritorious Service Unit Plaque and the ARC 10-year service pin.

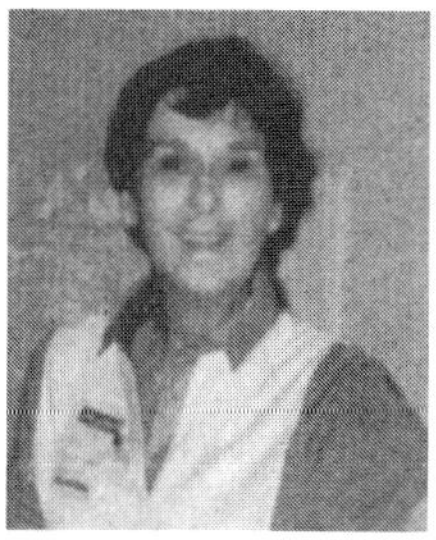

Rice married retired Col. Banner P. Rice in 1987, and they have a son, Jeff, in CA; two granddaughters and a step-son, David in GA. Rice is currently retired.

WONEVA M. RICHARDSON attended business college in Rapid City, SD from 1934-35, and served with Nursing Services and the Blood Program from 1954-77 at the Multnomah Chapter, Portland, OR. Richardson remembers recruiting volunteers to teach classes, serve in shelters and donate blood. Her RC experiences were very gratifying. She is married to James O. Richardson (1987), and they have a two sons, James O., Jr., and Michael L.; a daughter, Janice (deceased) and six grandchildren. Her best award received was to be the parent of two college graduates.

JAMES "JIM" F. RIVES was born in Louisville, KY on April 16, 1924. He received his AB from Carson Newman in 1949, and served in the RC after service in the Army in WWII and Korea. His RC assignments were at Ft. Benning, GA; many other US military bases; Europe; Thule, Greenland; HI, Korea (twice); Vietnam with the 3rd Marine Division, 1st Air Cavalry Division (Vietnam, 1970) and 23rd Americal Division (1970-71).

He is currently retired after 30 years of service in RC SMI. He is married with two daughters and one son. One daughter, Carol Lee was in the ARC, asst. field dir., Ft. Knox, KY for a short time. He has four grandchildren.

JOHN "JACK" BURNS ROBERTS graduated from Western MD College with a BA, 1950. He served as an asst. field dir. at Keesler AFB, MS, 1956-69; field dir., ARC Natl. Aquatic School, 1959-60 and field dir., Frankfurt, Germany. His best memory is being thanked by Capt. Carl Johnson for having found his father whom he had only known as a child in Guam, 1964.

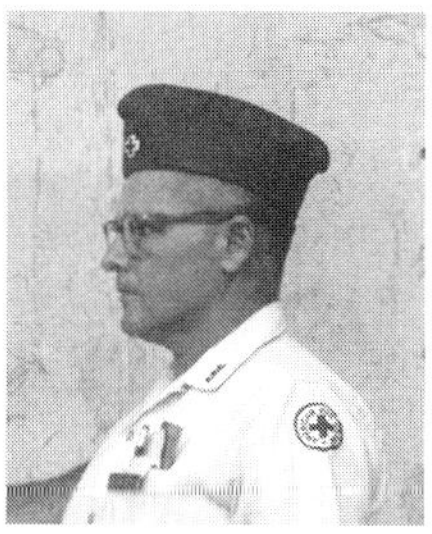

He received the USA Medal for Civilian Service in Vietnam. Roberts passed away Jul. 28, 1998 in Asheville, NC. He is survived by his wife, Mildred Burghardt Roberts and three sons, John B. Roberts II, Fred Roberts, and Herbert C. Roberts.

JACQUELINE "JACKIE" HAUSON ROBBINS was born Oct. 1, 1916 in Osawatomie, KS, and attended the Univ. of MO, 1935-38. She was assigned with the RC in Manhattan, KS; HI; Saigon; Japan and Baltimore, MD, from 1944-75. She is currently retired and lives with her husband, James W. Robbins in TX.

MELBERN "JOE" ROBINSON was born April 26, 1914 in Osecola, MO. He graduated from MO Univ., 1942. Robinson married Bobby Cash Sutter in 1943. After serving on the USS *Canberra*, WWII, he joined the ARC and was sent to Germany, spending the next thirty-two years serving in the following capacities: asst. field dir., Oberpfaffenhoffen, West Germany, 1941-49; Nuremburg, West Germany, 1947-49; Camp Pendleton, CA-1950; field dir., Edwards AFB, CA, 1951-52; Ft. Richardson, AK, 1953; Harlington, TX, 1955, Ft. Smith, AR, 1955; disaster relief, Hungarian Refugee Program, 1956; asst. dir. of Service to Military Installations, St. Louis, MO, 1956-62; asst. dir. of personnel, Midwestern Area, 1962-66; dir. of personnel, European Theater, 1966-71; asst. dir., SMI, St. Louis, MO and Ft. Riley, KS, 1971-73; field dir., Ft. Leonard Wood, MO, 1973-77.

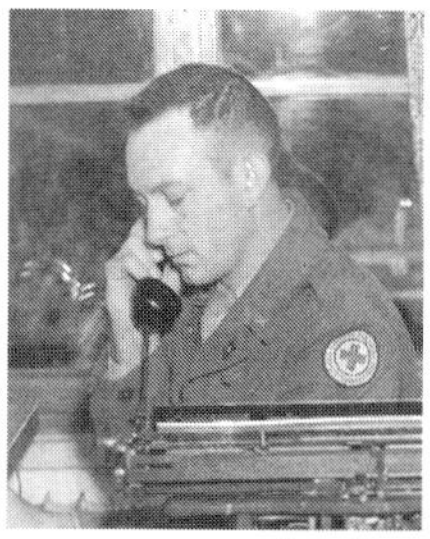

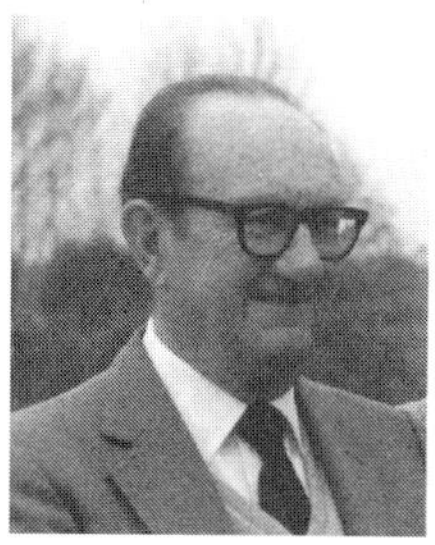

Robinson retired to the life of gentleman farmer near Bobby's birthplace, Guthrie, MO. Since 1977, he has served as an active member of several help associations for retired persons in Callaway county, such as Meals On Wheels. He also served two terms in the MO Silvered Hair Legislature in Jefferson City, MO, and is a member of The Retired Officer's Association. He is a member of Ft. Leonard Wood Retiree Council, advising the Commander of the Maneuver Center on retiree issues. He and Bobby have two sons, Daniel, an information management specialist; and Scott, a major in the US Army.

DALE "RED" EVANS ROE graduated from high school, Preston, ID, 1933 and obtained a BS, UT State Agricultural College, 1937.

RC assignments included: field rep. and asst. dir., Pacific Area ARC, FAWSAP HQ, San Francisco, 1941-45; Safety Services, Disaster Services and mgr., Oakland-South Alameda Co., Oakland, CA, 1946-82.

Memorable experiences were associations with and help from natl. and area Safety Services officials, including Commodore Wilbert E. Longfellow. Working with volunteers helped build a good life for himself. Also memorable were military assignments including Doolittle's Raiders and the Atomic Bombing Group, Sendover field, UT and serving at military hospitals to help shape swim programs for rehabilitation of disabled veterans.

Among the awards he has received are: Commodore Longfellow Society, 50-year recognition certificate, 1994 and Silver Beaver, 1982.

Currently, Row is a freelance writer, having edited the book, *Flood Fighters 1983-1984*, and produced *Bountiful, UT, 100th Anniversary*, a souvenir magazine. He was an ARC volunteer, Salt Lake City ARC 1983-86.

He is married to Lela Allen, and they have a son, Michael (deceased), and two daughters, Frances Moulton and Elgena Roe Brenning.

ANTONECE BERTRAND ROGERS, born Oct. 7, 1920, in Purmela, Coryell Co., TX, and a John Tarleton Agricultural College graduate, was employed there during WWII, then transferred to TAM Univ. post WWII. Married to a veteran, Rogers became a homemaker and community volunteer.

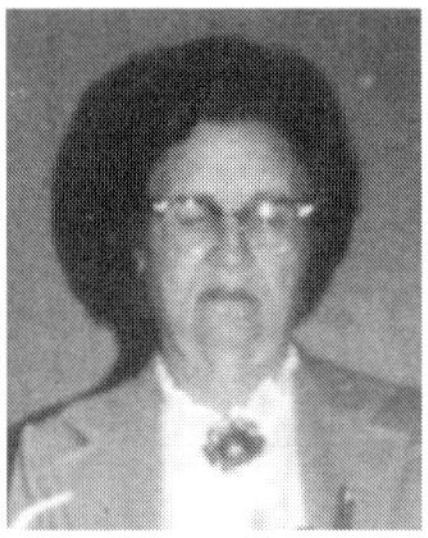

Later during Vietnam she became exec. secretary, Coryell Co. Chapter ARC, adjacent to Ft. Hood. She retired 20 years later after directing the Chapter including fiscal management, casework for SMF&V, Health Services, Disaster, Blood Service along with myriad mgr.ial responsibilities including supervising a small paid staff and hundreds of volunteers and attending out of town meetings. Endless record keeping and reporting was required, serving at a Grant Chapter doing an abundant SMF caseload. We were dedicated to rendering complete service or making proper referral, taking seriously the Mission of RC. Hers was a difficult position, but she is proud to have had the opportunity to be of service at a time which included the Vietnam years. Rogers receive many certificates, pins, media recognition, small gifts and various letters of commendation, including a certificate signed by Richard F. Schubert upon retirement.

She is the widow of Harmon Arch Rogers, Jr., who was a WWII veteran and a professional engineer. She has one daughter, Dr. Margaret Hale, DED and a son, Dr. Harmon A. Rogers, III, DVM, five grandchildren and two step-grandchildren.

CARL A. ROSS was born Aug. 23, 1904 in Miles City, MT and graduated from the Univ. of MT in 1931. His RC assignments included: 1925-1941, volunteer First Aid and Water Safety instructor; 1941, Natl. Staff field rep., First Aid & Water Safety, Mid-Western Area, St. Louis, MO. (territory of MT, WY, ND, SD and Western MN); 1944, India, survival and combat swimming program, ocean invasion of Japan; 1945, Germany, asst. dir., FAWS (territory of Bavaria and Austria); 1946-64, field rep, FAWS, Midwestern and Pacific Area; dir., Natl. Aquatic Schools, MN, AZ, WA, ID and CA; 1964-69, field rep for FAWS, Far Eastern Area, Camp Zama, Japan (covered Japan, Korea, Okinawa, Philippines, Guam, Vietnam, Thailand and Taiwan. In Vietnam, he set up Rest and Recreation Beaches and trained WS and Small Craft Instructors to man them.) During his time with Natl. Aquatic Schools, he was loaned to the Olympic Committee for the 1960 Squaw Valley Winter Olympics, planning the FA program and supervising the Ski Patrol.

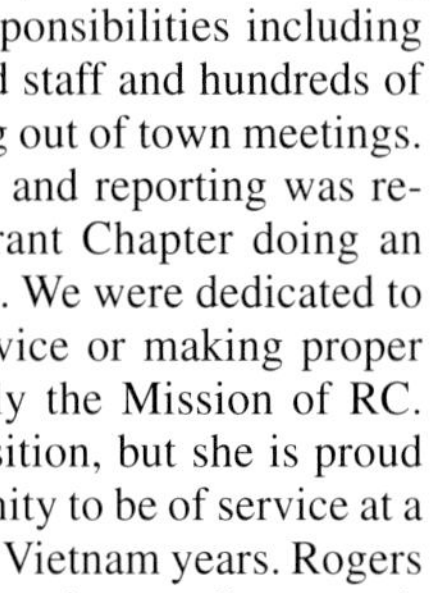

Carl retired in 1969 but continued his volunteer work with chapters in Reedsport, OR and Polson, MT until 1993. He received the following awards: letter of appreciation, Indian RC; letters of appreciation, Korean RC and Thailand RC; certificate, plaque and banner, Republic of China; banner presented by Madame Chiang Kai-shek, head of the Republic of China RC; letter of appreciation, Brigadier General Donald McGovern, Military Assistance Command, Vietnam; Intl. Order of the Golden Whale by the Commodore Longfellow Society.

He married Ethlyn Fowler Ross, Darby, MT in 1934. They were married for 61 years. She died in 1995. They had one daughter, Ann. Ross has completed 72 years of service to the ARC. He is currently retired. **See Red Cross Memories story, "World War II in India and Germany."*

MARTHA L. ROYSE received her Bachelor of education degree from ISNU, Normal, IL in 190. She taught school for two years, was with USO Club in TX, UT, and HI, and recruited in the RC as a hosp. recreation worker in Oct. 1953. Her many assignments included: MASH in Korea; two years at Elmendorf, AK; a year in AF Hosp., Tripoli, Libya (very interesting!); three years at Wurzburg, Germany Army Hosp.; two assignments at Clark AFB, Philippines; Vietnam and six months on the hosp. ship. Her most memorable times were sanctuary and the next six years at Army hosp. in Saigon. She started as a hosp. recreation worker, then became hosp. field dir. in one-worker stations. Her last assignment was at David Grant Medical Center, Travis AFB, CA, where she still resides. Working with many wonderful people, and assisting patients and their families gave her much satisfaction through the years. She salutes the organization and all it stands for and does.

Royse is currently retired, after 31 years, active with Meals on Wheels, Friends of the Library and Tele-Care. She is single with very little family, but is blessed with lots of friends.

JOHN ROBERT RUSSELL, born Nov. 27, 1915, holds a BS and MA from IN Univ. He began his RC career June 14, 1943 in Alexandria, VA. His other assignments included: Camp Claiborne, LA; Camp Campbell, KY (now Ft. Campbell); Northern Field, Tullahoma, TN; Esler Field, LA; SE Area Office, Atlanta, GA; Natl. HQ, Washington, DC; Hartford, CT Chapter; Indianapolis Chapter. He also assisted in many disasters.

Among his most memorable experiences was the RC office at Esler, a tar paper covered building, open to the outside by a double door and a window on each side of a single room. They had a lone damaged eight-inch fan and no water cooler. The area office, at his request, granted $10 to purchase a water cooler which he found at a local store: a 10 gallon wooden keg with a spout. Each day he got ice from the mess hall across the street, and day after day, the little thermometer on the office wall registered 108 degrees in mid-afternoon. Added to the physical discomfort was the job demand to be at the Alexandria railroad station at 2:00 a.m. almost every day to write loans or grants to soldiers leaving on the train. It was the most physically demanding job he had in his 37 years with the RC.

He received the Sagamore of the Wabash Award, the highest civilian award in the state of IN. He is currently retired in 1980, after 37 years, residing with his wife Dorothy. They have four children and 10 grandchildren. **See Red Cross Memories stories, "A Memorable Red Cross Experience" and "A Red Cross Career."*

LORICE SALEM was born Jan. 25, 1928, in Pawtucket, RI. Salem was the 1946 salutatorian at Central Falls High School. Salem began a RC career as part-time bookkeeper/full charge, replacing the full-time person, thus saving the Chapter money. The most memorable experience was working and understanding the basic four computer system, when they did not have access to home computers. Salem was featured in ARC 1993-94 "Do-ers," Lifestyle Profiles, and is currently retired.

DORIS MARGARET JOHNSON SATRE was born June 27, 1910 in Seattle, WA. She holds a Master's in social work, which she obtained in 1944. She worked as a social worker with the RC in Menlo Park, CA from 1944-46 and at the OR Trail Chapter, 1952-75. She remembers working with seriously injured patients in need of plastic surgery and other reconstructive surgery, as well as with blind patients. All were combat injured. She is currently retired, the widow of the late Arthur Satre, who passed away Oct. 19, 1946.

LILLIAN SCHEFFELS was born in St. Louis, MO on Sept. 6, 1905. She is a high school graduate who began serving with the RC as typist and later was given the title of admin. asst. with the Fund Campaign Division in the Accounting department of the Midwestern Area Office, St. Louis, MO, 1944-70. This office was comprised of 17 states, and is now the local St. Louis Chapter office. Scheffels worked with two asst.s until retirement at age 65, which was the age limit in 1970. She had served 26 years with the RC. She enjoyed every minute of her employment with the ARC office.

ELINOR BRAWNER SEEVERS, born Feb. 2, 1919, Dumfries, VA, attended elementary and secondary schools, Prince William Co. VA.

Her RC Assignments were: Personnel Services, Eastern Area Office, 1944-46; receptionist, Eastern Area Office, 1946-62; asst. to building supervisor, EAO, 1962-64; receptionist/transportation clerk, EAO, 1964-1980.

Her favorite memories are watching staff members, many of whom she met when they came into EAO for their pre-employment interview, depart for overseas assignments, and whether in peacetime or war, greeting them upon their safe return. Also her "retirement" party in Eastern Area Mgr.'s office in 1980 is a special memory.

GENE FAULKNER SEEVERS, born Oct. 24, 1925, Pleasant Hill, MO, was educated in Pleasant Hill, MO, and also at WA Univ., St. Louis, MO, (Anny Air Corps Pre-Flight/ ASTRP), 1944; SD State College, Brookings, SD and Central MO State Univ., Warrensburg, MO, 1949-51 (BS, history).

ARC Assignments were: Ft. Hood, TX, 1955; Ft. Polk, LA, 1955; Ft. Riley, KS, 1956; Midwestern & Eastern Area HQ, 1956-59; Andrews AFB, MD, 1959; Bolling AFB, DC, 1959-60; US Naval Receiving Station, DC 1959-60; Ft. Belvoir, VA, 1960-62; Natl. HQ, Alexandria, VA., 1962-1985.

His memorable experiences include: "Operation Sagebrush," Ft. Polk, LA, 1955; the then largest post WWII "wargames;" the Hungarian Refugee Operation, Camp Kilmer, NJ, 1956-57; his first "real" disaster operation, a tornado in Dallas TX, 1957. Most memorable of all is the lovely brunette at Eastern Area's reception desk, who "in a moment of weakness accepted my plea to matrimony in 1958, and who still puts up with me after more than 40 years."

Seevers is currently retired and an active antique collector; past president of Pewter Collectors Club of America, currently member of its board of governors; life member Historic Dumfries, VA, Inc., past member of its board of directors; artifacts contributor to its exhibits at Weems-Botts Museum; avid reader and occasional golfer.

JESSE FRANK SHOUSE born in Brookfield, MO on Feb. 11, 1939, holds a BS in education from Bob Jones Univ., Greenville, SC, which he obtained in 1967.

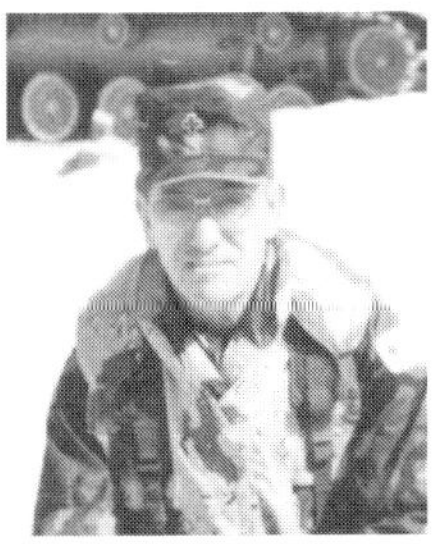

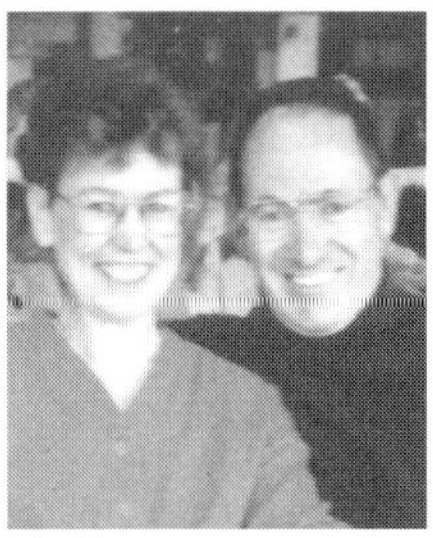

He began his RC career at Western Area HQ, San Francisco, CA in Mar. 1969. His assignments were: training at Ft. Lewis, WA; Service to Military Installations; Oakland Army Terminal, CA Travis AFB, CA; Quang Tri, Vietnam; Da Nang AB, Vietnam; Naval Air Station, Oak Harbor, WA; Clark AB, Philippines; Fitzsimmons Army Medical Center, Aurora, CO; Bamberg, Germany; Operation Desert Shield/ Storm, Saudi Arabia; RAF Lakenheath. He took an early retirement in Mar. 1995.

The experiences he remembers best are the ones he had in Vietnam and Saudi Arabia. On Christmas Day, 1970, he taking a RC "Donut Dolly" and a jeep full of ditty bags to every military unit assigned to Quang Tri. While delivering the ditty bags he met Admiral John McCain, Commander of Pacific Forces who had come to the DMZ to look out over North Vietnam and wonder about his son John who was then a POW. We were able to give him a ditty bag and some pictures were taken.

Shouse received the Civilian Service Medal for serving in Vietnam; the Service Medal for Desert Shield/Desert Storm and the Fundraising Award for small military installations in Western Area.

Shouse currently works part-time in collections for Roper Pontiac, GMC, Buick, Honda, & Subaru. Most of my time is spent in volunteer activities at church and as Scripture Chairman for the Joplin Camp of Gideons Intl. He was married to Marie Anna Bohonos for 29 years, who died in England shortly before he retired. They had one daughter Maria who graduated from college and is now teaching English in Beijing, China. He has remarried Jean Marie Fullerton, who is employed at St. John's Regional Medical Clenter in Joplin, MO.

SYLVAN SILVER was born Aug. 18, 1914 in Baltimore, MD, and is a graduate of Univ. of Baltimore Law School, LLB, 1938. His assignments with the RC included: dir. of Public Relations, DE Chapter, Wilmington, DE, 17 years (June 1959-April 1976); Atlantic Coast Disaster, 1966; minor disasters; fundraising; disaster fund appeals. Silver received citations from Eastern Area Public Relations for outstanding news coverage and publications.

Currently Silver is retired, after 33 years of news correspondence, reporting and editing. He served with four newspapers and five publications. He was married for 51 years, when his wife, Ruth, died in April 1996. He has two sons in Rockville, MD and Timonium, MD, and four grandchildren.

VIVIAN GRAY PARTIN SIMMONS was born Jul. 15, 1913 in Franklin county, Decherd, TN. She took business courses 1941-42, and served with the RC from 1942-77 in the following capacities: clerk-typist, field dir. office, Camp Forrest, TN; clerk-steno, SVAO, Nashville, TN and SVAO, St. Petersburg, FL. She married Richard Simmons on Feb. 16, 1963. He passed away on Dec. 31, 1976.

Simmons received a token of high esteem in recognition of faithful performance of service for 32 years, and is enjoying retirement.

PALMER M. SIMPSON was born Aug. 18, 1914 in Brownsville, TN, and is a 1939 graduate of Southwestern (Rhodes) College, TN. He was a professor at Hampden Sydney College, VA, 1939-46. His RC career from 1946-68 included: Military Service dir., Atlantic Command, St. Johns, Newfoundland; general field rep., Midwestern Area office, Forrest City, AR; Little Rock, AR; disaster dir., St. Louis Midwest Area office; deputy natl. disaster dir., DC; area dir., Midwest office, St. Louis, MO; mgr., Houston Gulf Coast Chapter.

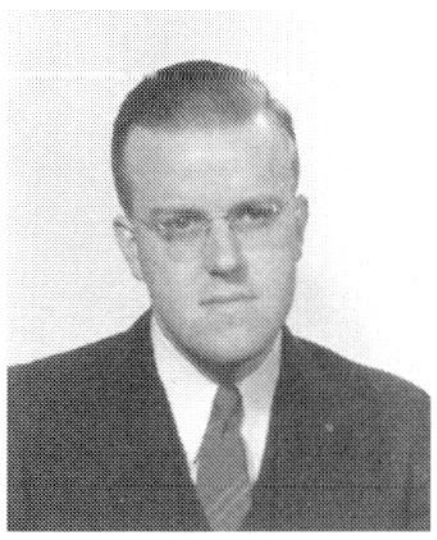

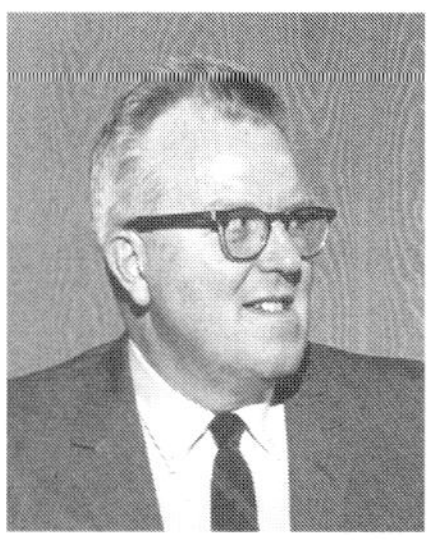

Simpson married Eloise Whitley April 11, 1941, and they had a daughter, Katherine Simpson McCarty; a son, Palmer Martin Simpson, Jr. and two grandchildren, Sarah W. McCarty and Ryan McCarty. Simpson died June 24, 1999.

E.M. "MAC" SLEE, former newspaperman, began his career with the ARC as Public Information dir. with the Oakland, CA Chapter, 1962. In 1966, he accepted the position of asst. dir. of Public Information for the Western Area HQ, San Francisco. In 1968 he was named dir. of that office, and in 1971, was appointed dir. of Public Relations, European Area, Stuttgart, Germany.

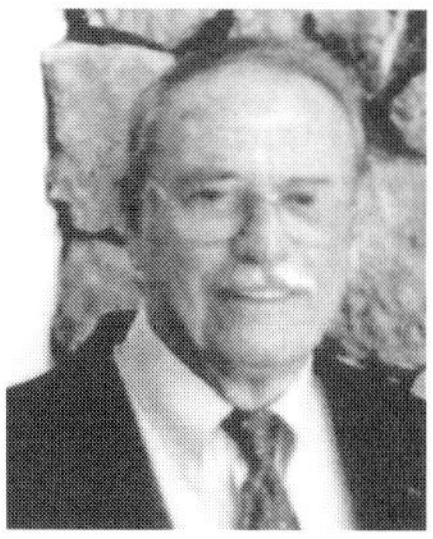

During his European tour he represented the ARC at conferences conducted by the League of RC Societies and the Intl. Committee of the RC both HQ in Geneva, Switzerland. It was during this period that he was assigned to document the relief work of the internatl. bodies in India and Bangeldesh where he worked with Mother Teresa and her Sisters at Charity. He also worked closely with the German RC in programs of service to both the American Military community and local German communities in Ludwigsburg and Kornwestheim, and represented the ARC at meetings of Western and Eastern societies in Geneva; Copenhagen; Koln and Varna, Bulgaria.

Upon his return to the United States in 1975, he was appointed natl. dir. of public relations at the organization's HQ in DC. In 1977 he again served in San Francisco Bay Area as exec. dir., Solano Co. Chapter of the RC until his retirement for medical reasons in 1987.

Slee was a native of DC and attended DC Public Schools, Randall's Naval Academy Prep School and George WA Univ. He served in the United States Navy during the WWII. His stories and photos have appeared in numerous publications in this country and abroad, and most recently he was elected to the Intl. Poetry Hall of Fame. He died Feb. 28, 1998.

JANE SLOSS started as a RC volunteer in the Motor Corp of the San Francisco RC during WWII. She did look good in that handsome "RC Motor Corp" uniform, complete with Sam Brown belt. She was promoted to lieutenant and later became chairman of the program in San Francisco. During those years RC Motor Corps fleet was over 100 "woodie" station wagons, used to transport military dependents and provide canteen service at the San Francisco docks ad US troop ships departed and arrived.

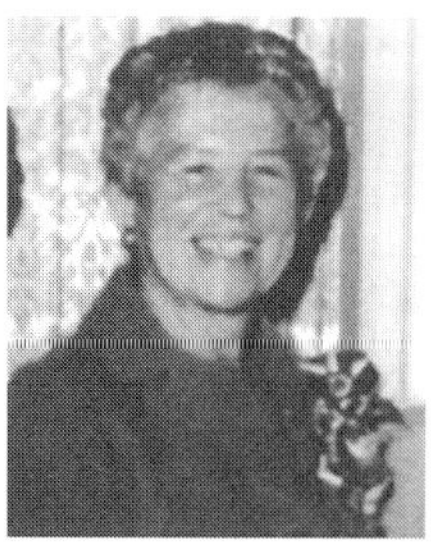

Sloss' organizational skills got her promoted to chairman of volunteers, San Francisco Chapter and from 1960 to 1973 went on to be chairman of volunteers, Western Area office, ANRC. Her first disaster assignment was the 1964, 8.4 AK Earthquake. In 1980 she also served on 7.0 Earthquake in Eureka, CA.

In 1973 a big retirement party was held for her at San Francisco Marines Memorial Hall with hundreds in attendance, including a large group from DC. She was called back on duty, as the natl. consultant for the Blood Program. Sloss received the prestigious RC Harriman Award. She worked on the ARC History and Education project to create a Museum at DC HQ. She and her husband Richard Sloss, had two daughters, and now have five grandchildren and five great grandchildren. Jane died April 15, 1998.

ESTHER HERVEY SMITH was born in Dover, NH, Mar. 9 1908. She graduated from Dover High School, 1925 and graduated Univ. of NH, 1929 with a BA. She received her Master's degree from Brown Univ. while recorder (registrar) at Penbroke College in Brown Univ.

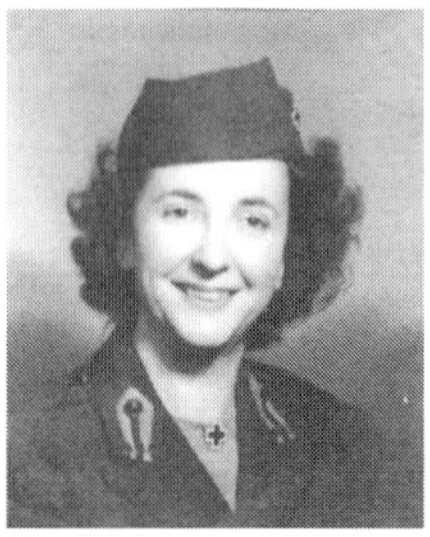

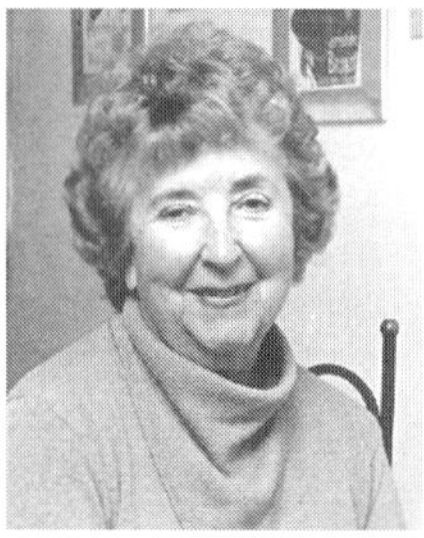

Smith entered RC service May 6, 1944, and after basic training was assigned to a 1,000 bed Army Hosp. at Erlestoke Park, England in charge of recreation. She was redeployed across USA to Japan. She did not get to Japan in 1945 because the war ended. She spent one year at Ft. Lewis as head recreation worker in Convalescent Hosp. From 1946-51 she was assigned to Veterans Hosp. in Framingham, MA and Providence, RI as asst. field dir. and field dir.

After a cut in budget, she was head recreation worker in hospitals in the USA, Guam and Tachikawa, Japan, and upon her return from Japan, became personnel asst. in charge of recruitment, Eastern Area Office. From 1957-65 she was assigned to field service and center dir. in France and Morocco, and from 1965-73 she was exec. dir., Greenwich Chapter, CT. Smith retired in Mar. 1973. **See Red Cross Memories story, "Recreation."*

RICHARD N. SMITH began his career with the ARC in 1960 in the Nashville-Davidson Co. Chapter, Nashville, TN, his home town. In 1967 he transferred to the natl. sector as an asst. field dir. in Service at Military Installations, with assignments in SCand HI. In 1968 he volunteered for a 12 month Intl. Services assignment in Southeast Asia. He supervised a joint refugee relief team of the ARC and the RC Society of the Republic of South Vietnam and managed liaison relationships with South Vietnamese and United States government officials in Quang Tin province.

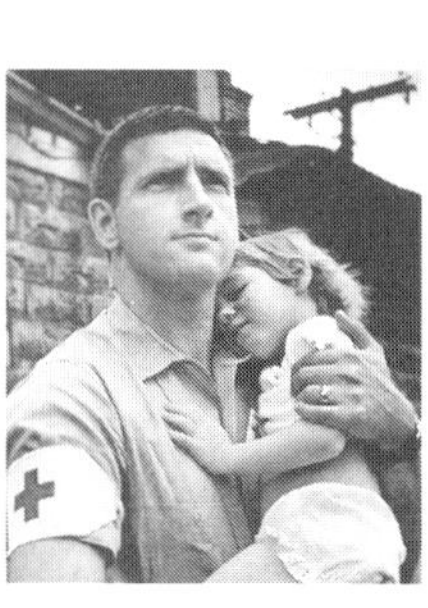

Over the next six years Richard held positions in disaster services, blood donor recruitment, field service, division management, and financial development, serving in chapters and in the Southeastern Area Office. In 1975, he was appointed dir., financial development, Eastern Area, and was subsequently promoted to deputy mgr. and then vice president/general mgr. in that HQ. In 1990 he was awarded the President's Tiffany Award for Employee Excellence.

In Oct. 1991, he was assigned responsibility for managing the transition planning to implement the SD21 Field Service System and the creation of state service councils, a major organizational restructuring. He was appointed general mgr., Chapter operations admin. at Natl. HQ in 1992, where he served until his retirement in Jan. 1998. He now resides in Mount Vernon, VA with his wife Lynda, a former RC nurse.

JAMES MARVIN SMYTH, born Aug. 17, 1897 at Dexter, MO. He was a RC volunteer for 20 years, and became a staff member Jul. 1942. He served as field dir. on Army stations in KY and around DC. Following WWII, he was assigned to the Southeastern Area office as asst. dir., Jr. RC, based on a Master's degree in education. This assignment provided opportunity for me to lead two special projects in Germany: to assist the German RC in organizing its Jr. RC and to assist them in operating it. In the early 50s Smyth became the SE dir., Jr. RC and in the late 50s became the SE dir. of personnel. He retired in Aug. 1962.

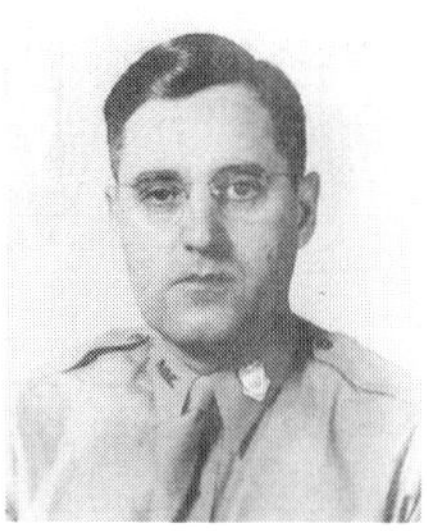

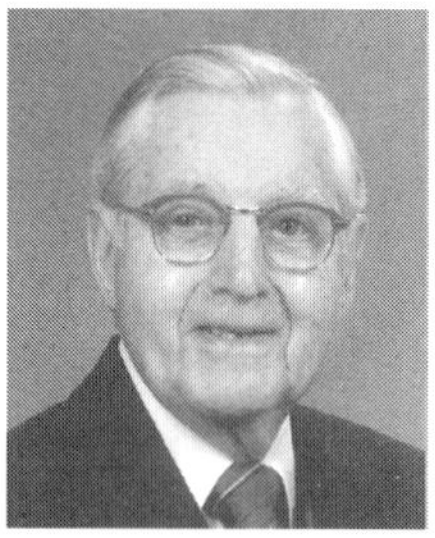

In 1957 he married VA McIntire, also a RCer. They reside in Decatur, GA. He enjoyed a fabulous 100th birthday party and was also privileged to enjoy #101. He is still enjoying life.

PATRICIA A. MACPHERSON SNYDER was born at Hollywood Presbyterian Hosp. (HPH) where she took her nurse's training, and graduated as an RN in 1952. While working as a student nurse, she met her husband Tom Snyder, who was visiting his father, one of her patients.

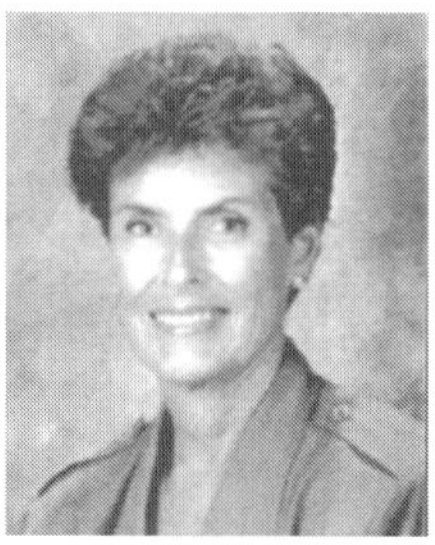

Her RC Disaster assignments included: a plane crash into a Pacomia school yard, 1955; volunteer nurse teaching "Mother-Baby Care" classes; nurse, Sylmar Earthquake; San Fernando Valley Disaster Action team; many other local disasters; Appalachian Floods, KY; Los Angeles Chapter Disaster chairman. She served as natl. chairman, Disaster Services, 1989-92; Hurricane Hugo, Loma Prieta and Northridge Earthquakes, typhoons on Guam, floods; Mexico City Earthquake and numerous other disasters. She also served as Intl. League of RC Societies delegate, establishing a program for earthquake victims who had become amputees; leader, Northern and Southern CA Disaster Institutes and as Disaster Service natl. instructor and monitor. She was appointed by the governor to the CA Seismic Safety Commission, 1989, and named chairman, 1997.

In 1984, she was awarded the prestigious "Harriman Award", for developing the first RC Earthquake preparedness program "Safety and Survival in an Earthquake".

Snyder and her husband shared the hobby of sport fishing and she holds three Intl. Records for women's light tackle sport fishing. They had two daughters Christia, and Kathy, who provided five grandchildren: Sharon, Trisha, Heather, Brian and Kendall. Her husband died in 1997 of Lou Gehrig's Disease (ALS) after their marriage of 45 years. She continues her volunteer activities with the Los Angeles Chapter of the RC, and Amyotrophic Lateral Sclerosis (ALS) Association.

PHOEBE STEFFEY was born in Williamsport, MD, attended public schools there, and graduated from the Univ. of MD, 1933 with a BA. Following two years in "exploratory positions" she taught school in her hometown. She became a member of the natl. staff of the ARC in 1942. Her RC assignments included: 1942-44, head recreation worker, Service in Military Hosps. (SMH), Natl. HQ.

Naval Medical Center, Bethesda, MD; 1944-46, recreation consultant, SNM, Natl. HQ, DC; 1944, ARC rep., US Army Hosp. Ship, Mediterranean; 1945, ARC rep., Brideship Operation (5 Trans-Atlantic voyages); 1946-47, recreation consultant, SMaine, Europe; 1949-76, natl. staff; 1949-50, head recreation worker, Letennan Army Hosp., San Francisco; 1950-52, asst. dir., Volunteer Special Services Western Area; 1952-54, asst. dir., Volunteer Services, Eastern Area, Alexandria, VA; 1954-76, asst. dir., Volunteer Services; asst. dir., Volunteer Program Development; dir., Community Volunteer Programs Natl. HQ, DC; 1956, RC rep., US Transport Eltiniz; 1973, caseworker, RC refugee operation, Guam (5 months).

Steffey retired from the RC in 1976, and resides with her sister, Jane, in Sykesville, MD. **See Red Cross Memories story, "Hospital Ship."*

JUNE J. STRATE was born in Spokane, WA, and attended Eastern WA Univ., 1961-64. She served with the RC in the Inland Empire Division, Spokane, WA, 1964-74; Louisville, KY, 1977-78; Broward Co., 1979-81; DC Chapter, 1986-87; Office of Volunteer Personnel (dir.). Her most memorable experiences were in disaster work, which was limited. She received the usual staff awards: pins and appreciation. Strate is currently retired, enjoying her four children and six grandchildren.

JOHN D. STROUD began his service with RC in the Los Angeles Chapter, Jan. 1, 1965 as the asst. dir. of the San Fernando Valley District, the largest district of the Chapter, serving over one million people. Paul Gillis was the mgr. when he started but was killed that same day in an accident on a major disaster relief operation in Happy Valley, CA.

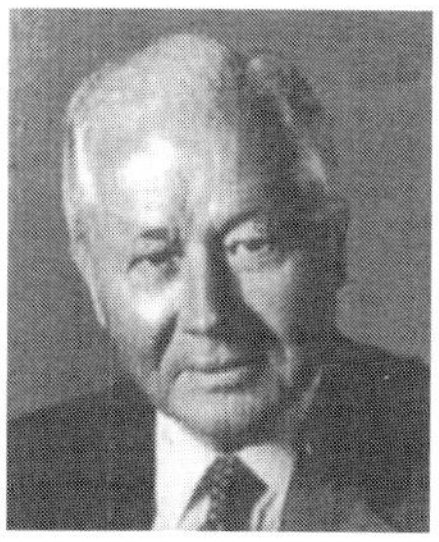

John Martin succeeded Paul Gillis as district mgr. and served for four years. He had been transferred from running one of the most successful youth programs in RC for the entire chapter in Los Angeles Co.

During his years with RC, Stroud also served as the San Fernando Valley Area campaign dir., United Crusade, a partnership of the United Way and the RC; West District mgr., San Fernando Valley; asst. mgr., Operations, Los Angeles Chapter; Chapter/Division mgr., Los Angeles Chapter, Southern CA Division; center Chapter mgr., Los Angeles-Orange Counties Regional Blood Services (Chapter exec. officer).

Stroud also served on many natl. committees such as the President's Advisory Council and was the only paid staff member of the search committee that selected Mrs. Dole as the President of the ARC. He retired in 1991 and has continued to serve in many volunteer positions.

ELAINE M. SWEET was born Mar. 30, 1929, and served as dir., CT Valley East Brach, Greater Hartford Chapter, 1956-91; dir., North Central Brach, 1991-92 and dir., Northeast Branch, 1992-94. Her best RC memory was making a special doll for a young heart patient, with whom she kept contact until the girl became and adult, and later passed away. Sweet is currently retired. **See Red Cross Memories story, "I Remember."*

DOROTHY B. TAAFFE was born in Albany, NY, and holds a BA from College of St. Rose, 1936 and an MA from Columbia Univ., 1939. Her assignments with the RC included: England General Hosp., Atlantic City; Tilton General Hosp., Ft. Dix, NJ; St. Albans' Naval Hosp., St. Albans, NY; San Francisco, CA; American Recreation Society, Natl. Association of Recreation Professionals; RC Youth, Natl. HQ, DC; internatl. services, Natl. HQ, DC.

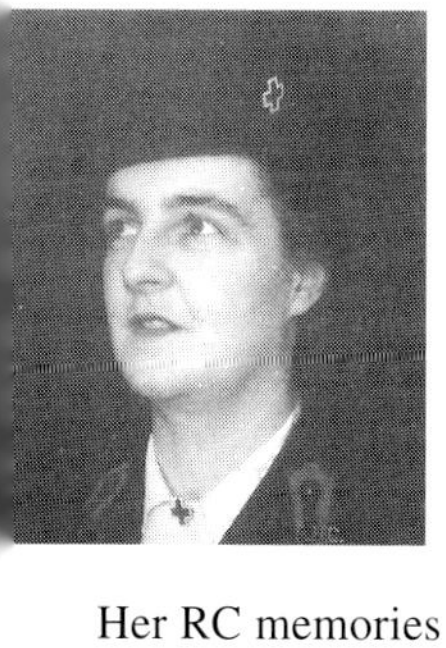

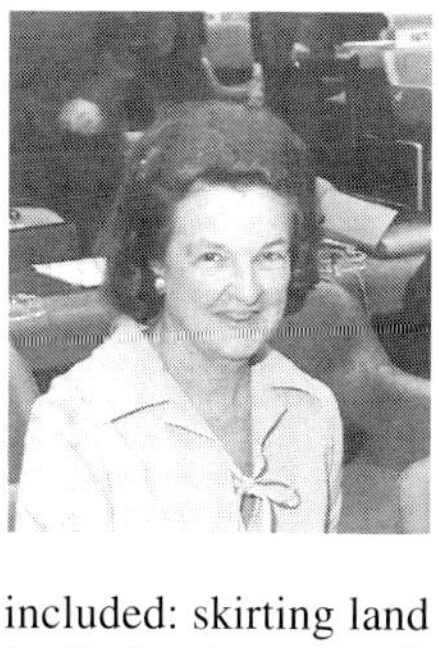

Her RC memories included: skirting land mines at Thailand-Cambodia border to reach ICRC field hosp., headed by Dr. Jim Cobey, RC volunteer; meeting planes of evacuated wounded, many midnights at Ft. Dix; rejoicing with ARC Youth volunteers who trained hundreds of First Aid and Health instructors in foreign countries; introducing a joint resolution of governments and RC societies with Dr. Frank Stanton, ARC chairman, and Goerge Elsey, ARC president, at RC Intl. Conference in 1977, Bucharest, Romania — "to improve the health and well-being of people, particularly women and children, in developing countries" (it was passed by 107 countries); the sheer excitement of shaking hands with Emporer Hirohito of Japan and figuratively swimming in many seas, but literally in seas from the Baltic to the Indian.

Taaffe's brother Jim is former natl. deputy dir., Veterans Admin., often aided in ARC "Reunion of Families." Her sister Miriam collaborated. Taaffe is currently retired.

DONNA E. MCCULLOUGH TAYLOR, born Nov. 2, 1929 in Chicago, IL, obtained her BA from Cornell College, 1951. She began as WSI at Cornell College. In 1952, she became Safety Service specialist in the Chicago Chapter. After marrying and raising a family, Taylor returned in 1972 as Safety Service dir. for the Boise, ID Chapter, holding that position until 1980. In 1982, she became the exec. dir., Morgantown, WV, remaining in that position until her retirement in 1994. Under her leadership, the Chapter became the State Coordinating Chapter in 1992. In 1986, she was awarded the Tiffany Award at the Vice Presidential level.

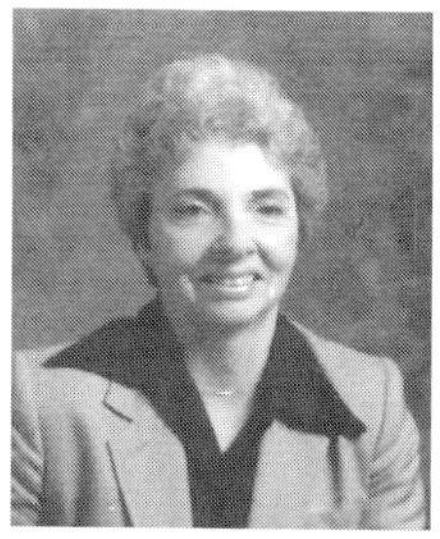

After retirement, Taylor and her husband returned to Boise, where she chairs the State Disaster Committee, and with the DSHR system, presently serves as dir. of level IV disaster operations. She was awarded the Clara Barton volunteer award in 1996. She and her husband have four children and seven grandchildren.

BRYCE TORRENCE started his career with the ARC at the Los Angeles, CA Chapter in 1964, after he retired as lieutenant colonel from the US Army. Torrence had enlisted in 1942 in the Natl. Guard, attended Officer Candidate School at Ft. Lee, VA in 1943, and served in India during WWII, Germany from 1947-51, PR, 1944-58, and Vietnam, 1962-63.

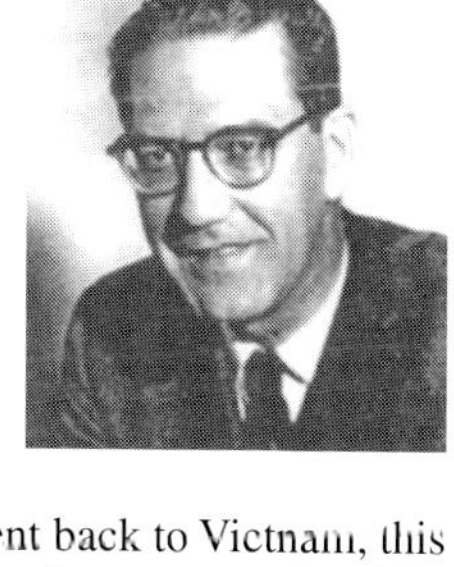

In 1966, he was sent back to Vietnam, this time to help RC manage refugee centers. In 1969, when he returned to the US, he joined the natl. staff at the Western Field Office in San Francisco, CA. As dir. of Disaster Services, he headed up Operation New Life, the ARC support of the government's refugee operation at Camp Pendleton, CA, where over 150,00 Vietnamese refugees were processed and welcomed into the US. During Torrence's years of service to the organization, he is especially remembered for establishing cooperative relationships with the US government and helping to establish the Federal Emergency Management Agency (FEMA) as well as embracing member organizations into the Natl. Voluntary Organizations Active in Disaster (NVOAD).

Torrence retired in 1979, continuing to volunteer on disaster relief operations and consulting with the disaster leadership. He died on Jan. 12, 1984 and is survived by wife June; children Tom, Terryann, and Kelly, from his first marriage; and children Raymond, Kathleen, and Deborah with June, as well as eleven grandchildren.

NAOMI L. TOWERS graduated from Columbus State in 1952 and J.L. Kellogg Graduate School of Management, Northwestern Univ. in 1962. Her RC service was from 1960-95 and was all in Columbus, OH with Blood Services and Chapter Services. Her last position was chief operating officer. She fondly remembers meeting so many fine people, serving on President George Elsey's Advisory Committee, representing Blood Services, serving as a peer reviewer of Blood Centers for National HQ, and teaching the new asst. and Blood administrator courses. She was awarded the local Tiffany Excellence Award, developed in her honor for diversity excellence, and the Region II Tiffany Award for mgr. excellence.

Towers married J. Ambrose Towers in 1956, and they have one daughter, Brenda Rivers, who has two children; Steven Rivers, age 14; and Lauren Rivers, age 12. Towers retired after 35 years of RC service and is presently caring for her two grandchildren after school.

MARIE TULLY's RC service included: US Naval Hosp., Houston, TX; US Army Hosp., Ft. Riley, KS; Great Lakes Navy Hosp., IL; Ft. Smith Army Hosp., AR; US Air Force Hosp., Fairbanks, AK; Ft. Richardson, Anchorage, AK; Brooke Army Medical Center, San Antonio, TX; Madigan General Hosp., Tacoma, WA; Travis Air Force Hosp., Fairfield, CA; Parks Air Force Hosp., Pleasanton, CA; Mar. Air Force Hosp., Riverside, CA; US Naval Hosp., San Diego, CA; US Naval Hosp., Ft. Pendleton, CA; US Army Hosp., Heidelberg, Germany; US Air Force Hosp., Spangeahalm?, Germany; Oak Knoll Naval Hosp., Oakland, CA; Ft. Ord Army Hosp., Monterey, CA; Camp Pendleton Marine Hosp., Oceanside, CA; Lefterman Naval Hosp., San Francisco, CA; US Naval Hosp., San Diego, CA; Clarke AFB, Manila, Philippines. Her titles were hosp. recreation worker, hosp. recreation supervisor and hosp. field dir.

After her retirement in 1973, until 1992, she served as a volunteer, Concord and Solano Co., CA Chapters and as chairman, Volunteers for Service to Military Families (SMF), Board of Dirs., Solano Co.. She received awards from many of the above listed hosp. commanders; an award from USAF Chaplains Services for assistance with choir and as organist; recognition from Korean Army, Clark AFB, Philippines; was Guest of Honor, Stockton Chapter 100th Anniversary Celebration, 1990; was guest instructor, Natl. ARC Training Center, Univ. of VA (several times) and received the "Emerald" Volunteer Service Pin, Solano Co., CA Chapter.

MARY DILLARD TUTOR was born Jul. 19, 1919 in Toccopola, MS. She graduated from high school and served as RC switchboard operator a total of 14 years and two weeks. She enjoyed it all.

Tutor is the widow of Rouble Tutor, who passed away Jan. 28, 1999. They were married 64 years. She has three sons, six grandsons, one granddaughter and four great grandchildren.

KATHERINE HARRIS VAN HOGENDORP *(see Red Cross Memories story, "Katie.")*

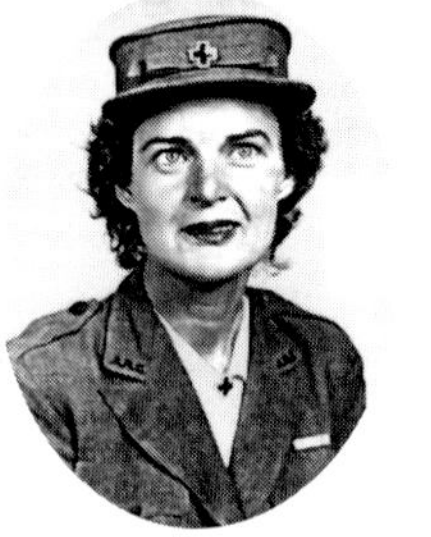

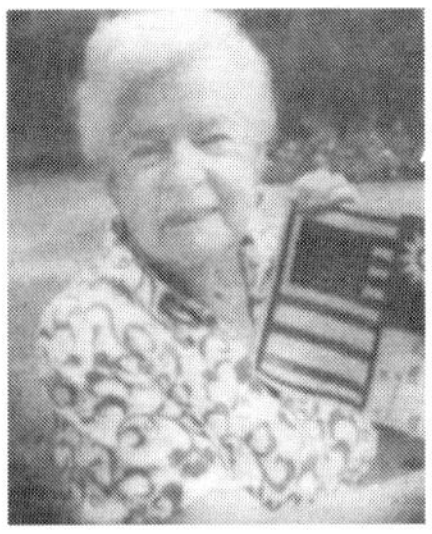

EDGAR LEIGH VENZKE, born April 30, 1920, holds both BA (1941) and MA (1947) from Johns Hopkins Univ. His RC positions were: traffic mgr., General Supply Office, 1971-72; asst. general supply officer, DC HQ and Alexandria, VA, 1972-74. His memorable experiences were managing the warehouse and distribution operations for two months following Hurricane Agnes and arranging supply shipments after destruction of Managua. Venzke received four letters of commendation and a letter of thanks from Brazilian RC for arranging an emergency shipment of medicine which saved a child's life.

Venzke is currently retired, and resides with his wife in VA. They have four children, and four grandchildren.

MAE LOUISE CULLER VIOLA, born June 21, 1919 in Orangeburg, SC, received her AB from Coker College, Hartsville, SCand MA from Syracuse Univ., NY, 1951.

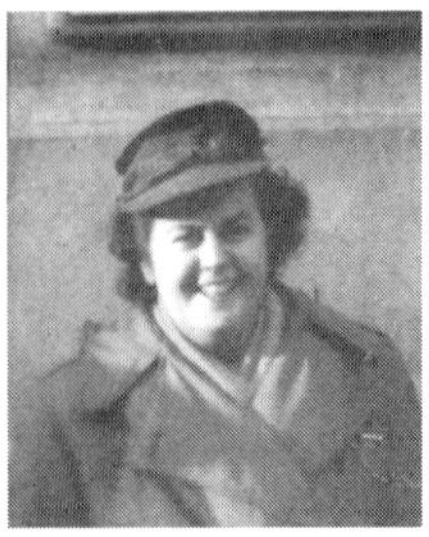

She served five years with the RC as senior hosp. recreation worker. Her assignments included: CAW, Livingston, LA, 1942-43; Ft.Jackson, SC, 1943-44; 68th General Hosp., ETO (ENGLAND), 1944; London HQ, 1944; LeHavre, France, 1944; Paris, 1944; Hosp. Train 38 to Belgium (whisked off train by Mps outside Liege, Belgium); 56th General Hosp., 1944-45; 77th Evac. Namur, Belgium, 1945; 21st General Hosp., Mirecourt, France, 1945; Ft. Jackson, SC, 1946; ETO, 1946; Frankfurt, Germany; 385th Station Hosp., Nuremburg, Germany, 1946. Viola retired in Feb. 1947.

After her marriage, she moved to Syracuse, NY and became education dir. of the YWCA, a guidance counselor and asst. principal in Liverpool & North Syracuse Schools. She is listed in Who's Who in American Education, 1958. She is now retired and lives from May to Nov. in Cape Vincent, NY, and Nov. to May in The Methodist Oaks Retirement Community, Orangeburg, SC. She is currently writing ARC experiences and her family history.

MERIDITH B. WAGNER, born in Boston, MA, on Nov. 8, 1921, graduated from Nursery Training School of Boston in 1944. She was a volunteer with the Boston ARC Motor Corps, 1944-45, and joined Club Services in April 1945, serving with hosp. services and recreation services in HI; Korea; Japan (to her delight, during which time she visited Shanghai, Nanking, Canton and Hong Kong); Germany; AK; France; Long Island, NY; Ft. Meade, MD; Bethesda, MD; Newport, RI. She was assigned to all military services except the US Coast Guard. Wagner enjoyed overseas assignments and travel in Europe, the Far East, AK and HI. She attended Korea's Independence Event, traveled the length of Japan and saw China.

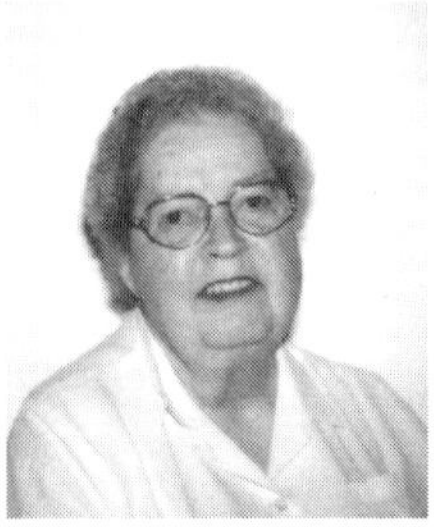

Wagner retired in 1969, after which she served as dir. of volunteers in Salem, MA and Melrose, MA. She served a total of 20 years as a volunteer, and completely retired in 1990. She visits family often in MA and CT.

ROBERT HARVEY WATSON (1895-1998), centenarian, was a special supporter of the ARC. He was helped by RC, worked for RC, and watched the RC grow.

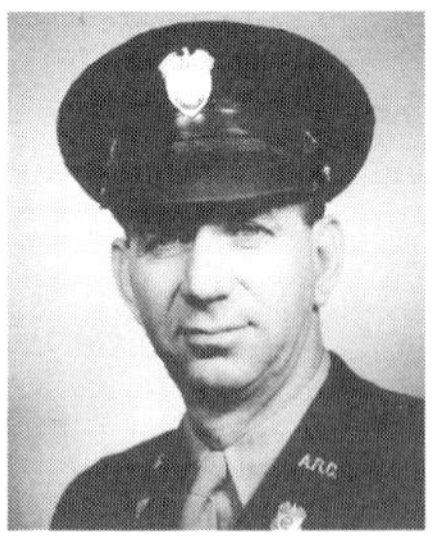

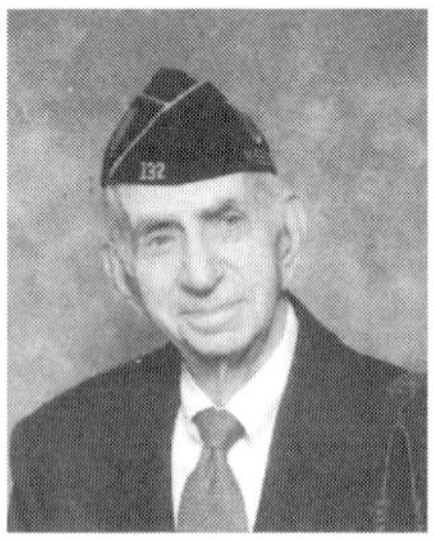

Watson's first RC contact came during WWI when as a member of the First Army Division he was hosp.ized in ARC Hosp. #1 in France. During his hosp.ization his life of "volunteerism" began with cutting and folding bandages for ARC nurses. Honorably discharged in 1919, he was the recipient of the Silver Star, Purple Heart with Oak Leaf Cluster, French Fourreguere, Victory Medal and a citation by his divisional commander. He was an 80-year member of the American Legion.

In 1942, Watson began an 18-year ARC career as field dir. in several TX military installations, including Ft. Hood where he directed an staff of 55. Later assignments included veterans claims work in KS City, Milwaukee and Wichita, and field dir. at Wichita's McConnell AFB. After retirement in 1960, he spent summers as field dir. in Natl. Guard camps. He continued to volunteer with the local VA Hosp. and Chapter, and in 1994 received a special citation from ARC President Elizabeth Dole during her Wichita visit.

Watson's 100th birthday was designated as Robert H. Watson Day by Wichita's mayor. He was also designated by The Retiree (ARARC newsletter) as the oldest retiree with the most years of service. On his 102nd birthday he received special birthday greetings from Willard Scott on natl. television. He is featured in the book, *More Larry Hatteberg's KS People*, and on the Internet in the ARC Registry. Shortly before his death, Watson was designated as a Chevalier of the Natl. Order of the Legion of Honor (the *Legion d'honneur*), the highest award made by the French government, to express the gratitude of the French people for the American valor during WWI.

ED H. WEBB, born in Tacoma, WA on Sept. 20, 1928, obtained his BTh degree in 1951. He served with the RC at the HI State Chapter, Honolulu as Health and Safety dir., 1975-80, as asst. chapter mgr., 1981-82, and asst. district dir., 1983-84. In Fairbanks, AK, he served as chapter mgr./station mgr., 1985-86, and in Anchorage, AK, as field service mgr./hub station mgr., 1987-93. He retired Oct. 1, 1993, and received the 50 year pin and the CA Golden Bear Award in 1998. He is currently a volunteer interim chapter mgr. and disaster services instructor/monitor.

ROBERT B. WEEKLEY, JR., born Aug. 31, 1921 in Mt. Clare, WV, attended Barrackville High School, Barrackville, WV, 1937-1940. He was trained in SAGE Radar Operations Course, Keesler AF Base, MS, 1959 and Senior NColorado Academy, Hamilton AF Base, CA, 1963. He served in US Army Air Corps, 1940-45, with 34 months in the South Pacific. He reenlisted in 1948 and retired 1967 with 25 years. service.

He started with RC five days later as asst. field dir. at Ft. Hood, TX and also served at Camp Enari, Vietnam (4th Infantry Division), 1968; Phu Cat Air Base, Vietnam, 1969; Ft. Hood, TX, 1970; as field dir., Minot AFB, ND, 1970-74; station dir. 1, US Naval Station, Keflavik, Iceland, 1974-78; SD 1, Tyndall AFB, FL, 1978-81; SD 1, Homestead AFB, FL, 1981; SD 1, Hahn AFB, Germany, 1981-84. He returned to the US with 17 years RC service.

DORIS DIANE WHEELER, was born in Austin, TX, Feb. 5, 1934. An AS graduate, she attended UT. Married 44 years to Bill Wheeler who supported her efforts with RC, they had two children, Robby and Diana.

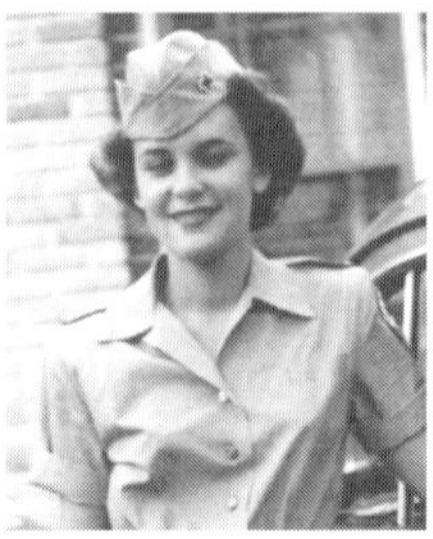

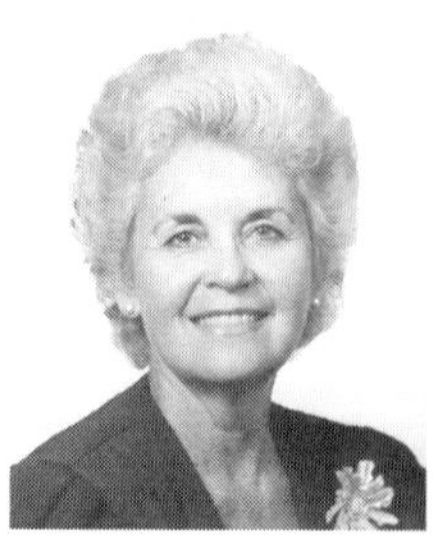

Her career with RC began as a secretary/receptionist in 1951. In June 1956, with the arrival of Robby, she quit working. Her RC career began anew in Feb. 1962 when she returned to the Centex Chapter as Philippines dir. From 1962-84, under various titles, Wheeler oversaw nursing, youth, volunteers, even bookkeeping. She was also asst. to the chapter mgr. In 1984, Wheeler became PR dir., asst. mgr. and responsible for fundraising. These duties cottoned until fall 1990 when she was named deputy mgr./PR dir. for the Chapter. She continued in this capacity until her retirement Aug. 1, 1992.

Wheeler was awarded the highest honor for RC employees, the ARC Tiffany Award, and also received the prestigious Austin Star Award from the PRSA chapter in Austin for dedication.

Her friends say Wheeler brought to the ARC immeasurable energy, infinite dedication and an uplifting personality and she will always embody what RC is all about. "People helping people, that's RC and that's Diane Wheeler." She served 35 years and is still active as a RC volunteer.

LUCIA GARDNER WHITTEMORE, a Springfield, IL native, was born Dec. 7, 1906. She received her BS from the Univ. of IL in 1929 and her MS in social work from Columbia Univ. in 1946. In Nov. 1943 she interrupted her child welfare career to become RC asst. field dir., 40th General Army Hosp.

The 40th General operated in Cirencester, England until Aug. 1944 when it was moved by ship to Normandy, France. After six weeks under "tentage" and black-out conditions, it was put aboard the first train to Paris on repaired tracks, damaged earlier by the Germans. It functioned in LeVesinet, outside Paris.

In Feb. 1945, Whittemore was transferred to the 21st General Hosp., a WA Univ. Medical School reserve unit operating in Mirecourt, France. That hosp. was soon treating 4,000 patients.

Whittemore was awarded the Army's Medal of Freedom. She and her husband, Howard Whittemore, also assigned to the 21st General, were married in 1950. Now retired, they reside in Falls Church, VA.

ELIZABETH HULDA WOMER, born Jul. 27, 1912 in Agra, KS, graduated as RN, from St. Luke's Hosp., KS City, MO. She served at the 1948 Galveston, TX Polio Epidemic and later in the Blood Program in Wichita, KS. She retired as asst. chief nurse. Her memories include trying a new drug for polio that did no good, travels in parts of six states to take blood and sending blood to two wars, first in bottles, then in bags. Several times she went to St. Louis, MO and DC to staff meetings. She received a thank you letter from Natl. Foundation for Inf. Paralysis in 1949, and is in the ARC Legacy Society.

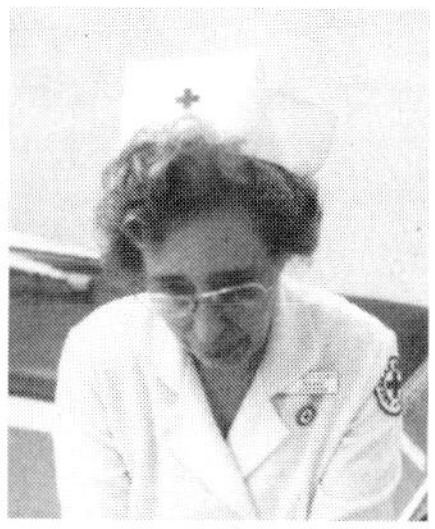

Womer retired after 23 years, after which she continued to volunteer. She has two sister, one niece, one nephew, one great niece and one great nephew.

NORMA G. YOUNG was born Feb. 20, 1923 at Lakemba, NSouthwestern, Australia, and educated at St. George Girls High School, Kogarah, NSouthwestern, 1934-38. Serving as exec. dir., Lincoln Co. Chapter, North Platte, NE, 1965-82, she has too many memorable experiences to write about. Young received Appreciation Award for 17 years of outstanding, dedicated service, Cornhusker Division; Certificate of Appreciation, Mid-Plains Community College and Certificate of Appreciation, "Project Find."

She is married to Vernon W. Young, and they have one daughter, VA J. Bullis, a school teacher, and one son, Terry W. Young, project mgr., Northrop Corp; six grandsons, two granddaughters, and three great grandsons.

DICK ZAMJAHN is from Waukesha, WI, and is a graduate of WI State Univ. in River Falls. During his 29 year career with the RC, he served as FASouth CarolinaWS Representative traveling MN and parts of WI and ND starting in 1962 for three years. After a short stint as a faculty member at Bemidji State College in MN, he joined the staff of the Greater KS City Chapter as dir. of Safety Services for three years followed by three years as dir. of Public Relations. He left KS City in 1971 to take the position of Chapter mgr. of the Tacoma-Pierce Co. Chapter, WA until 1991 when he retired.

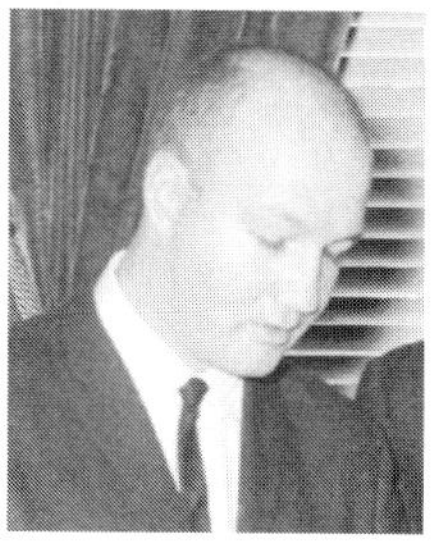

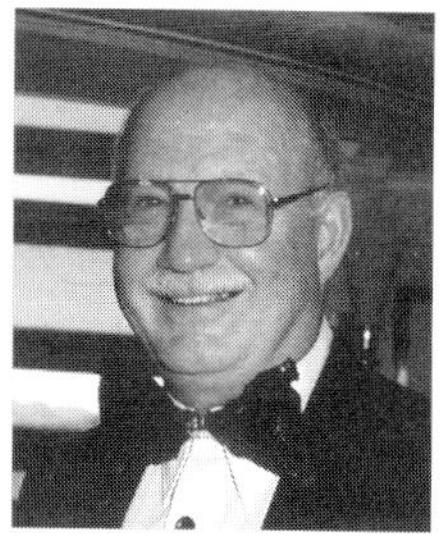

In retirement, he edits the Commodore Longfellow Society newsletter, is interim mgr. for chapters, works for FEMA as a Community Relations Specialist, operates his business Island Images, for a local community college and on cruise ships.

LINDA ESTHER MAJUL-ZAYEK was born in Cuba on April 9, 1934, and entered the ARC on Mar. 16, 1972. She graduated from high school in 1950 and business college in 1971. She was assigned as admin. clerk to the ARC Mission Service Center. The ARC Mission Service Center was established in Sept. 1971. The population that it serves is mostly the Spanish community from all the Latin countries. Her assignment was to help provide the general public with vital English and citizenship classes, working with the senior citizens, information and referrals on community resources. Zayek retired, and is now a volunteer. She has a brother, Edward, and a sister, Blanca.

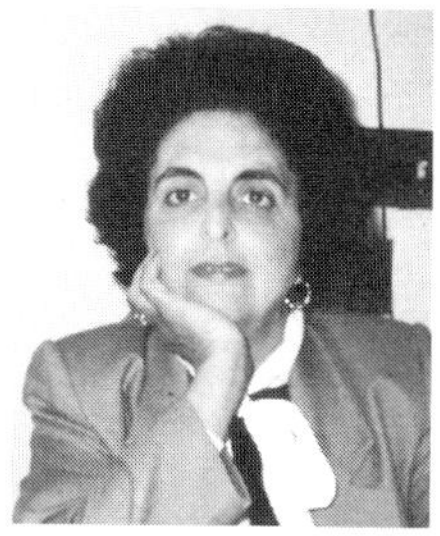

Index

A

Allen, Lucile 66, 72, 73, 83, 88, 89
Anderson-Savage, Gayle 54
Antoinette, Margo 17
Ascensio, Connie 30

B

Bain, M. Victoria 70
Balane, Ozv Hornyak 53
Banks, Carolyne N. 84
Barton, Clara 17, 65, 96
Barton, Clarissa Harlowe 16
Boardman, Mabel 17, 18, 65, 97
Boatright, Margaret 83
Boyer, Charles 44
Bradshaw, Homer V. 72, 73, 74, 75
Bradshaw, Wilda H. 74
Bradshaw, William A. 74, 75

C

Colle, Gaylord W. 64, 65
Conn, Wilber Daniel 70
Cooper, E. 73
Cosby, Bill 52
Crawford, Joan 52
Culler, Mae Louise 77, 83

D

Darnell, Linda 52
Davidson, Lucie 62, 63
Delano, Jane 20
Denman, Elizabeth Reed 62
Dietrich, Marlene 52
Dole, Elizabeth 90, 101
Drew, Charles R. 21
Duncan, Robert 64

E

Elick, Chet 72
Elsey, George M. 100
English, Neal T. 61
Enlows, Harold E. 65
Ettlin, Helen L. 68
Evans, Byron W. 60

F

Fannin, Doye 59, 60, 83, 85
Ferrar, Marjorie 25
Flynn, Erol 44
Foley, James 80
Foley, Jim 81
Forsythe, Emmit 83
Fredericksen, Melvin 57
Furse, Ruth 71
Fylee, Carroll 84

G

Gaddis, Phil 72
Gallant, Richard 84
Gates, John 64
Grandcolas, Helen M. 72
Guenther, Alfred M. 69, 99
Guy, Erna M. 76

H

Hamelau, Bill 55
Harriman, E. Roland 98
Harriman, E.H. 19
Healy, Bernadine 1xs02
Hogendorp, Katherine van 26
Holland, Jerome 22
Hope, Bob 52
Hubbell, Julian B. 17
Hutchins, George 55

I

Irving, Tom 54, 55

J

Joel, Peter 48
Johnson, Walt 83
Jones, Linda 77
Joyal, Margaret Truitt 52, 53

K

Kilbourn, Charlotte 81
Klass, Marge 72
Kohlman, Eleanor Harriet 58
Kostalanetz, Andre 38

L

Lewis, Robert L. 72
Longfellow, Wilbert E. 64
Longoria, Gladys L. 67
Lou, Laura 44, 73

M

Mallory, Pearl Duty 25
Marshall, Cleo 81
Marshall, Mindy 90
Meadows, Cindy 63
Mel Fredricksen 14
Minamoto, Mary 71
Moore, Samuel 74

N

Nicholson, James T. 74, 75

P

Patterne, Carlos 56
Payne, John Barton 20
Pons, Lily 38
Powell, Mildred 83
Priem, Ann Woessner 13
Pulley, Rebecca 84

R

Robinson, Melbern 55
Roosevelt, Franklin D. 18
Roosevelt, Theodore 17
Ross, Carla 56
Rundstedt, Marshal von 58
Russell, John R. 55, 68

S

Sage, Russell 19
Salon, Elizabeth Arden 50
Sanders, Kyoko 71
Saunders, A.L. 44
Saunders, John 46
Schenkenberg, Philip 72
Schilman, Amy 90
Scrymser, James A. 19
Shaeffer, Ray 55
Shaw, Darrell 21
Shouse, Frank 86
Smith, Esther H. 54
Smyth, James M. 84
Steffey, Phoebe 53
Swanson, Steve R. 57
Sweet, Elaine M. 67
Szhertnere, Fribyesene 53

T

Thelma Radden 4
Thomas, Jesse O. 21
Throop, Josh V. 17

W

Waite, Eloise B. 66
Waldrop, Mary 72
Watson, Robert H. 90
Wiese, Harry 19
Willicombe Jr., Joseph 58
Wilson, Woodrow 19
Woessner, Ann 79

Y

Yagos, Joe 31

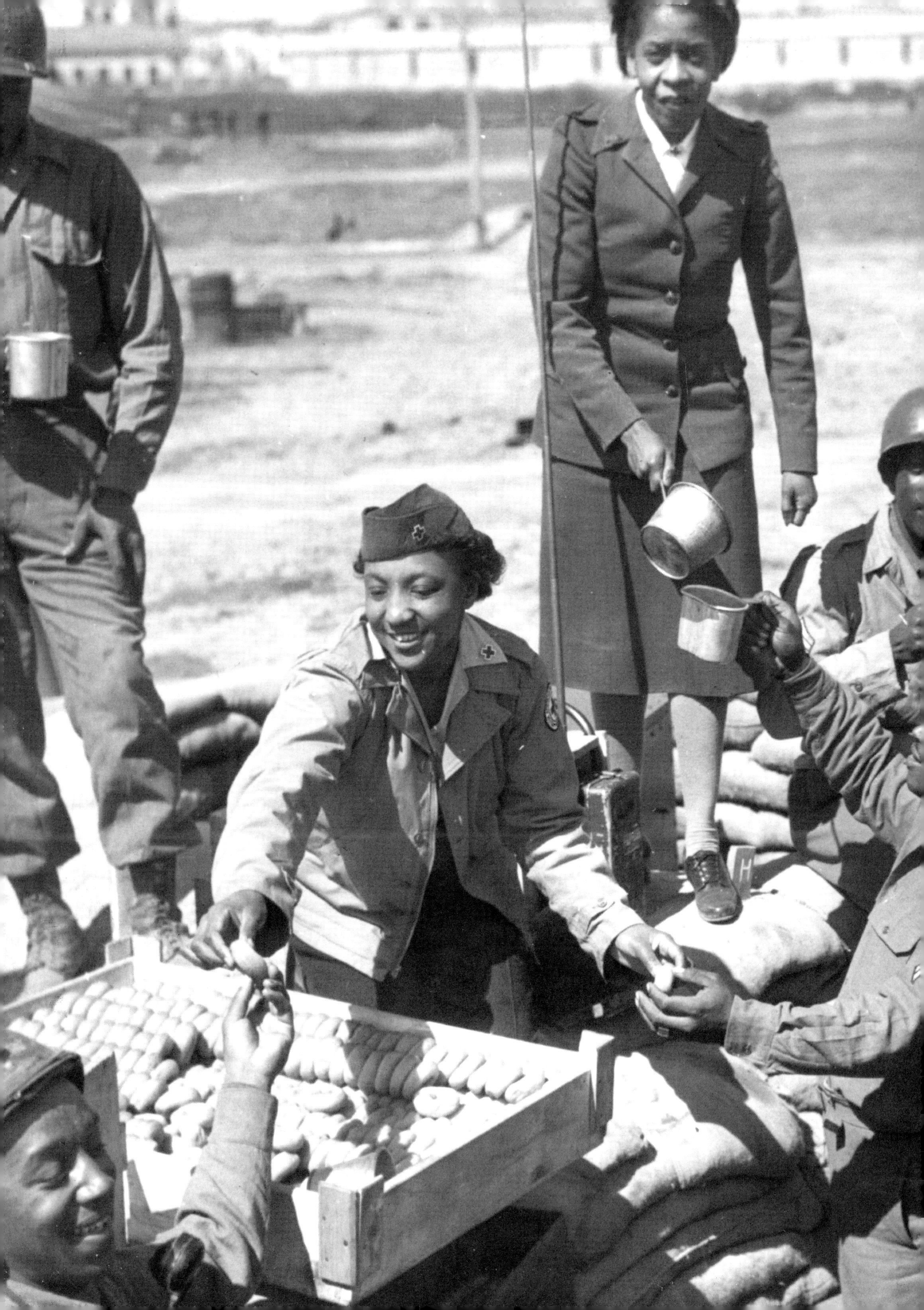
H